Dr. Cass Ingram's

How to Eat Right and Live Longer

KNOWLEDGE HOUSE PUBLISHERS

Buffalo Grove, Illinois

First Revised Edition

This book was formerly published under the title *Eat Right to Live Long* and under the title of its original edition, *Eat Right or Die Young.*

Printed in the United States of America on recycled paper

Disclaimer: The information in this book is not intended as a substitute for medical diagnosis or treatment. Anyone who has a serious disease should consult a physician before initiating any change in treatment or before beginning any new treatment.

Ordering information
This book may be ordered from any bookstore by using the title or ISBN number: 0-911119-21-3. For prompt mail order call: **1-800-243-5242.**

To pay by money order enclose $21.95 plus $5.00 S & H to: Knowledge House P.O. Box 4885 Buffalo Grove, IL 60089. Add $1.00 postage for each additional book. For orders of 3 to 5 books postage is free. For orders of 6 to12 books the price is $18.00 each plus postage (as above). Delivery is prompt (within 2 weeks). For bulk or case orders call: 1-800-243-5242.

To view other book titles by Dr. Ingram see the Web site **NutritionTest.com**.

Dr. Cass Ingram's Web Contribution

An important, monumental Web site is now available. This site will assist the individual in determining precisely what are his/her nutritional needs. Using a highly sophisticated and accurate technology, this system greatly aids in the correct determination of nutritional deficiencies. The objective is to help the individual rebuild his/her health through accurate nutritional and biochemical assessment. This is followed by extensive corrective recommendations. This is a completely individualized system. It offers two components: dietary analysis and specific tests for a wide range of nutrients. The site includes regular nutritional updates by Dr. Ingram. It is a pay-for-service site. Look for it on the World Wide Web. It is called:

NutritionTest.com
Test yourself for nutritional deficiencies

The cost is $29.95 for over 30 tests, or approximately $1.00 per test.

Contents

PART I

Principles

Introduction

What does it mean to live long? The human body is designed to live—up to 120 years or more. Yet, tens of millions of people are dying young, and people living in the Western world are far from immune.

Cancer and infectious diseases such as AIDS and pneumonia are major killers. However, heart and circulatory diseases remain number one. This is despite the use of the most advanced methods of lifesaving intervention known in the world. So, why is there still such a problem? Surely, it is diet related.

Wherever the typical American diet exists, there also exists a high incidence of heart disease, diabetes, Alzheimer's disease, and cancer as well as a wide range of other degenerative diseases. Poor diet creates illness. A lack of nutrients impairs the function of the human body. Poor nutrition disrupts immunity, impairs circulation, and disturbs hormonal balance, resulting in disorders ranging from heart disease and arthritis to cancer. Faulty dietary habits predispose the body to awide range of degenerative diseases, which are descriptively called diseases of civilization.

Poor diet is the primary cause of heart disease, stroke, heart attack, hardening of the arteries, high blood pressure, cancer, diabetes, and arthritis as well as numerous other "modern" diseases. The longer an individual is on a poor diet, the more rapidly such diseases will occur.

A nutritionally depleted diet affects the gene pool as well. If your ancestors had a poor diet—a diet rich in refined sugars, white flour, processed foods, and refined fats—your genes were/are negatively affected. Then you will be even more vulnerable than they were to the development of the diseases of civilization. Your children or future offspring are at a greater risk if you indulge in a poor diet. Eventually, the

I

gene pool will become so depleted that civilization itself will be at risk for survival.

The question is, why have a heart attack or stroke or develop heart disease, Alzheimer's disease, diabetes, or cancer if you can avoid it? Isn't it better to prevent these illnesses from happening? If you already have an illness, why not do something to attempt to cure it?

The proponents of modern medicine have led us to believe that there is no cure for the majority of diseases. Heart disease is a case in point. Most doctors claim the only thing that can be done is to "treat the symptoms." Or, they state that eventually the patient will succumb to a heart attack or stroke, and the only known and effective treatment is bypass surgery or medication. Regarding nutrition they claim, "Diet and nutritional supplements play a minor role, if any role at all." If you have heart disease, the same has probably been said to you.

The medical profession takes the same stance for a variety of other disorders. Those afflicted with arthritis, cancer, skin diseases, colitis, peptic ulcer, asthma, emphysema, lupus, and mental diseases are given a similar dictum: "No cure exists except medications or surgery. Diet and nutrition play no significant role."

This fatalistic approach is highly destructive, and the harmful results are apparent in the appallingly high rate of degenerative disease afflicting Americans. Virtually every illness can be successfully treated through nutrition and dietary alterations. What may be even more important is the fact that the development of these diseases can be prevented by making specific dietary changes and by taking herbal and nutritional supplements.

Medical doctors occasionally dabble in prevention. In the case of heart disease some physicians stress the importance of exercise. Others insist that avoiding naturally occurring substances such as cholesterol, salt, and saturated fat is protective. With cancer, a diet emphasizing fruits and vegetables may be recommended. However, few physicians offer any hope for a cure.

At most, all of these measures are merely palliative. The real causes behind disease and its development are not being addressed.

Surgeons frequently offer the ability to cure. They claim that by removing the "diseased organ" they are providing a cure. Thus, an individual with an inflamed or stone-filled gallbladder is "cured" once the gallbladder is surgically removed. No mention is made to the patient that there are nonsurgical methods for curing gallstones or gallbladder disease. Nor is any mention made of the significant side effects and illnesses which can occur after the gallbladder is removed. The gallbladder was put there for a reason. Removing it *does* compromise bodily functions.

The cardiovascular surgeon and the cardiologist are particularly prone to proclaim curative powers. They actually make the claim to cure heart disease. The surgeon attempts to cure the angina and arterial blockage with bypass surgery, and the cardiologist performs the special "curative" procedure known as angioplasty. Here, cardiologists thread a tiny plastic tube (catheter) into the heart's arteries in an attempt to remove blockages.

There is no need for me to exert my personal opinion about the supposed curative power of these procedures. The statistics speak for themselves. On average patients who refuse to undergo these procedures live longer than those who do.

Internists also claim to cure. Drugs are given to patients who have high blood pressure in an attempt to artificially lower it. Ironically, artificially lowering the blood pressure can cause strokes. Yet, this is the very thing these doctors are trying to prevent. A government study showed that patients with moderately high blood pressure who were taking blood pressure drugs died at a more rapid rate than those with high blood pressure who took no drugs. Blood pressure drugs exert their effects in part by a bizarre mechanism of action. They remove minerals from the body which are necessary to maintain normal blood pressure. Incredibly, standard high blood pressure drugs deplete potassium, magnesium, sodium, chloride, and zinc, as well as nerve-calming B vitamins, such as thiamine and riboflavin, all of which are required for keeping the blood pressure normal. Why physicians would even consider prescribing a treatment that upsets the body's natural defenses defies common sense. The fact is if the body is properly nourished, high blood pressure, as well as heart disease, cannot exist.

Drug-Free Doctoring

Can a doctor practice medicine in the United States without using drugs? The answer is yes. For over fifteen years I treated people with a wide range of conditions. My prescription pad was used more often to write notes to airlines or for school excuses than for drug prescriptions. Also, I never used a hospital once during that period. There are many countries where drugs play a secondary role to natural, safe remedies such as herbs, diet, vitamins, minerals, etc. The same could be accomplished here. Unfortunately, much of the medical education is influenced by the pharmaceutical industry, although the medical school professors and administrators would never admit it. The fact is these schools are given grants, as well as gifts, by the drug industry. However, some effort is being made to introduce nutrition into the medical curriculum, but the results are rather feeble. Even so, if both the public and professionals would work together, eventually, drug-free doctoring could become a mainstay.

It is critical that physicians be trained in the use of nutritional therapy. If this is done, each person plagued with a serious illness will have the option to choose—to try safe, nontoxic therapies, or to sucumb to the route of modern medical care. Freedom of choice should be available.

A life free of the need for medications and/or aggressive, invasive procedures is a critical element in the attempt to live a longer and happier life. Death from overmedication can and does occur. The ill-advised use of potentially toxic medications or dangerous surgical procedures is a major cause of premature death.

Medications and surgery are often useful and may even be life-saving, particularly during emergencies. However, drugs and surgery rarely cure disease. Rather, it is the natural substances found in food, herbs, spices, and water which truly have curative powers. It is reasonable to state that for every malady that exists, there also exists within nature its cure, prevention, or treatment. For those who might be skeptical about this, understand that 80% of all medications currently being developed or used were originally derived from herbs. Many of these drugs are nothing more than humanity's attempt to synthesize (meaning "create" in a laboratory) what nature has already created.

The chemist cannot produce exact replicas of these natural healing agents. Vitamin E provides an excellent illustration. Researchers have found that natural vitamin E is far more potent and effective than its synthetic counterpart. Plus, the chemical structure of the natural vitamin E compounds is different than synthetic E. what's more, it works better and stays in the body longer.

An excellent example of medical oversight concerns the treatment of the heart attack patient. Recently, it was discovered that the majority of hospitalized heart attack patients are deficient in magnesium. Most of the body's magnesium is found within the cells, so the usual blood tests which evaluate only serum levels are inaccurate. This is why magnesium deficiency in heart attack patients was not discovered earlier. Studies have shown that magnesium injections alone reduced the death rate by more than 90%. What a travesty it is that this is not common knowledge in our medical centers. As a result of this oversight hundreds—perhaps thousands—of lives are needlessly lost every year. Just think. Magnesium is only one of many naturally-occurring substances. Imagine how healthy cardiac patients could become if all of their deficiencies were corrected. Each health condition has its own specific nutritional deficits, as will be shown later in this book.

Research indicates that high blood pressure is due largely to a potassium and magnesium deficiency. Does it make sense to take a drug which depletes the body of these minerals? It makes better sense to restore the body's reservoirs of these critical nutrients.

Arthritis is another example of erroneous treatment practices by the medical profession. Potent anti-inflammatory drugs are the common treatment, but these drugs damage the digestive tract and destroy nutrients. Arthritis is often the result of a combination of weakened intestinal walls and intestinal toxicity. It makes no sense to treat arthritis with drugs which further damage the intestinal walls and increase the toxicity. Intestinal damage and, particularly, sudden intestinal or gastric bleeding are the major side effects from arthritis drugs. Medical journals unanimously agree that arthritis medicines, such as aspirin, Motrin, Indocin, Naprosyn, and similar drugs, are the primary cause of emergency gastrointestinal bleeding, resulting in thousands of deaths yearly. This is a travesty, because it is largely preventable.

In the case of hardening of the arteries the arterial blockage and damage affects every artery within the body. The body contains approximately 60,000 miles of blood vessels. It makes no sense to cleanse only the coronary arteries—a mere few inches. The sensible approach is to treat all of the arteries in the body.

Address the cause of whatever your condition is, and you will feel better. Eat right and you will likely improve. Treat only the symptoms, and you may well die prematurely.

CHAPTER ONE

What Is Eating Right?

It is just as easy to eat right as it is to eat wrong. The reason this is mentioned is that many individuals fear the changes necessary to eat right. The majority of people feel that eating in a nutritious manner requires more discipline than they can muster. They are afraid that eating right is synonymous with boredom and self-denial. Eating right does not imply these things at all. It means consuming only those foods or drinks which nourish the body and help it to function better. It means avoiding the consumption of anything which is harmful to the body. In fact, you are denying yourself to a greater extent by eating what is harmful to you than by eating what is good for you. Wouldn't it be disappointing to have planned a wonderful vacation and fail to accomplish it because of falling ill? How about getting a new wardrobe and becoming too fat to use it? What about being too tired to function to your greatest potential or to enjoy yourself at work or home? This is a heavy price to pay, and yet, all of these ill effects are a consequence of eating wrong.

It is ironic that we often take better care of our vehicles or our pets than we do our own bodies. Would you purposely feed your cat or dog French fries knowing full well that it could hurt it? If you wouldn't do this to your pet, then you most certainly shouldn't do it to yourself or your children. Yet, most people do eat harmful things.

Eating right, in essence, means not hurting yourself with YOUR OWN TWO HANDS. You are the one who chooses what you eat. Only you operate the controls. This book will help guide you to make the right choices so you can live a productive life and retain your health—forever.

Which Choice is Right for You?

What is nutritionally correct for you may not be the same as what is needed by friends or relatives. Each person is genetically different, and the body's needs for certain nutrients may differ dramatically for each individual. For example, some people need 50 times as much vitamin B_6 as is usually required just to function properly. Vitamin C is another example. The daily needs vary dramatically, with some individuals requiring 10 to 20 times the "normal" amount.

Even so, certain rules apply to virtually everyone. Throughout this book these rules have been clearly outlined. Certainly, there are exceptions to the rules, but in general 90% of all people will benefit by following these simple dietary principles that follow.

Knowledge is the Key

The key is to know which dietary habits can hurt you and understand why substances found in the diet are harmful.

Warning: Once you gain such knowledge, it becomes your responsibility to act upon it. Ignorance is not bliss, nor is premature death from a heart attack, stroke, diabetes, Alzheimer's disease, lupus, cancer, or any other debilitating disease.

Eat Right: Change Old Habits

Now you know the secret: knowledge. Use this book to your advantage, and learn what is good or bad for you. Once you understand why certain things are harmful, it will be much easier to change old eating habits. You will find these habits easier to eliminate than you could have ever believed.

Make the Commitment

Commit yourself immediately to changing any self-destructive habits. To do so, just follow these simple principles:

1. You are not responsible for ignorance, but as soon as you know right from wrong, you are responsible.

2. Do not hurt yourself with your own two hands.

3. Eating right is just as easy as eating wrong.

4. Since eating wrong is harmful, you are denying yourself to a greater extent by eating wrong than by eating right. Food is your fuel. Use only premium fuel.

5. Don't procrastinate about eating correctly. Your health is your most valuable asset. Start eating right immediately.

Maintain the Commitment

6. If you are chronically ill or feel constantly tired or sluggish, commit yourself to a new way of living. Take charge of your eating habits so you can feel like a human being should—healthy, vital, vigorous, strong, and full of life.

7. Treat yourself to nourishing, healthy, and tasty food. Refuse to feel cheated when you avoid the junk food and sweets. Remember, you are the one who operates the controls. Don't make excuses for bad eating.

8. Get into the habit of eating right. Habits are hard to change, so establish healthy ones right from the beginning. Don't allow yourself to develop noxious eating habits.

9. Even if you have a disease with a poor prognosis, don't give up. In other words, don't give in to continuing destructive habits. Change damaging habits now to give your body the chance to heal. You owe yourself at least that much. Remember, the length and quality of your life depends upon the choices you make.

10. Once you start in the right direction, never stop. Keep the momentum moving in your favor. That's the best advice for giving yourself the ultimate reward: excellent health.

Practice these principles. The rest of this book will give you the knowledge you need to adhere to them. This knowledge will enable you to incorporate these principles into your lifestyle—immediately.

CHAPTER TWO
How To Eat Right

Eating right doesn't have to be difficult. It simply means to consume all food and drink as close to the natural state as possible. It means eating food that will not damage the body. What's more, it means eating food for nourishment, not just for taste and pleasure.

You might think you eat "right" now. However, you probably don't. The common belief is that as long as an individual adheres to the government guidelines he or she will be reasonably well nourished. Yet, what are these guidelines? Few individuals could list them. The impression is that the standard American diet of breads, grains, packaged foods, milk products, meats, vegetables, and fruits is entirely balanced in the nutritional elements we need. This is certainly what Americans have been told by the media and medical profession as well as the food processors. At first, this system was called the four basic food groups, a concept developed by food industry in the the 1940s. This has recently been abandoned, and the government currently endorses a seven-tier food pyramid. This pyramid emphasizes starchy foods such as beans, legumes, grains, pasta, and fruit while restricting the intake of whole milk products, eggs, natural fats, and fresh meats. Neither of these approaches is nutritionally adequate, but the new one is actually worse. What's more, no account has been made for the method by which these foods are grown or processed. Plus, it is possible to eat junk food and "qualify" for fulfilling the pyramid or four basics. A hot dog with pickle relish, glass of skim milk, and French fries fills the daily requirement for several of the groups. What's more, if an individual strictly follows the current seven-tier pyramid, he or she will summarily become a carbohydrate, that is, sugar addict.

Also, the pyramid de-emphasizes foods naturally rich in animal fats such as eggs, whole milk products, whole fat cheese, fatty fish, and fresh meat. This places the population at a high risk for developing deficiencies of certain vitamins, notably vitamins A and D, as well as riboflavin and pantothenic acid, because fat-rich foods are the best sources of these nutrients. Furthermore, the severe reduction or elimination of fresh red meat places the masses at risk for developing trace mineral deficiencies, since red meat represents an ideal source of potassium, magnesium, copper, iron, and zinc.

A 1998 article in *Sports Medicine* illustrated how adolescent girls who adhere to this pyramid are developing severe, perhaps life-threatening, mineral deficiencies. Iron and zinc were the minerals most severely deficient. However, the greatest atrocity of the seven-tier food pyramid is the fact that it lists sugar as a food requirement, a statement which belies the most thorough findings of research and defies common sense. The government-endorsed requirement for the consumption of sugar is disastrous. This was proven by a scientific study done in the fall of 1998 at the Minnesota School of Public Health. Surprisingly, the researchers, who studied the dietary intake of thousands of women in Iowa, discovered that the government or perhaps, more correctly, "industry" emphasis upon eating starchy and sugary foods increased the risks for certain diseases, notably heart disease and diabetes. In other words, adhering to this highly touted and advertised dietary food pyramid is making people sick. For instance, women who were free of heart disease when the study began in 1986 developed evidence of disease by the time it ended. This caused renowned nutritional experts, such as Harvard's Walter Willet, Ph.D.,to call for the pyramid to be overhauled.

To illustrate the nutritional travesty of this pyramid, candy, ice cream, and other sweets are legitimized as appropriate dietary substances. What's more, both ends of this pyramid, that is the base as well as the tip, specify sugars/carbohydrates. This high-carbohydrate load is linked to a wide range of health problems, including severe fatigue, irritable digestion, fungal infestation, chronic headaches, mental disorders, and blood sugar problems. Regarding the latter, common symptoms include irritability, inability to concentrate, mood swings, agitation, fatigue, tiredness after meals, dizziness, insomnia, ravenous appetite, and fainting spells. Diseases directly related to excessive carbohydrate and sugar consumption include obesity, heart disease, high blood pressure, diabetes, and cancer. Interestingly, it is not just simple sugar that is the culprit. The so-called complex carbohydrates are also at fault.

In this era of vested interests and industry meddling, it is rather dangerous to rely upon the government for nutritional advice. Perhaps the federal government's greatest sin is the apathy it has created within the population. During talk show interviews I frequently hear comments from the public such as, "I eat correctly," or "I follow what is supposed to be right." Yet, these individuals usually fail to comprehend what they are following. Test yourself. Try to construct the seven-tier food pyramid by yourself on a piece of paper. If you can do so, list underneath each category the foods contained within it. Except for an occasional registered dietitian, hardly anyone knows this.

Another problem is that no attempt has been made to account for the variability of nutrient content as related to soil and growing conditions. As first described by Judy Kay Gray, M.S., renowned nutritionist, there is no standardized type of food in terms of nutrient content. A carrot grown in Colorado is actually significantly different in terms of nutritional density and composition compared to a Michigan carrot or one grown in a garden. Furthermore, the damaging effects on nutrient content caused by food shipping and processing has not been addressed.

You are not eating right if you regularly eat fast foods, deep fried foods, processed, packaged, or canned foods, white flour, pasta, pastries, or sweets. You are not drinking right if you regularly consume pop, sugar-sweetened fruit drinks, commercial cow's milk (versus pure organic milk), or alcoholic beverages. What's more, you are not eating right if you follow the current government guidelines of a high starch/low protein diet. Nor are you eating right if you adhere to the typical low-fat diet. It is impossible to achieve a proper intake of the critical nutrients, that is, the vitamins, minerals, and amino acids, with a diet consisting primarily of beans, grains, rice, pasta, or similar foods.

Are You Nutritionally Deficient?

If you adhere to the standard American diet, your eating habits are creating severe nutritional deficiencies. Here are the consequences of the typical American diet:

- 80% chance you are deficient in folic acid
- 70% chance you are deficient in niacin
- 62% chance you are deficient in vitamin B_6
- 70% chance you are deficient in thiamine
- 65% chance you are deficient in riboflavin
- 43% chance you are deficient in vitamin B_{12}
- 100% chance you are deficient in chromium
- 100% chance you are deficient in manganese
- 65% chance you are deficient in calcium
- 80% chance you are deficient in magnesium

- 75% chance you are deficient in selenium
- 100% chance you are deficient in essential fatty acids
- 50% chance you are deficient in vitamin C
- 40% chance you are deficient in biotin
- 65% chance you are deficient in zinc

The myth that the American diet is nutritionally sufficient is finally exposed. How can we be so deficient? It is, in fact, very easy to understand why this is so. Food processing destroys nutrients. For example, heating and boiling food can destroy over 90% of the folic acid content. You can be assured there is little or no folic acid left in canned vegetables or in French fries which are cooked at searing temperatures of up to 400 degrees. The same is true for most other nutrients. Furthermore, the soil is depleted in nutrients, especially minerals. If there are no minerals in the soil, obviously the food will be nutritionally deficient. Plus, food grown in deficient soil is considerably lower in enzymes and vitamins than food grown in intact soil.

Genetic alterations, that is genetic engineering, are the latest assault upon human health by the chemical magnates. This approach entirely fails to account for the nutritional value of the food. In other words, the engineering is rarely, if ever, aimed at increasing the food's inherent nutritional value. Rather, profit is the motive. What's more, these procedures are highly experimental; in other words, proof for the value, nutritional strength, and safety is nonexistent. In fact, the nutrient content of numerous genetically engineered foods, such as the now withdrawn "Flavor-Saver" tomatoes, is greatly diminished. Avoid all genetically engineered foods. Eat foods engineered by the powers of nature: natural God-given foods, which have been proven safe and nutritious by the test of time. For a listing of wild or naturally-grown food guaranteed to be free of genetically engineered ingredients, see Appendix B.

What About Fortification?

There is little value to food fortification. The only commonly eaten processed foods which are fortified are the grains. In addition, the fortification process itself is incomplete. Only a few of the nutrients destroyed by processing are replaced. For example, in the process of converting whole wheat grain to white flour, some 24 nutrients are destroyed. Of these, the only ones replaced are thiamine, niacin, riboflavin, and iron, although folic acid is now added as well. Few individuals are aware that much of the vitamin E, vitamin C, and the minerals copper, chromium, manganese, magnesium, selenium, and zinc are destroyed or left behind in the bran and germ during the milling process. The same is true for other refined foods such as white rice, corn meal, rye flour, oats, or barley. Let's look at this in terms of percentages:

Vitamin Losses in the Refining of Whole Wheat into White Flour

B$_1$ (Thiamine) ......77% is lost

B$_2$ (Riboflavin) .....80% is lost

B$_3$ (Niacin) ....81% is lost

B$_6$ (Pyridoxine) .....71% is lost

Pantothenic acid ....50% is lost

Folic acid ....67% is lost

Vitamin E ....86% is lost

Mineral Losses in the Refining of Whole Wheat into White Flour

Chromium ....87% is lost

Manganese ....90% is lost

Copper ....66% is lost

Zinc ....82% is lost

Iron ....81% is lost

Magnesium ....83% is lost

This chart makes it obvious that the majority of Americans have significant nutritional deficiencies. This is because refined wheat and wheat products form a major part of the typical American diet. Foods containing large percentages of nutrient-depleted refined wheat, such as bread, pasta, pastries, cookies, crackers, and cereals, make up as much as 60% of the daily calories. Add to this the consumption of vitamin or mineral destroyers, and the deficiencies can become profound or even life-threatening. This is because a number of serious diseases result from extreme mineral deficiency. Plus, a relatively minor illness, such as a bout of diarrhea or a sudden infection, may cause enough mineral loss in a depleted individual to lead to sudden death.

Vitamin-Mineral Destroyers

Are you using vitamin-mineral destroyers? This test will tell.

Answer "Yes" or "No" to the Following: Do You Use...

- alcohol
- aspirin
- caffeine
- coffee
- drugs
- mineral oil
- white flour
- cholesterol-lowering drugs
- antihistamines
- antibiotics
- birth control pills
- cigarettes
- cortisone
- laxatives
- water pills (diuretics)
- diet pills
- chewing tobacco

Count the number of times you answered yes. If you only use one or two of these and your use is occasional, then you are probably destroying only a small amount of nutrients. However, if you regularly use any of these substances, you are at risk for severe nutritional depletion. If you use most or all of them, you are severely deficient. In this instance you have a high risk for developing a variety of diseases due to extreme nutritional deficiencies.

Medications Rob Specific Nutrients

If you take prescription or nonprescription drugs, it is important that you carefully read this section. The medication(s) you take may be causing deficiencies of specific nutrients.

The mechanism of action of each drug is different. Most drugs are highly specific according to where they act in the cellular chemistry and in how they inactivate or destroy certain nutrients. The result is that medications can be the primary cause of nutritional deficiencies. Here are some of the ways medications do this:

1. By increasing urinary excretion of the nutrient

2. By blocking the site where the nutrient attaches within the cell

3. By blocking absorption of the nutrient

4. By binding to the nutrient and, therefore, inactivating it

5. By causing the nutrient to be used up more rapidly

6. By actually destroying the nutrient

7. By increasing the loss of the nutrient in the stool

Table for Common Medication-Induced Deficiencies

This chart provides a comprehensive list of the major nutrients and the drugs which negatively affect them. There are hundreds of other drugs which cause these nutritional deficiencies—only the more commonly used ones have been included. The more drugs that are taken, the greater the odds that nutrients are deficient. Individuals taking a preponderance of medications, such as nursing home occupants, heart disease patients, diabetics, etc., are likely to be deficient in most if not all of these nutrients.

Deficient Nutrient	**Medication**
Vitamin A	antacids, aspirin, cholesterol-lowering meds, Coumadin, mineral oil
Vitamin B_{12}	antibiotics, aspirin, birth control pills (BCPs), cortisone, Mycolog, Stelazine, Tagamet, Zantac, Pepcid, Axid, Prozac
Vitamin C	antihistamines, aspirin, BCPs, cortisone, Coumadin, Naprosyn, Motrin, Indocin, Clinoril, Butazoladin, theophylline, tetracyclines
Calcium	aspirin, Phenobarbital, tetracyclines, caffeine
Vitamin D	barbituates (Phenobarbital, Seconal, etc.), cholesterol-lowering meds, mineral oil, cortisone, Dilantin, BCPs
Vitamin E	BCPs, Tamoxafen, cholesterol-lowering meds, mineral oil
Folic acid	antacids, antibiotics, aspirin, BCPs, Dilantin, Macrodantin, Methotrexate, sulfa drugs (especially Septra and Bactrim), Tagamet, Zantac, Pepcid, Axid, caffeine
Iron	aspirin, Clinoril, Coumadin, Indocin, tetracyclines, Motrin, Naprosyn
Vitamin K	antibiotics (all types), barbituates, cortisone, Coumadin, Dilantin, Pro-Banthine, cholesterol-lowering meds, tetracyclines, BCPs, mineral oil
Magnesium	diuretics (including Lasix, Diuril, and thiazides), laxatives, tetracyclines, aspirin, caffeine, antacids

Potassium .aspirin, cortisone, diuretics,
caffeine, laxatives

Pyridoxine (vitamin B$_6$) . . . . .BCPs, cortisone, Dilantin,
Penicillamine, antibiotics, Prozac,
caffeine

Riboflavin (vitamin B$_2$) . . . . .antacids, antibiotics, BCPs,
diuretics, sulfa drugs

Thiamine (vitamin B$_1$) . . . . .antibiotics, aspirin, BCPs, drugs
containing caffeine, Indocin,
Motrin, Naprosyn, Clinoril,
antihistamines

Zinc . . . . .BCPs, cortisone, drugs containing
caffeine, diuretics

From this chart it becomes clear that many non-prescription drugs cause nutritional deficiencies. Aspirin is one of the worst offenders. Mineral oil is another example. It binds to fat-soluble vitamins, such as vitamins A, D, E, and K, causing their loss into the stool. Harsh laxatives cause deficiencies of vitamins and/or minerals. Regular use of antihistamines and cough syrups results in vitamin C and B vitamin deficiencies.

Most people who take drugs are already nutritionally compromised. It is obvious that drugs greatly aggravate the deficiencies. With drug therapy there are great risks, and often, little is gained. In contrast, nutritional therapy along with proper diet is safe, and the gains are usually immense.

Dr. Ingram's 10 Worry-Free Principles for Eating Right

You can now see how important it is to begin eating right as soon as possible. Through an improved diet, the body's nutritional reservoirs are refurbished, and the result is improved health. There are hundreds of opinions regarding what is the most nutritious diet. You are probably wondering how you can sort through all of these opinions and the confusion they generate so you can learn to eat right. Following these principles will help simplify your task:

1. Do not fret over what you have eaten in the past. Just eat right from now on.

2. Do not be concerned about eating out. Simply eat around the unhealthy foods.

3. Cooking foods is OK as long as you do not heat them excessively. Just try not to overcook meats or vegetables.

4. Do not be concerned about eating all raw foods. Just eat some raw fruits and vegetables every day.

5. Do not worry about eating too much meat. Just avoid eating smoked, processed, and preserved meat (bacon and other meats containing added nitrates, food dyes, MSG, and flavorings).

6. You don't have to completely avoid canned or packaged food, since certain of these foods are healthy. Simply try to eat as much food in its original natural state as possible (for example, fresh beets versus canned, even though canned beets are healthy).

7. Do not become fixated about food-combining or food groups. Just eat a variety of healthy, chemical-free foods. Listen to your body. If certain foods or combinations there of don't agree with you, avoid them.

8. Do not become obsessed about fat consumption. Simply avoid all synthetic fats. That means margarine, shortening, and refined liquid vegetable oils.

9. Concentrate as much as possible on eating natural organic foods or chemical-free foods.

10. Avoid the white stuff, that is, white flour, rice, and sugar as found in pasta, bread, crackers, cookies, and similar processed foods.

CHAPTER THREE
What Does It Mean
To Die Young?

Dying young is something most of us fear. There is nothing more scary than the thought of dying in a fiery car accident or in a plane crash. Though we don't usually think about it, most of us would like to live a normal lifespan—perhaps longer than normal. Virtually everyone would like to live to be 80, 90, or 100 years old, perhaps even older, if the quality of life is excellent.

The degree of anxiety with regard to premature death depends upon the type of illness a person has and also the severity of that illness. For those afflicted with heart disease, there is often a constant apprehension about suddenly dying from a heart attack. Those who have cancer are concerned that the condition will eventually or rapidly lead to their demise. For those with severe infections the concern is will the infection become toxic enough to cause organ damage or death?

Dying young doesn't mean merely living a shortened lifespan. It means living in a way that disrupts optimal productivity, both mentally and physically. By this definition, most individuals in nursing homes have "died young."

Living in a semi-vegetative state with no purpose or function is a form of death. A person placed in a nursing home at, for example, age 60, despite existing there until 80 years old, is dead spiritually, emotionally, and, to a large degree, physically at age 60. Are these the cold hard facts? Perhaps they are. Yet, this is precisely what happens.

Is there any difference between death and a state of living death? Probably not. Examine how you feel about it. Chances are you dread the thought of living in a nursing home no matter what the circumstances or provisions.

Modern medicine and emergency lifesaving care are setting the stage for the elderly to live in this manner. I have seen individuals hooked up to tubes on respirators, merely existing for up to two years or more, only to die as soon as the breathing tubes are removed. There is no purpose in such "living." Dying young is just that: the loss of all quality of life. Thus, a morbidly ill cancer victim is an example of dying young; a patient permanently disabled by a stroke or neurological disease, such as multiple sclerosis, has died young; an individual whose brain is destroyed by Alzheimer's or Parkinson's disease has been lost before his/her time.

Premature death due to disease is dying young. The death of all children who have contracted cancer and were killed by either the cancer or the therapy, the death of all youths from alcohol and drug-related accidents, the loss of all women who, in the prime of their lives, developed breast, ovarian, uterine, or cervical cancer, and the loss of vital, valuable men from heart attacks and strokes are all examples of premature death.

Perhaps even more devastating is the fact that there are sudden deaths of youngsters due to corrupt foods and/or medicines, and these are deaths that are completely preventable. In Pennsylvania a 19 year old died after being injected with a genetically engineered drug: the drug directly caused his death. A dear friend, who was at the prime of her little life, died suddenly after the ingestion of processed/chemicalized food. The fact is thousands of children and teenagers suffer disability or death as a result of the poor quality foods they eat. Toxic and/or allergic reactions to foods happen every day. Millions are negatively affected, and many die.

What makes this subject so important? After all, these people are dead and gone. Nothing can be done about it. While this is true, the fact remains that many of these deaths could have been prevented. Also, it is important that we learn from these events so that terrible mishaps can be prevented in the future. Believe me, most of these horrible deaths could have been averted. If you are grieving for one of these precious souls, you will appreciate what I have to say.

Modern medicine is directly responsible for a certain percentage of premature deaths. It is well known that many medications can be toxic, especially if they are given in improper dosages. Hundreds of thousands of individuals die or are permanently disabled every year as a result of the side effects of prescription medications. Up to 40% of the admissions in major medical centers across the country are due to the side effects of drugs. Thousands of others die as a consequence of unnecessary surgical procedures. The irony is that many of these illnesses could have been treated with much safer and less toxic therapies. If caught early enough, most diseases are treatable by methods other than drugs, surgery, or other invasive procedures.

For those afflicted with a condition for which no treatment has yet been discovered, such as the loss of limb or spinal paralysis, I extend to you my love and support. For anyone else who is ill I extend only this: do your utmost to get back your health. Continue to search for a solution. If you find the solution, you will unchain your inner spirit, and what an excellent feeling that will be. This is because it is likely that you will live life to its fullest and avoid the plague of dying young.

Causes of Premature Death

The individual can live life to the fullest without the risk of diseases which shorten lifespan. A list of the more common conditions which cause premature death and/or significantly reduce the quality of life includes:

- alcoholism
- Alzheimer's disease
- cancer
- diabetes
- drug addiction
- rheumatoid arthritis
- AIDS
- emphysema
- tuberculosis
- Crohn's disease
- heart disease
- neuromuscular diseases
  (i.e. multiple sclerosis, ALS,
  and muscular dystrophy)
- Parkinson's disease
- stroke
- hepatitis
- asthma
- lupus
- colitis

All of these diseases are preventable. This is because they are all caused by environmental factors, errant lifestyle, and poor diet. By removing the causative factors and taking the appropriate treatment, the individual can expect to avoid becoming a victim of any of these diseases. Some of these illnesses are so severe that a major effort is required to halt the progression, let alone reverse them. Yet, everything can be done to prevent them from happening. Let's concentrate on how you can stop serious diseases from striking you. There are many pearls of wisdom throughout this book on how to avoid disease, disability, or premature death which results from poor diet and negligent lifestyle habits.

CHAPTER FOUR
Is Your Body Giving You Signals?

Now it is clear how poor diet leads to nutritional deficiencies. Once these deficiencies become severe enough, the body may manifest certain warnings or signals. The human body is wonderfully constructed, and one of its miracles is to provide warnings of impending danger. Unfortunately, these signs of disease and/or deficiency are frequently overlooked by both the patient and the doctor.

There are hundreds of warning signs of nutritional deficiency, many of which seem rather innocuous. Dandruff is an excellent example. While usually regarded as only a cosmetic problem, surprisingly, this is a complex symptom, signaling a number of nutritional deficiencies. In its most severe form dandruff is known by the medical term *seborrhea* or *seborrheic dermatitis*. This term is derived from the name of the oil-secreting sebaceous glands located in great numbers on the scalp. To make an adequate supply of their protective oils these glands are reliant on a generous supply of substances known as *essential fatty acids*. In addition, their proper function depends on adequate amounts of the B vitamins, especially B_6, niacin, and biotin. Dandruff is a reliable indicator of vitamin and essential fatty acid deficiencies.

As the deficiencies within the scalp become prolonged and severe, the local, as well as systemic, immunity is disrupted. The weakened immunity increases the risks of infection, which may readily develop in the hair follicles as well as sebaceous glands. The causative organism is usually a fungus. The nutritional deficiencies which particularly increase the risks of infection include a lack of vitamin B_6, biotin, zinc, selenium, and the essential fatty acids, all of which are required to maintain the normal structural integrity, as well as immunity, of the scalp.

In summary, dandruff or seborrhea is associated with deficiencies in the following nutrients:

1. essential fatty acids
   (linoleic and linoleic acid)
2. vitamin B_2 (riboflavin)
3. vitamin B_3 (niacin)
4. vitamin B_5 (pantothenic acid)
5. vitamin B_6 (pyridoxine)
6. biotin
7. vitamin A
8. selenium
9. zinc

Recently, it was discovered, primarily as a result of the research of Dr. Rosenburg and colleagues at the University of Tennessee, that scalp disorders, notably seborrhea, psoriasis, and simple dandruff, are associated with the overgrowth of a fungus. This fungus, which normally inhabits the scalp, only invades if the body is deficient in key nutrients such as essential fatty acids, B vitamins, and trace minerals. Nutritional deficiency leads to a breakdown in the immunity, and as a result the fungus aggressively invades the scalp and hair follicles. Other microbes, such as strep and staph, may also play a role. A diet high in sugar worsens this condition. The sugar encourages the growth of yeasts, plus it depletes the B vitamins and trace minerals needed for the health of the skin of the scalp. Those little flakes of dandruff may be a warning that your nutritional state has gone awry.

The body may provide other warnings. Changes in the texture and color of the hair warn of essential fatty acid and protein deficiency. Dry and oily hair are indicative of essential fatty acid deficiency. The hair is a barometer of the nutritional state of the body. It is particularly sensitive to changes in fatty acid and protein nutrition. Changes in hair can be noticed shortly after a period of intense emotional stress. In susceptible individuals just eating a few servings of deep fried foods can lead to noticeable changes in the health of the hair and scalp. This is because vegetable oils, especially hydrogenated and partially hydrogenated oils, greatly interfere with essential fatty acid metabolism and may even block the absorption of these critical compounds.

Unmanageable hair which stiffens and stands on end is a classic sign of poor fatty acid nutrition. Those absolutely unmanageable tufts of hair are reversible by improving fatty acid nutrition. Greasy hair is telltale evidence of essential fatty acid as well as magnesium and vitamin B_6 deficiencies. Coarse or brittle hair may warn of vitamin A deficiency and may also indicate sluggish thyroid function. Hair loss is indicative of vitamin-mineral malnutrition along with poor digestion and absorption of fatty acids and proteins. Excessive hair loss may also be a signal of impaired blood flow to the scalp. Yet, according to recent research fungal and/or parasitic invasion may be the primary cause of hair loss, especially in men.

Although most people eat plenty of protein, that doesn't mean it is being digested and absorbed properly. Many fail to eat enough of the high-quality proteins, that is those which are rich in all eight essential amino acids. To have healthy hair, all eight essential amino acids are required. The hair, being mostly protein, will readily reflect poor protein status by signals such as hair loss, split ends, slow-growing hair, and brittle hair. The health of hair is also dependent on another group of nutrients: the minerals. Most important in this regard are zinc, sulfur, and silicon.

Though representing a small surface area, the fingernails, provide a wide range of indications about nutritional developments, as well as disease, within the body. Ridges on the nails which run across the nail bed often indicate hormonal disturbances. Vertical ridges, that is those which run up and down the nail bed, indicate mineral deficiency (especially calcium and iron), protein malabsorption, and possibly vitamin A deficiency. White spots on the fingernails warn of zinc deficiency. Nails that look like spoons, that is they have a scooped-out appearance, are accurate indicators of iron deficiency and, therefore, anemia.

The skin can be revealing. Patches of dry scaly skin particularly on the face and cheeks indicate poor fatty acid, zinc, and B vitamin nutrition. Biotin deficiency may also be involved. Easy bruising without trauma may signal a deficiency of essential fatty acids, vitamin K, bioflavonoids (found in fruits and vegetables, especially the rinds of citrus fruit), and vitamin C.

There are, of course, signs of a more serious nature. Pain in the chest, arm (particularly the left one), shoulder, or jaw may precede a heart attack. A hardened, fixed mass in the breasts may forewarn of breast cancer. Dramatic, persistent changes in bowel habits may be an early warning of bowel cancer, although other causes, such as intestinal parasite infection and yeast infestation, must be considered. These *medical* signs require medical diagnosis and treatment. Is your body giving you signals that you are developing significant nutritional deficiencies? Take the following test to find out:

Check the appropriate response   YES   NO

1. Do you have dandruff or seborrhea of the scalp?   ____ ____

2. Is your hair dry or brittle?   ____ ____

3. Do you have premature graying of the hair?   ____ ____

4. Is your hair losing its texture or shine?   ____ ____

5. Is your hair excessively oily?   ____ ____

6. Do you have alopecia or significant hair loss?   ____ ____

7. Do you have coarse hair?   ____ ____

8. Does your skin crack open easily, especially
   during the winter?   ____ ____

9. Do you have acne?   ____ ____

10. Do you have dry patches of skin
    on your face and cheeks?   ____ ____

11. Is your skin dry and flaky?   ____ ____

12. Do your fingernails grow slowly?   ____ ____

13. Do your fingernails break or peel?   ____ ____

14. Do you have white spots on your fingernails?   ____ ____

15. Do you have horizontal ridges on your fingernails? ____ ____

16. Do you have vertical ridges on your fingernails?   ____ ____

17. Do you have hangnails?   ____ ____

18. Are your hands and feet always cold?   ____ ____

19. Are the hairs on your eyebrows falling out
    (especially the outer third)?   ____ ____

20. Are you developing growths on the skin such as
    moles, skin tags, raised brown spots, etc.?   ____ ____

21. Do you bruise easily?   ____ ____

22. Do your gums bleed easily, or do they bleed
    when you brush?   ____ ____

23. Do you have receding gums and/or gum infections?   ____ ____

24. Are you developing age or liver spots?   ____ ____

If you answered yes to any of these signals, you have nutritional deficiencies. Some of these deficiency symptoms are more serious than others. If you answered 10 or more as yes, then you have severe nutritional deficiencies. A score of 15-plus indicates massive nutritional deficits. The following is a listing of what each means medically and nutritionally. For a more extensive approach to self-testing for nutritional deficiency see the Web site, **NutritionTest.com.** This site offers a method for systematically evaluating nutritional deficiencies.

Interpretation of Results

#1. As stated earlier, you may have an overgrowth of fungi and bacteria in the scalp, secondary to both nutritional deficiency and a breakdown in immunity. Most of the B vitamins are lacking, especially riboflavin, B_6, niacin, biotin, and folic acid. Deficient minerals include zinc and selenium (many dandruff shampoos contain selenium as the active ingredient). Essential fatty acid deficiency is a major issue, and protein maldigestion is likely.

#2. Major factors: protein maldigestion/deficiency and essential fatty acid deficiency. Vitamin A is also probably lacking. Brittle hair indicates mineral deficit, especially sulfur, silicon, and zinc.

#3. Major factors: stress is a prime culprit, and B-vitamin deficiencies are likely, especially vitamin B_5, PABA, and folic acid. Recently, vitamin D deficiency has been implicated. A hormonal imbalance should also be considered.

#4. Major factors: a lack of essential fatty acids seems to be the key. Deficiencies of B_6, magnesium, and zinc are also associated.

#5. Major factors: both oily and dry hair are associated with a malabsorption and/or deficiency of essential fatty acids. Zinc, B_6, riboflavin, and folic acid are also lacking.

#6. Major factors: poor circulation to the scalp is a common causative factor. Alopecia (patchy hair loss) may be a sign of substantial metal poisoning. Alopecia is also associated with deficiencies of folic acid, zinc, and inositol (a natural substance not technically listed as a vitamin or mineral). Hair loss and/or balding is a sign of severe deficiency of a wide range of nutrients, including protein, essential fatty acids, B vitamins, silicon, and zinc. Certain essential oils may aid in the reversal of alopecia, notably oils of myrtle, rosemary, lavender, and oregano. These oils are available in a formula called Scalp Clenz. For virtually any scalp condition, simply rub Scalp Clenz essential oil formula into the scalp once daily. It's completely safe for all age groups.

#7. Major factors: vitamin A deficiency is automatic. Coarse hair may also signal hypothyroidism (sluggish thyroid function). Thyroid hormone is needed for vitamin A metabolism. Protein deficiency may also play a role.

#8. Major factors: a severe deficiency of essential fatty acids is almost certain. Zinc, which is needed for essential fatty acid metabolism, is also lacking. There may be a malabsorption or deficiency of essential amino acids. This symptom may also be a sign of adrenal dysfunction.

#9. Major factors: nutritional deficiency and acne are directly connected. This is especially true in teenagers. It is likely that the diet is poor, being high in fried foods, saturated fats, hydrogenated fats, chocolate, refined flour, and sugar. Food allergies also play an important role. Vitamins that are deficient include B_2, B_3, B_5, A, C, and E. Improving essential fatty acid nutrition will help clear the acne, as will supplementing with minerals, especially zinc, magnesium, and selenium. Herbal oils, especially those from rosemary, myrtle, and oregano, would prove valuable.

#10. Major factors: this is a sign of essential fatty acid, zinc, and B_6 deficiency.

#11. Major factors: this is a classic indication of severe essential fatty acid, zinc, and B_6 deficiency. When fatty acid nutrition becomes this deranged, other internal problems develop. Metabolically active organs become damaged, and they may actually degenerate or shrink in size. The highly active organs include the liver, thyroid, and adrenal glands. The heart and arteries are also affected. Without an adequate supply of these fatty acids, circulation is impaired. The cells lining the digestive tract are dependent upon a plentiful supply of essential fatty acids. These cells die and are renewed every five to seven days. Without the nutrients they need, they will fail to develop properly, will be malformed and, therefore, metabolically inefficient. As a result, malabsorption of nutrients will result. If your skin is poor in quality and/or is dry and peeling, just think about how your insides look. The same degenerative process is likely occurring within you as well.

#12. Major factors: this is indicative of protein, fatty acid, and mineral malnutrition. The minerals most commonly lacking are calcium, magnesium, sulfur, silicon, copper, and zinc. Vitamin A also plays an important role.

#13. Major factors: calcium deficiency is definite, although essential fatty acids play an important role. The latter make the nails pliable. Zinc, silicon, magnesium, and iron are also required for strengthening the nails. Brittle nails in women may signal iron deficiency anemia. A severe vitamin A deficiency is also likely.

#14. This indicates zinc deficiency. Malabsorption of zinc due to a lack of pancreatic enzymes is also probable. Vitamin A deficiency can also lead to zinc malabsorption, since a healthy intestinal absorptive surface is dependent upon an adequate supply of it.

#15. Horizontal ridges are an indication of severe nutrient malabsorption, especially protein and minerals (sulfur and calcium), although hormonal imbalances are also involved. If the horizontal ridges are numerous, this is a signal of severe stress either induced by health problems or prolonged psychological/emotional distress. The ultimate cause is stress-induced collapse of the adrenal glands. Numerous, that is dozens, of horizontal ridges may warn of hidden cancerous tumors. However, the usual cause is stress. Crude royal jelly is a potent anti-stress tonic. To reverse the stress-induced damage, take 3 to 4 capsules of Royal Kick twice daily.

#16. Ridges which are vertical, meaning they run up and down, are a warning of severe mineral deficiency. They may also warn of a lack of protein and vitamin A. It is important to note that mineral absorption is greatly dependent upon adequate vitamin A nutriture. Thus, if both vitamin A and minerals are lacking, the ridges will be severe.

#17. Major factors: folic acid and vitamin A are the most important deficiencies indicated by this sign. Hangnails are usually cured when these two nutrients are taken in sufficient dosages. In essence, hangnails are an indication that the body is unable to synthesize the cells which line the inside and outside of the body fast enough. That's why the skin around the nail bed fails to grow completely. These skin cells are known medically as *epithelial cells*. Vitamin A and folic acid help restore the rate of synthesis of these cells to normal. Zinc may also be necessary to maximize the rate of cellular repair.

#18. Major factors: it is likely that the thyroid and adrenals are malfunctioning. This may also be a clue of vitamin E or essential fatty acid deficiency. Patients with yeast infections often have cold extremities. So do patients who are deficient in vitamin A and/or niacin (vitamin B_3).

#19. Hypothyroidism is guaranteed if you have this. If prolonged or left untreated, this condition results in a variety of health problems, including fatigue, weight problems (too heavy or too thin), elevated cholesterol, cardiac arrhythmia, chronic fungal infection (in the intestine, vagina, or on the skin), digestive disturbances, cold extremities, hair loss, swollen/thick skin, etc. Hypothyroidism can even lead to heart attacks, particularly in obese women.

#20. The development of new growths on the skin is a sign to take seriously. While it may not mean you have cancer, such growths are a warning that serious problems, such as cancer or rapid aging, could occur. This is particularly true if you are developing new moles or if an old mole is changing color or shape. Skin cancer is the modern plague, and the incidence of melanoma, the most dangerous and life-threatening form of skin cancer, has risen in young adults over 1,200 fold in the last 20 years. These new skin growths are the most important signal I have listed. This is because they are the body's outward signals of severe nutritional deficiency, which leads to organ dysfunction and premature aging, as well as serious disease. Moles and brown spots indicate disturbed antioxidant function, with deficiencies of selenium, vitamin E, pantothenic acid, vitamin C, and beta carotene, and glutathione being most important (see Chapter Six). Skin tags are associated with severe blood sugar disturbances (hypoglycemia). Some researchers note that they are a type of "skin tumor," and that they may indicate the existence of excessive cell growth (i.e. precancerous lesions). Do not get overly concerned. Skin tags which have existed for years that remain unchanged are relatively harmless. The cancer connection is in individuals virtually covered in certain areas, like around the neck. Multiple brown spots, moles, or skin tags are a sign of a severe deficiency in antioxidants. In addition, the organs controlling the blood sugar metabolism are malfunctioning (the pancreas, liver, and adrenal glands). For natural blood sugar control use DiabaGon and Herbsorb (see Appendix B). If you have multiple skin tags, take extra doses of anti-cancer antioxidants such as selenium, vitamin E, chromium, manganese, and beta carotene.

Antioxidant herbs and spices possess even more powerful antioxidant and anti-aging actions than vitamins and minerals. These herbs and spices included cumin, rosemary, fenugreek, turmeric, and oregano. Fenugreek offers the additional benefit of aiding in blood sugar control. For direct action against skin tags, rub the tags with oil of oregano and oil of rosemary, but also take edible spice oils internally. Taintu and other researchers discovered that certain edible spice oils, particularly sage, oregano, cumin, rosemary, and clove oils, are the most powerful natural antioxidants known. Myrtle oil is yet another valuable tonic for damaged skin, especially on the face. If you are developing age spots or other disfiguring lesions, rub oil of myrtle on the facial skin morning and night. This lovely tonic has been relied upon since antiquity as a skin rejuvenator. The Romans applied it for beautification and during medieval times it was famous for skin conditions. Brown spots may be erased using aromatic oils, particularly oil of myrtle and oil of oregano. Use only the pure, wild oregano and myrtle. Or, use Skin Clenz, a special topical formula containing a mixture of wild myrtle, oregano, rosemary and more. Do not use Thymus capitus or Spanish oregano. When using essential oils, be sure the source is pure and chemical free. This is especially true of oil of oregano. Thus, read the label carefully. If you see the words marjoram, thyme, thymus (or Thymus capitus), or thymol or if it states Product of Spain or Mexico, it cannot be a true oregano. In other words, it is an imitation. According to Julia Lawless, author of *The Encyclopedia of Essential Oils*, the vast majority of the commercially available oils are not true oreganos but are instead marjoram and/or Spanish thyme. This is crucial to know, because industrial and/or commercial marjoram and thyme should not be taken internally. What's more, industrially produced thymus oils, often falsely labeled as oregano oils, may not be safe if applied topically. I have documented dozens of cases of harmful effects from the topical use of such industrial oils. While such false labeling is certainly atrocious, currently there are no laws against this. The point is without assurance and/or proof from the manufacturer that the product is a true wild oregano, do not use it. However, a true oil of oregano from the edible wild species, that is, the same species used as a Mediterranean spice, is listed by the federal government as a safe food additive and is safe for human use. Oreganol™ oil of oregano is the P73 Mediterranean source and is researched, tested, and guaranteed wild; plus it is free of thymus additives. Look for P73 on the label.

Brownish lesions which are raised are usually a form of skin tumor. Most often they are nonmalignant. Yet, they are an indication that a disturbance in your anticancer mechanisms exists. It is likely that your immune system is sluggish and that there is a deficiency in protective nutrients. Here again, if you suffer from multiple brown/age spots, take plenty of antioxidant minerals and vitamins; also, take antioxidant herbs/spices, especially the edible/emulsified oil of oregano, oil of cumin, oil of sage, and oil of rosemary.

In summary, skin tags indicate blood sugar problems, chromium deficiency, and a lack of antioxidant nutrients. New or changing moles indicate a profound need for antioxidants and anticancer nutrients such as selenium, vitamin E, beta carotene, vitamin C, and antioxidant spices such as oregano, cumin, sage, and rosemary. Garlic's high selenium and sulfur content assists the body in the synthesis of an enzyme known as glutathione peroxidase, discussed in more depth in Chapter Six. I have seen moles disappear upon adding selenium and garlic to the diet. What's more, I dissolved my own mole using SuperStrength oil of oregano (in olive oil) topically.

Melanomas are a more serious condition. However, nutrition is the most important additional element in their treatment. Melanomas may be related to certain vitamin deficiencies. A lack of vitamin B_6 (particularly in the form of pyridoxal-5-phosphate), vitamin D, vitamin E, and riboflavin have been correlated with an increased risk. Colorado researchers have discovered that topical application of vitamin E also helps. Ideally, boost your antimelanoma defenses with a regular intake of these vitamins. Better yet, saturate the region with oil of wild oregano and oil of wild rosemary. Research shows that these oils dramatically increase the skin's resistance to cancerous invasion. For best results also take these oils internally. Use only edible oil of oregano and rosemary emulsified in extra virgin olive oil. I do not recommend self-treatment alone of any of these lesions, but I do believe you should find a physician who is open-minded enough to support any treatment you desire. After all, it is your body. You have the right to seek whatever treatment you desire.

#21. Easy bruising can indicate a variety of dysfunctions. First, it signals a deficiency of vitamin C and bioflavonoids. Bioflavonoids are a family of natural chemicals found primarily in fruits and vegetables, although many herbs are rich in them. In citrus fruits bioflavonoids are concentrated primarily in the rind. Thus, eating the inner rinds of citrus fruits may prove helpful in strengthening the blood vessels and halting the bruising. However, you can only do this if the fruit is organically grown, because the rind is where the pesticides are concentrated. Flavin-C is a convenient means to consume these flavonoids. This is a unique supplement providing unprocessed natural vitamin C and flavonoids, including the rinds of chemical-free immature oranges and tangerines. For relief from easy bruising or for building blood vessel strength, take two or more capsules daily. Crude, unprocessed vitamin C and bioflavonoids are invaluable for strengthening the body. In contrast, synthetic vitamin C is weaker, perhaps relatively ineffective. It was Dr. Szent Gyorgi, the Hungarian Nobel Prize winner, who proved categorically that the natural, unprocessed vitamin C was infinitely more effective than the synthetic vitamin. Dr. Szent Gyorgi found that a crude extract of certain foods rich in vitamin C cured animals and humans of certain diseases. When he finally isolated and refined the supposedly active component, the ascorbic acid, he gave it to the sick individuals. However, it failed to work. He was forced to utilize the unprocessed food source to aid his patients.

Bioflavonoids strengthen the inner lining of the blood vessel walls, thus keeping the arteries strong and preventing their degeneration. Bruising and bleeding tendencies, such as nosebleeds and hemorrhoids, may also may be caused by impaired liver function. A variety of blood-clotting factors are synthesized in the liver. If this organ malfunctions, blood vessels will become weakened and bruising results. The liver also produces albumin, which is the main protein required for transporting calcium. This mineral is essential for blood clotting, and without albumin, calcium can't be adequately delivered where it is needed. Thus, my research reveals that liver disorders may be the cause behind nosebleeds, blood in the urine, bleeding hemorrhoids, and easy bruising; that is, bruises which occur without obvious trauma.

The intestines serve as the primary source of vitamin K, where it is synthesized by intestinal bacteria. Vitamin K is needed for blood to clot normally. If you bruise easily, you may have a vitamin K deficiency secondary to the overgrowth of organisms such as yeasts in the intestines, which crowd out the useful bacteria. Thus, easy bruising may be the result of using too many antibiotics. Antibiotics destroy the naturally occurring microbes in the bowel. These helpful microbes are then replaced by organisms which serve no useful function. In fact, the noxious microbes actually consume rather than provide nutrients. Diet may predispose to this microbial imbalance. Eating sugar and other refined carbohydrates, such as pasta, white bread, and white rice, encourages the growth of excessive amounts of yeasts in the bowel. Remember, yeasts are fungi, and they thrive on sugar and starch as food.

People who were not breastfed tend to suffer from a deficiency of the helpful intestinal bacteria. This is because breast milk is loaded with the healthy bacteria, while formula and cow's milk contain little or none. These delicate, microbial creatures are known as *Lactobacillus acidophilus and bifidus*. The bifidus bacteria are particularly vulnerable and can easily be destroyed by a wide variety of substances such as toxins in the environment, chlorine in the water, aspirin, and, of course, antibiotics. The reason this is so important is that many societies get extra acidophilus and bifidus bacteria in their diet. As a rule, Americans do not. Strong concoctions of fermented milk products rich in these bacteria form a regular part of the diet of Ukrainians, Rumanians, Hungarians, Russians, Indians, Pakistanis, Armenians, Syrians, Turks, Lebanese, etc. Such groups make special efforts to prepare and eat acidophilus/bifidus-rich fermented foods. Thus, these people are continually rebuilding their intestinal flora, plus they do not take antibiotics. Antiseptic herbs, such as wild oregano, and cumin, may also help curtail the problem.

#22. Bleeding gums are also an indication of vitamin C and bioflavonoid deficiencies. However, this is also a signal of a number of other problems, such as folic acid deficiency, intestinal fungal infection, poor immunity, and infection within the gums themselves. Severe bleeding gums may also warn of liver disease, with the resultant lack of vitamin K and albumin. A deficiency of a special nutrient known as *coenzyme Q-10* can also lead to gum disease. While not technically listed as a vitamin or mineral, coenzyme Q-10 is critically important for proper functioning of gum tissue and many other cells and organs. Bleeding gums may also warn of chronic infection within both the teeth and gums.

#23. Receding gums are a classic signal of nutritional deficiency. Here, the gums can't grow fast enough to meet the proper alignment with the teeth. Deficient nutrients include coenzyme Q-10, zinc, vitamin C, vitamin K, riboflavin, and folic acid. Coenzyme Q-10 and folic acid appear to be the most critical, since supplementation with these two nutrients alone usually reverses the problem.

Gum infection warns of widespread nutritional deficiency as well as compromised immunity. However, taking the nutrients alone often fails to resolve this problem. I have seen great success in eradicating tooth/gum infections with potent natural antiseptics. The supreme treatment is Oreganol oil of oregano, which is very aggressive in eradicating dental infections. Simply apply this antiseptic oil on the gums and teeth twice daily. Add it to toothpaste or apply it on the toothbrush whenever brushing. Plus, it keeps the toothbrush from harboring germs.

#24. The existence of age spots means the body is undergoing a process known medically as *lipid peroxidation*. Be concerned if there is an increase in the number or size of these spots. This means the fatty acids in the body are decomposing at a rapid rate and that the individual is susceptible to a variety of degenerative diseases, including cancer, Alzheimer's disease, and rapid aging.

Peroxides are fatty acids which have undergone a process known as *oxidation*. A good example of this is butter that is heated excessively. Butter is easily oxidized when heated, and this is manifested by it turning dark brown. This is, in a sense, what happens in the body when fatty acids lining the membranes of the cells become "oxidized." In the case of living tissue, heat is usually not the factor initiating the oxidative changes. Brown spots are caused by radiation, toxic chemicals, toxic oils, and poor diet low in antioxidants, all of which initiate the oxidation of tissue fats. It has now been proven that the body's lipids degenerate more rapidly if deficiencies of selenium, vitamin E, beta carotene, vitamin C, pantothenic acid, and vitamin B_6 exist. A word of caution: poor quality fatty acids are worse for you than no fatty acids at all. Eating oils which are overheated (including butter), deep fried foods, highly processed fats, such as commercial vegetable oils, margarine, and lard, only leads to an increase in the rate at which the fatty acids in our bodies degenerate (see Chapter Five). Anything which so greatly affects our cell membranes, the guardians and protectors of the cells, will also increase the risks of degenerative disease, infection, and/ or cancer.

The degeneration of the fatty acid coating, whether it be the skin or the outer membrane of, say, a liver cell, is one of the major factors predisposing individuals to cancer and immune decline. Avoid all substances which cause lipid peroxidation (see Chapters Five and Six). Furthermore, take antioxidant herbal oils. These substances act as powerful antioxidants, protecting the fatty acids within our cells from degenerating. Rosemary, oregano, sage, clove, cinnamon, myrtle, and cumin oils are among the most potent, effective herbal antioxidants known and are even more powerful in antioxidant action than the synthetic chemicals used for this purpose. However, guaranteed quality of these edible essential oils is mandatory. The manufacturer should be willing to verify that the product is wild, edible, and/or 100% pure, as does the North American Herb & Spice Company which invented and developed the emulsification process for the finest edible herbal oils available.

Some Serious Warnings

If any of the following symptoms exist, something vitally important may be developing. These warnings must be heeded, and the individual must become more aware of what the body is revealing. This is not to create paranoia. It is only to help the individual aggressively change the way he/she lives in order to prevent health disasters. Here are the serious warning signs:

1. chest pains, particularly left-sided, which worsen upon exertion

2. severe leg pains or cramps, which worsen when you exercise or walk

3. a noticeable decrease in memory or mental sharpness

4. moles and other growths which are growing in size or number

5. a noticeable decline in how fast wounds heal

6. increased sensitivity to hot or cold, noises, or smells

7. lowered resistance to colds or flu

8. poor or slow recovery from illness, especially infections

9. a noticeable alteration in bowel habits

10. severe depression, anxiety, or agitation

If you suffer from any of these signals, it may be necessary to seek medical help, ideally from a physician skilled in preventive/nutritional medicine. Change the way you eat, quit eating harmful foods, quit smoking, and curtail alcohol consumption. Above all, don't neglect your health. Do whatever it takes to get well and stay well. Remember, natural medicine is the safest of all types of medicine.

CHAPTER FIVE

What Are The Time Bombs?

The time bombs are defined as those substances found in the diet and in the environment which have a potentially devastating effect upon the human body. They are so named because their regular consumption is likely to reduce lifespan. Here is a list of the major time bombs:

1. refined sugar

2. white flour

3. alcoholic beverages

4. processed or cured meats

5. deep-fried foods

6. refined vegetable oils such as corn, sunflower, safflower, rapeseed, and soybean oil

7. margarine and other hydrogenated vegetable oils such as Crisco or shortening

8. pesticides and herbicides

9. industrial chemicals

10. radioactive chemicals

11. exposure to heavy (toxic) metals

12. cigarettes

The time bombs are frightening, because they threaten lives and destroy human cells. Every day virtually every American receives a dose of not one but many of these time bombs. However, there is no need to despair. Although it is impossible to entirely avoid exposure to these substances, you can largely control the first seven. If you at least remove these seven dietary time bombs from your lifestyle, you will enjoy better health.

The first seven items on the time bomb list can be largely controlled by dietary and lifestyle alterations. This chapter focuses primarily on five of these; item #1 (refined sugar), item #4 (processed and cured meats) and items #5, 6, & 7 (deep fried foods, refined vegetable oils, margarine, and other hydrogenated fats). Let's see how much exposure YOU are getting.

Your Refined Sugar Time Bomb Quotient

Refined sugar is a toxic substance. By definition this category includes white sugar, table sugar, brown sugar, corn syrup, malt syrup, glucose, commercial molasses, and dextrose. The latter names are what are usually listed on food labels. Most of the refined sugar intake in North America is in the form of white sugar and corn syrup.

Refined sugar has many negative effects and no positive ones. Its consumption is associated with an increased incidence of diabetes, heart disease, cancer, high blood pressure, Alzheimer's disease, yeast infections, gum disease, and many other maladies. In children, behavioral disorders, obesity, heart disease, high cholesterol, asthma, ear infections, sore throats, tonsillitis, visual problems, and dental disease are directly correlated with high sugar consumption.

Even a small amount may be too much for the body to handle. As little as a teaspoonful per day can be harmful. Just think about the damage being done to those who are consuming it by the handful. Determine your sugar quotient by taking the following test.

Circle the appropriate response. On the average do you consume:

POINTS

1. Doughnuts, cupcakes, and/or sweet rolls

1-2 per week 5

3-5 per week 10

1 per day 15

2 or more per day 20

2. Cakes, pies, and/or brownies

1-2 pieces per week. 5

3-5 pieces per week. 10

1 piece per day 15

2 or more pieces per day 20

3. Hot fruit pies and/or toaster-tarts

1 item per week. 5

2-5 items per week 10

1 item per day 15

2 or more items per day. 20

4. Pop (sweetened)

1 twelve oz. drink per week 5

2-5 twelve oz. drinks per week 10

1 twelve oz. drink per day 15

2 or more twelve oz. drinks per day 25

5. Coffee or tea (sugar added)

1-2 added teaspoons per week 5

3-5 added teaspoons per week 10

1-3 added teaspoons per day 15

4 or more added teaspoons per day 20

6. Other sugar-sweetened drinks (Kool-Aid, HI-C, etc.)

1-2 drinks per week 5

3-4 drinks per week 10

1 drink per day 15

2 or more drinks per day 20

7. Candy Bars

1 per week. 5

2-3 per week 10

1 per day 15

2 or more per day 20

8. Cookies

1-2 per week 5

3-4 per week 10

1 per day 15

2 or more per day 20

9. Hard candies and chocolates

2-5 pieces per week. 5

1 piece per day 10

2-3 pieces per day 15

4 or more pieces per day 20

10. Cereals (sugar-sweetened)

1 bowl per week 5

2-5 bowls per week 10

1 bowl per day. 15

2 or more bowls per day 20

11. Salad dressings, ketchup, and/or steak sauce

2-5 times per week 5

1-2 times per day 10

3 or more times per day. 15

12. Yogurt (sweetened), whipping cream, and/or non-dairy creamers

1-4 times per week 5

once per day 10

2 or more times per day. 15

13. Cured meats (bacon, ham, corned beef, bologna, hot dogs, etc.)

1-3 times per week 5

Once per day 10

2 or more times per day 15

14. Ice cream, malts, shakes, floats, and/or sherbet

1-2 servings per week 5

3-5 servings per week 10

1 serving per day 15

2 or more servings per day 20

YOUR SCORE _____

5-30 Points You are consuming a small but significant amount of sugar. Reducing your sugar intake could lead to a noticeable improvement in your health.

35-70 Points You are consuming sugar at a rate of a heaping teaspoon or more per day. It would be wise to slow down before the sugar slows you down.

75-130 Points You are consuming sugar by the heaping tablespoonful daily. Damage is being done. Curtail this excessive sugar intake immediately.

135-Above You are eating sugar every day by the handful. As a result, you are inducing widespread damage to your body. The fact is you are in the category of consuming 100 to 200 pounds-plus of sugar per year. If you continue at this pace, you will likely develop diabetes, high blood pressure, heart disease, or cancer. Stop now, and you will recover much of your health.

Anyone with a score of 75 and above is living in the danger zone. At this level of sugar intake there is a risk of damaging or even destroying the adrenal and thyroid glands. These delicate glands must work overtime to help the body deal with the excess sugar. Under the pressure of constant bombardment of refined sugar, these glands literally burn out. Certainly, the glands are capable of regenerating and their function can return *if you make the appropriate dietary changes and get off the sugar.* However, there is a risk for permanent damage if you continue this massive sugar consumption. The more sugar that is consumed over the years, the more likely it is that you will have decimated a portion of your pancreas, adrenal and thyroid glands. Remember, the average American consumes approximately 150 pounds of sugar each year. That is enough to damage even the pancreas, adrenal, and thyroid glands. The following case history is an example of how this happens:

> Mr. M. was a long-standing lover of sweets. He not only ate them on a daily basis, but also gave various sweets, such as cheesecake, chocolates, and candies, to all of his friends. Needless to say, Mr. M. is a sweet man. Although Mr. M. presented with the primary complaint of angina and hardening of the arteries, his underlying problem was *adrenal insufficiency* secondary to his sugar-laden diet. Interestingly, his heart trouble improved dramatically when he was placed on a diet free of all refined sugar. Plus, he lost a great deal of weight just by eating right. However, he continued to buy chocolates for his "friends," including his doctor, who graciously received them but secretly disposed of them in the trash.

Your Hydrogenated Fat Time Bomb Quotient

Hydrogenated oils are the most commonly consumed types of fats in the American diet. These fats are found everywhere in commercial foods. Next time you go into the supermarket, look at the labels. You will see the terms hydrogenated oils and partially hydrogenated oils on hundreds of supermarket items. The fact is, at least one of three packaged foods contain these noxious ingredients. As delineated by the Harvard School of Public Health, margarine and hydrogenated oils are unfit for human consumption.

Because of the toxicity of these fats you must know your degree of consumption. Another major reason is that the most common overall deficiency in this country is that of the essential fatty acids. These fatty acids are just as the term suggests—they are essential to life itself. In the typical American diet these fats are being displaced by unhealthy ones, particularly hydrogenated and partially hydrogenated oils. In other words, the hydrogenated/partially hydrogenated oils induce a deficiency of the essential fatty acids. In fact, in North America they are the number one cause of this deficiency. Take this test to find out where you stand regarding hydrogenated oil consumption.

Circle the correct response. On the average do you consume:

POINTS

1. **Deep-fried foods (French fries, fried chicken, chicken nuggets, fish sticks, egg rolls, potato skins, corn dogs, fried mushrooms, hush puppies, fish 'n' chips, etc.)**

   1-2 times per week 5

   3-4 times per week 10

   Once per day 15

   2 or more times per day 25

2. **Bakery items cooked with shortening (cookies, pies, pastries, cakes, etc.)**

   1-2 times per week 5

   3-4 times per week 10

   Once per day 15

   2 or more times per day 20

3. **Margarine (used as a spread or in cooking)**

   1-2 servings (tablespoons) per week 5

   3-4 servings per week 10

   1-2 servings per day 15

   3 or more servings per day 20

4. **Crackers or snacks containing hydrogenated or partially hydrogenated oils, lard, or shortening**

   1-2 servings per week 5

   3-5 servings per week 10

   1-2 servings per day 15

   3 or more servings per day 20

5. Breads or buns containing hydrogenated or partially hydrogenated oils, lard, or shortening

2-5 servings per week 5

1 serving per day. 10

2-3 servings per day 15

4 or more servings per day 20

6. Imitation ice cream, whipping cream, non-dairy creamers, and various coated ice cream bars

1-2 servings per week 5

3-4 servings per week 10

1-2 times per day. 15

3 or more servings per day 20

7. Candy bars, chocolates, and hard candies

1-2 servings per week 5

3-4 servings per week 10

1 serving per day. 15

2 or more servings per day 20

8. Frozen or packaged dinners, frozen hash browns, pizzas, or French fries

1-3 times per week 5

4-6 times per week 10

1-2 times per day. 15

3 or more times per day. 20

9. Mayonnaise and foods made with mayonnaise (potato salad, cole slaw, etc.)

1-3 times per week 5

4-6 times per week 10

1-2 times per day. 15

3 or more times per day. 20

10. **Tortilla chips, corn chips, taco shells, cheese puffs, and similar corn meal snacks**

     1-3 times per week 5

     4-6 times per week 10

     1-2 times per day. 15

     3 or more times per day. 20

11. **Potato chips and/or potato sticks**

     1-3 times per week 5

     4-6 times per week 10

     1-2 times per day. 15

     3 or more times per day. 20

12. **Toaster pastries, granola bars, and similar quick breakfast snacks**

     1-3 times per week 5

     4-6 times per week 10

     1-2 times per day. 15

     3 or more times per day. 20

YOUR SCORE _____

5-35 Points You are getting a small but significant amount of hydrogenated or harmful fats in your diet. Avoid the foods you are eating which contain these fats.

40-80 Points You are eating harmful fats by the teaspoonful every day. These hydrogenated fats are harming you, your cells, your organs, and your immune system. Avoid all foods containing these fats.

85-130 Points You are eating harmful fats by the tablespoonful every day. Significant damage to your internal organs and immune system is likely if you continue. Curtail the consumption of these noxious hydrogenated fats immediately. Read labels!

135 and above—Danger Zone You are eating hydrogenated fats by the tubful every day. Your risk for developing heart disease, cancer, or some other life-threatening disease is exceptionally high. It is crucial that you change your diet immediately. To help heal the damage it is necessary to eat foods rich in natural essential fatty acids and take fatty acid supplements.

How Margarine and Hydrogenated Fats Originated

The large scale production of margarine was partly the result of a food shortage. During World War II butter was scarce. Chemists had long before found an alternative. They discovered as early as the late 1800s that liquid vegetable oils could be turned into solid fat through a process known as *hydrogenation*. During this process hydrogen gas is bubbled into the oil, which is heated to a high temperature. Nickel is then added to catalyze (speed up) the reaction. These hydrogenated fats are what make up margarine and shortening. In addition, in an attempt to mimic butter, synthetic dyes are often added to turn the whitish-colored hydrogenated fats into margarine.

If you think about it, you will be able to understand how unnatural and unhealthy hydrogenated fats really are. True, margarine is touted as being low in cholesterol and saturated fats. Yet, it is high in unnatural fats, toxic fats, and cancer-causing chemicals.

Is There a Safe Amount?

Even a small amount of hydrogenated fats and oils is too much. Hardened fats should be eliminated entirely from the diet. While butter is a solid fat, it is an acceptable food, since it is natural and unaltered in its chemistry. However, one problem with butter is that it may contain Butter Yellow, a cancer-causing dye. So, be sure to read labels and purchase farm fresh natural butter or butter-colored with natural substances, like carotenes and annato.

Even the typical refined liquid vegetable oils found in the supermarket must be used sparingly, if at all. Researchers have proven that their consumption is associated with an increased cancer risk.

Why Processed Fats are so Bad

If you are getting the wrong kinds of fats in your diet, beware. The body needs a certain amount of fat every day, but it needs the "good" fats. If you eat only the processed kinds, your body has no option but to make use of them. Processed fats, especially the hydrogenated variety, confuse the body, because the chemical structure of these bizarre fats is different than the structure of naturally occurring fats, the kinds which are normally recognized and utilized by the digestive organs and cells of the body.

Once the "bad" fats are absorbed, they are taken to the liver, where they are stored or converted into energy. The chemistry of these fats is abnormal and, thus, it is difficult for the liver to determine what to do with them. When a cell is damaged and needs fatty acids for repair or other purposes, these abnormal fats will be made available to the cell, especially if there is a lack of natural essential fats. The cell will attempt to insert the abnormal fat into its membrane, resulting in a weakened, malfunctioning cell. Thus, synthetic fats damage cells. Yet, unprocessed or unaltered fats which naturally occur in whole foods, such as butter, milk fat, nut fats, oily fish, and even the fat marbled in meat, fail to cause any type of organ or cell damage. On the contrary, a lack of them is a primary cause of cellular damage.

Have Your Cells Become "Hydrogenated"?

Would you believe that in all probability you are "partially hydrogenated?" Over the years you have developed untold thousands of hardened (hydrogenated) cells. This is because these cells have inserted into their membranes trans fats from a dose of margarine or from some French fries cooked in a deep fryer, etc.

An example of this is what happens to white blood cells exposed to hydrogenated and partially hydrogenated oils. These cells incorporate the hydrogenated fats you eat into their membranes. When this happens, their membranes actually become stiff, and, thus, the white cells become sluggish in function. Such white blood cells are incapable of defending the body against infection. This leaves the body highly vulnerable to all sorts of derangements of the immune system. Cancer, as well as infections by yeasts, bacteria, parasites, and viruses, can more readily gain a foothold. Furthermore, susceptibility to allergic reactions is greatly heightened.

Chemically altered and hydrogenated fats are no longer a food. They, in effect, become a poison, polluting the body's cells and organs. Once deposited within the tissues, these fats may induce widespread damage in the cells and organs. In fact, one of the quickest ways to paralyze the immune system is to eat on a daily basis significant quantities of deep-fried foods or fats such as margarine, partially hydrogenated cottonseed/palm/corn/soybean/sunflower/rapeseed/saf-flower oil, or lard.

Recently, it has become fashionable to consume the so-called cholesterol-lowering margarines. Another debacle is the addition of fat substitutes such as Olestra and Olean. None of these substances provide food value, and all of them are inferior nutritionally to the true natural fats such as pure extra virgin olive oil, butter, crude pumpkinseed oil, and nut oils. The point is avoid the consumption of synthetic fats. Ideal natural oils which help cleanse the body of bad or toxic fats include primrose oil and cold-pressed Austrian pumpkinseed oil. Recently, a stabilized type of Austrian pumpkinseed oil has become available. Known as *Pumpkinol*, it contains only the finest grade of crude extra virgin Austrian pumpkinseed oil stabilized with powerful antioxidant edible essential oils. Crude Austrian pumpkinseed oil (Pumpkinol) is an excellent source of essential fatty acids, which are direly needed for fat and protein metabolism.

How Fats Become Hydrogenated
(The Trans Fat Story)

Trans fats result from the chemical process of hydrogenation. As described previously, chemists take oils, such as corn, cottonseed, soy, rapeseed, and safflower, which are normally liquid at room temperature and heat them to a very high temperature. They then add chemicals, including the metal nickel, to cause a twisting in the oils' molecular bonds. This causes the chemical structure to be altered from the normal *cis* configuration to the *trans* structure. These trans fatty acids are *not found in nature*. Thus, the human body is unable to properly utilize them. In fact, because the body fails to recognize and utilize these unnatural fats, it forces them into abnormal places within the tissues. This causes tremendous cellular distress and, ultimately, disease. In effect, what was once a food has now been transformed into a laboratory aberration—a freak, but not an accidental one.

All this is done for effect. Marketability, shelf life, and consumer appeal are the goals of the hydrogenated fat industry. These fats have an extended shelf life. Yet, your life may be shelved if you continue to eat them. While hydrogenated fats may not become easily rancid on the shelf, they induce a wide range of rancidity problems within the body. They waste antioxidants, such as vitamin E, glutathione, and selenium, which function to prevent fats from becoming rancid.

No wonder that a high consumption of margarine, shortening, and other hydrogenated fats is associated with a greater incidence of a variety of cancers. A list of conditions and diseases associated with their consumption includes:

1. Alzheimer's disease
2. atherosclerosis
3. autoimmune diseases
4. cancer
5. chronic candidiasis
6. diabetes
7. eczema
8. heart disease
9. high blood pressure
10. lupus
11. Parkinson's disease
12. PMS
13. psoriasis
14. Sjogren's syndrome

Avoid hydrogenated fats like you would avoid the plague.

Dr. Ingram's Five Simple Rules for
Avoiding Hydrogenated Fats

1. Shop in the outer aisles at the grocery store. Fresh foods, fruits, vegetables, fresh meats, eggs, milk, and cheese do not contain added oils.

2. Use only extra virgin olive oil, butter, Austrian pumpkinseed oil (Pumpkinol), or coconut oil in cooking or food preparation. Other cold-pressed vegetable oils are acceptable, particularly cold-pressed sesame, peanut, walnut, and avocado oils. Yet, the ideal and safest cooking oils are those low in polyunsaturated fats such as extra virgin olive oil, butter, coconut fat, tallow, and avocado oil. These are the types of oils which should be used in heating, since heat causes polyunsaturated oils, even those from cold-pressed oils, to become caustic.

3. Always ask your server what the restaurant is sautéing the food in. Most restaurants carry extra virgin olive oil or will carry it upon demand. If you forget to ask, *odds are the food will be cooked with margarine or hydrogenated fats.*

4. Tell your server as soon as you see him/her to hold the bread basket. This way your hunger will not overwhelm you. Most crackers and rolls contain hydrogenated fats.

5. Read all labels on canned, bottled, or packaged foods purchased at the grocery store. If you see the words hydrogenated, partially hydrogenated, or shortening, do not buy it or use it!

What are the Good Fats?

It is certainly insufficient to tell you only which fats to avoid. Fats and oils have been used in food preparation for centuries. Extra virgin olive oil is probably the most ancient cooking oil and has been used for thousands of years. Olive oil has proven itself with the test of time. Yet, only in the last decade has modern medical science recognized its healthful benefits. Flaxseed oil is another oil which has been used for centuries. This is also known as linseed oil (food grade). Europeans have extolled its health benefits since the Middle Ages.

The Inuits' high fat diet has been very beneficial to their health. It is modeled to fit their cold climate. Although Inuits eat a great deal of fat, they eat natural fats, primarily from fish, whale, and seal oils. Thus, they do not have the problems we do from eating altered or unnatural ones.

The oils of certain seeds/nuts, such as almonds, pumpkin, safflower, soybean, and sunflower seeds, also have healthy components. Yet, these oils are beneficial only if they are extracted under the appropriate conditions. The only way to insure the nutritional value of these oils is to extract them by cold-pressing, that is without the use of heat or chemicals. Commercial vegetable oils in the supermarket are extracted under conditions of very high temperatures and with the use of noxious chemicals such as dyes, degummers, and bleach. This process upsets the chemistry of the oils and destroys the naturally occurring antioxidants. For example, sunflower oil naturally contains a tremendous amount of vitamin E, the major antioxidant found in fats and oils. However, when sunflower oil is heat-extracted, all of the vitamin E is destroyed. This is why food processors add synthetic antioxidants, such as BHT, to their oils. BHT is a known carcinogen.

Most truly cold-pressed oils can be discerned by a simple fact: they contain a sediment at the bottom of the bottle. Extra virgin olive oil, while cold-pressed, does not usually contain a sediment, because it is usually filtered. Olives are up to 90% oil. They are one of the richest food sources of vegetable oil. Extra virgin olive oil is highly beneficial as a food, and it is the preferable cooking oil. It resists rancidity and can be heated to higher temperatures than other vegetable oils without being damaged. Extra virgin olive oil has beneficial effects upon the circulation, reducing cholesterol levels, increasing HDL cholesterol (the beneficial type), and improving blood flow. In addition, it is highly digestible, much more so than oils derived from grains, seeds, and beans such as soy, sunflower, or corn oil. Extra virgin olive oil is the major cooking oil you should use. Other vegetable oils, such as soy, sunflower, and safflower oils, can't withstand the cooking heat as well as the olive oil and tend to become rancid or toxic more easily. Crude coconut oil is another option, since it has a high tolerance and is readily digested.

Austrian pumpkinseed oil, that is Pumpkinol, can be consumed with any food. It is best to avoid heating it so add it to hot foods toward the end of cooking. The dark greenish-red color is a sign of purity and nutritional density. This oil is an excellent source of zinc and vitamin E, which are desperately needed for normal fatty acid metabolism. Thus, it is an ideal fatty acid supplement. Take a teaspoon or more daily.

Butter can also be used in cooking, but it should be cooked with low heat. Clarified butter is the best for cooking, since it withstands higher temperatures without discoloring or burning. At moderately high cooking temperatures the fatty acids in butter are damaged. If heated excessively, it becomes rancid and badly toxic. If you burn the butter, don't use it. Start again, and carefully heat it so it doesn't burn.

Cold-pressed almond, avocado, peanut, and sesame oils can also be used in cooking. However, use only moderate to low heat. Excessive heating damages the polyunsaturated oils, causing them to become toxic and potentially cancer promoting.

Which Foods are Rich in Essential Fatty Acids?

Only a few common foods are naturally rich in essential fatty acids. A partial list of them includes:

- avocado
- apricot kernels
- black currants
- eggs
- mustard seeds
- pine nuts
- pumpkin and squash seeds
- soybeans
- walnuts
- wheat germ
- whole wheat bread
- peanuts

- almonds
- beans
- Brazil nuts
- fish (fatty types)
- pecans
- poppy seeds
- rice germ or bran
- sunflower seeds
- watermelon seeds
- filberts
- caraway seeds
- wild game

Wild game is the richest meat source of essential fatty acids. This is due to the fatty acid-rich diet of these animals. The fatty acids within game are readily digested and assimilated. I highly recommend the addition of game such as pheasant, quail, deer, elk, duck, rabbit, and goose to your diet.

What About Essential Fatty Acid Supplements?

I believe firmly in the use of nutritional supplements. No area deserves more attention than the need to supplement the diet with essential fatty acids.

Essential fatty acids, by the strictest definition, are those fats which cannot be made in the body and must be consumed in the diet. Only two such fatty acids exist, namely *linoleic* and *linolenic* acid. Excellent supplemental sources of these fatty acids include flaxseed, evening primrose, borage, sunflower, and safflower oil. Other rich sources are sesame, corn, wheat germ, cod liver, almond, walnut, pumpkinseed oil, and soybean oil.

Note: Olive oil contains only small quantities of the essential fatty acids. However, it contains a number of other useful oils such as *oleic acid*.

For correcting deficiencies, flaxseed, borage, and primrose oils are ideal. A great deal of research has been done on the therapeutic benefits of these oils. In addition, both contain appreciable quantities of the rarer linolenic acid, while containing less linoleic acid than the other oils. Deficiency of linoleic acid is less common, since oils rich in it, such as corn, sunflower, soybean, and safflower, are more prevalent in the Western diet.

A deficiency of essential fatty acids can be caused by a variety of factors, including:

1. alcohol consumption

2. antibiotic overuse

3. chewing tobacco

4. cigarette smoking

5. all dietary hydrogenated, partially hydrogenated, and deep-fried fats (the number one cause in America today)

6. high intake of saturated fats, especially refined coconut fat

7. high sugar intake (the number two cause)

8. intestinal fungal or yeast infection

9. severe, prolonged emotional stress

10. toxic chemical exposure

11. regular intake of aspirin or non-steroidal antiinflammatory drugs (ibuprophen, naproxen sodium, etc.)

12. zinc, magnesium, vitamin C, vitamin B_6, niacin, or biotin deficiency

Diseases caused by or related to essential fatty acid deficiency include:

- Adrenal insufficiency
- Allergies
- Asthma
- Atherosclerosis
- Atopy
- Crohn's disease
- Diabetes
- Eczema and psoriasis
- Fungal infections
- Hypothyroidism
- Lupus
- Nephritis
- Prostatitis
- Ulcerative colitis

The Atopic Individual

Atopy, an illness occurring primarily in modern times, is an excellent example of how severe health problems can be induced by essential fatty acid deficiency. This term describes a condition related to defective genes, so it is hereditary. The defect lies in an inability to utilize essential fatty acids. Atopic individuals are unusually vulnerable to asthma, hay fever, food allergies, sinus problems, digestive disturbances, skin diseases, and PMS. In particular, atopic individuals are far more vulnerable than normal individuals to developing allergic reactions, both to foods and chemicals. They tend to be the ones who are "allergic to everything." They are also far more susceptible to the ill-effects of consuming processed or hydrogenated oils. Thus, they must be especially strict about the types of fats and oils they consume.

In most instances the symptoms and illnesses associated with the atopic state improve dramatically with fatty acid supplementation. A generous supply of vitamins and minerals, especially zinc, magnesium, pantothenic acid, pyridoxine, and biotin, also is necessary. For essential fatty acids, flaxseed is one of the best sources. However, since flaxseed oil turns rancid rapidly, it is preferable to consume the freshly ground seed as a more natural, less processed fatty acid source. Other excellent sources of essential fatty acids include lecithin, rice germ, and wheat germ. While the crushed flax is preferable, flaxseed oil may be a reliable source if it is truly cold-processed. After opening, keep it in the freezer.

Nutri-Sense is a B vitamin and essential fatty acid food supplement which is ideal for atopic patients. It contains three top essential fatty acid sources: stabilized ground flaxseed, lecithin, and rice bran/germ. However, usually flax oil or flaxseed is not enough to solve the atopic problem. There is another fatty acid missing called gamma linolenic acid, which is found primarily in primrose and borage oils. Here is an excellent protocol if you suffer from the symptoms of essential fatty acid deficiency and/or atopy: consume Nutri-Sense, three heaping tablespoons in juice or water every day, and take at least six capsules of evening primrose oil or borage oil daily.

Most people with atopic sensitivity have a condition known as the "toxic" colon. These individuals often suffer from a prolonged history of constipation. The overgrowth of yeasts and "unfriendly" bacteria in the colon helps maintain the constipation and toxic state. The fact is, yeast overgrowth is one of the most common causes of chronic constipation. It is also a major cause of eczema. To reverse bowel toxicity and eliminate constipation, take Nutri-Sense, three tablespoons twice daily in juice or water. Support this with three to six capsules per day of evening primrose or borage oil. Also, take acidophilus supplements on a daily basis. Removing the toxins is of little value unless the yeast overgrowth is resolved. To kill the yeasts and noxious bacteria, take wild oregano capsules (Oreganol gelcaps), two or three caps three times daily. Use also Oreganol oil of wild oregano, two to five drops twice daily. By eliminating the unhealthy germs and improving bowel function, the atopic condition invariably improves, and the improvement is usually rapid. This is because a healthy digestive tract and colon are vital for maintaining an excellent state of health.

Numerous other symptoms may signal essential fatty acid deficiency, including:

1. bleeding gums
2. brittle hair or nails
3. cold extremities
4. dryness of skin behind the ears
5. dry or flaky skin
6. dry or oily hair
7. dry patches of skin on the face
8. excessive thirst
9. excess oil on the face or hair
10. excess or lack of ear wax
11. hair loss
12. itchy ears
13. irritable or sluggish bowels
14. lowered resistance to infection
15. poor wound healing
16. slow-growing hair or nails
17. yeast infections
18. skin infections
19. lung infections
20. unmanageable hair

For more in depth test regarding the symptoms of essential fatty acid deficiency, see the Web site Nutrition Test.com

Immune Breakdown:
A Consequence of Essential Fatty Acid Deficiency

Essential fatty acid deficiency can result in a wide range of symptoms, many of them serious, as the previously mentioned chart illustrates. Let's concentrate on symptoms 14, 15, 17, and 18—symptoms indicating poor immune function. The immune system desperately needs essential fatty acids. It cannot function properly without them. Every immune cell and organ in the body requires a daily supply to stay in optimal working order. Furthermore, these cells and organs degenerate unless they get an adequate supply of essential fatty acids. This condition is known as *cellular atrophy*. This means that without essential fatty acids, cells shrivel and die.

The Skin: Our First Line of Defense

Essential fatty acids are necessary for maintaining the structural integrity of every cell and cell membrane in the body. The skin is the first defense against invasion by microbes. How does the skin remain taut and free of cracks despite aging, injury, and constant exposure? It is the essential fatty acids which are primarily responsible. They are required to help seal any cuts or wounds that occur and to help keep the skin pliable and soft. Tiny tears in the skin occur every day, although they are not always readily seen. The body heals these tears by mobilizing extra fatty acids from the liver and any that are stored in body fat. However, in the event of moderate to severe injuries or multiple wounds, these essential fatty acid reserves are rapidly depleted. In addition, zinc, selenium, biotin,   vitamin B_6, pantothenic acid, and riboflavin are required to aid in the utilization of these fatty acids. A steady supply of essential fatty acids is absolutely critical, and the organs of the human body are at a high risk for damage and disease in the event of a deficiency.

Fatty acids within the skin also protect us from the invasion of harmful germs. They not only help build a tough barrier against the microbes but also inhibit their growth. Therefore, they are truly the skin's natural antibiotics.

There is an even more insidious effect of this deficiency upon the immune system: damage to the cell membrane. Several nutrients are needed to keep cell membranes of the organs healthy. The list includes selenium, vitamin B_6, riboflavin, vitamin E, vitamin A, cholesterol (believe it or not, cholesterol has many useful functions), and essential fatty acids. If the cell membrane is not supplied with an adequate amount of any or all of these nutrients, it will degenerate. Obviously, if the membranes of immune cells, such as white blood cells and lymphocytes, begin to fracture, a wide range of serious problems will result. The body is left vulnerable to infection by all sorts of germs, not to mention cancer.

Do you know how much surface would be covered if all 70 trillion of your cell membranes were flattened out, end to end? Incredibly, these cell membranes would cover an area the size of Texas or even larger. This illustrates how important proper nutrition is to the health of human cells and organs. Imagine how readily such a huge surface area would degenerate if it was not supplied with the nutrients it needs to keep it strong. Remember, years of abuse caused by eating the wrong kinds of fats is not corrected overnight. It may take months or years to solve the problem. If you suffer from the warning signs of essential fatty acid deficiency, treat yourself to essential fatty acid supplements such as Nutri-Sense, Pumpkinol, and primrose oil, and use them regularly. Eat foods rich in essential fatty acids such as fresh nuts, seeds, the germ of grains, fatty fish, and wild game. Usually, it takes several months to resolve severe essential fatty acid deficiency, so be patient.

Your Processed/Cured Meat Time Bomb Quotient

Meat can be good for you, that is if it is fresh or if it is free of chemicals, hormones, pesticides, preservatives, or other additives. *Processed* meat, that is meat cured with nitrates, is a poor choice, especially when fresh meat is so readily available. Cured meats are loaded with chemical preservatives (nitrates, BHT, BHA), coloring agents, sugar, and other sweeteners such as dextrose and corn syrup. Take this test to find out how much exposure you are getting:

Circle the correct response. On the average do you consume:

POINTS

1. Hot dogs and/or corn dogs

1 per week 5

2-3 per week 10

4 per week. 15

1 or more daily 25

2. Pastrami, chipped beef, ham, and/or corned beef

1 serving per week 5

2-3 servings per week 10

4-6 servings per week 15

1 or more servings daily 20

3. Bologna, salami, and/or other deli meats

1 serving per week 5

2-3 servings per week 10

4-6 servings per week 15

1 or more servings daily 20

4. Sausages and/or bratwurst

1 serving per week 5

2-3 servings per week 10

4-6 servings per week 15

1 serving per day 20

2 or more servings per day 25

5. Turkey ham, turkey salami, and/or turkey pastrami

1-3 servings per week 5

4-6 servings per week 10

1 or more servings daily 15

6. Bacon and/or breakfast strips

1-2 slices per week 5

3-4 slices per week 10

1 slice per day 15

2-3 slices per day 20

4 or more slices per day 25

7. Beef jerky

1-2 sticks per week 5

3-4 sticks per week 10

5-6 sticks per week 15

1 or more sticks daily 20

8. Pork and beans or similar canned pork products

1-3 servings per week 5

4-6 servings per week 10

1-2 servings daily 15

3 or more servings daily 20

9. Pepperoni and/or Canadian bacon

1 serving per week 5

2-3 servings per week 10

4-6 servings per week 15

1 or more servings daily 20

YOUR SCORE _____

5-15 Points You are doing well. Considering how available and common these meats are, it is remarkable that your intake is so minimal. However, eliminating these meats entirely would help your overall health. "Zero" points is certainly what you should strive for.

20-50 Points Each week you are getting a significant dose of nitrates from eating processed meats. The nitrates in meats and the other noxious ingredients, such as coloring agents, sugar, etc., are bad for you. While you may not notice any obvious ill effects from eating these meats, eventually, it will catch up with you and have a negative bearing on your health.

55-85 Points It appears that you are getting a daily dose of nitrated and/or processed meats. This is extremely dangerous. Nitrates are curing agents, acting to retard spoilage of the meat. To be effective they must be added to the food in rather large amounts. At this level of exposure it is likely that you are experiencing at least two ill effects from the nitrates: 1) digestive disturbances, and 2) fatigue. The fatigue is caused by direct toxicity to the blood cells. Nitrates combine with hemoglobin in the blood and turn it into its inactive form. This is known medically as *methemoglobin*. Methemoglobin is useless to the body, since it cannot carry oxygen to the cells. The transport of oxygen is the primary function of the normal hemoglobin molecule. This lack of oxygen disrupts the cells' metabolism, resulting in symptoms ranging from fatigue to poor circulation and headaches.

90-125 Points You are eating significant amounts of nitrated and/or processed meats on a daily basis. Curtail the intake of these meats before they cause you to be curtailed. The continued consumption of nitrated meats greatly increases the risks for fatal diseases, including cancer, stroke, and heart attacks. This heavy consumption of nitrated foods is damaging to organs throughout the body, leading to problems such as allergies, immune system disorders, and even heart disease, heart attacks, and cancer. Cancer is the most ominous result. Nitrates combine in the stomach with proteins to form substances known as *nitrosamines*. Nitrosamines are proven carcinogens. In fact, they are among the most potent carcinogens known. They irritate the cells lining the stomach and intestines, causing inflammation. Nitrosamines interact with the genes of these cells, causing them to convert to cancerous cells. Certain nutrients help the body neutralize and detoxify nitrosamines. Vitamin C is perhaps most important, although bioflavonoids are also needed. To detoxify nitrosamines, take an unprocessed natural vitamin C/bioflavonoid supplement. Flavin-C offers raw, unprocessed vitamin C and bioflavonoids ideal for nitrosamine neutralization. Take two capsules three times daily.

The reduction in blood flow and blood oxygen content are largely why nitrates aggravate the heart, increasing heart-related symptoms. It is my contention that many a heart attack has been brought on by eating nitrate-laden meats.

130-Above You are eating an unbelievably large amount of nitrated and processed meats. Disaster is inevitable if it hasn't already occurred. These meats and the chemicals they contain are damaging the lining of your stomach and intestines. They are depressing your immune system and predisposing you to cancer of the digestive tract and possibly cancer of other organs as well. The liver, the body's factory for detoxifying noxious agents, is no doubt being crippled by the extra burden of additives and chemicals.

This degree of exposure to nitrates greatly increases cancer risks. Heed this warning seriously. Remove all of these meats from the diet, and when you eat meat, buy fresh meats such as hamburger, steaks, roasts, or chops.

If you do have health problems, they are most likely related to the consumption of processed meats. This will be confirmed by the increased sense of well-being and the improvement in energy and strength you will experience when they are eliminated from your diet.

The damaging effects of nitrates and nitrosamines is perhaps best described by the renowned cancer researcher, Kedar Prasad, Ph.D., who states: *"Nitrosamines, which result from the nitrosation of food constituents by ingested nitrites or nitrates, are one of the most potent human carcinogens."* He also states that the largest source of nitrite intake in the U.S.A. is from cured meats, although cigarette smoke is the primary source of direct exposure to nitrosamines.

To detoxify the nitrates and nitrosamines take a crude natural vitamin C supplement, such as Flavin-C, three capsules twice daily. It has been proven that the natural vitamins stay in the body longer than the synthetic. Natural vitamins are also absorbed and used more efficiently. They cause no stress on the body and only assist its functions. Also, take Gene's powerdrops (wild berry formula), a source of natural flavonoids and other anti-cancer nutrients, 20 drops daily. Smokers should take even larger dosages of both the Flavin-C and Gene's powerdrops. Multiple doses aid in the detoxification of poisons. Natural vitamin C and flavonoid molecules are effective protective agents against nitrates and nitrosamines. Rosemary extracts also block nitrosamine toxicity. Take the edible oil of wild rosemary or the Juice of Rosemary (North American Herb & Spice). The oil may be taken with meals or under the tongue such as five drops twice daily. The juice may be added to grapefruit juice or hot water as a tea such as an ounce in a cup of water or juice. Research has proven that rosemary contains potent antioxidants which effectively neutralize nitrosamine toxicity.

A high intake of or exposure to nitrates, nitrites, and nitrosamines initiates cancerous changes in the body. The organs receiving the brunt of the damage are the esophagus, stomach, large intestine, bladder, and lungs. Yet, these noxious compounds may also cause an even more sinister disease, illustrated by this case history:

> A two-year-old girl developed a variety of symptoms for which the cause was unknown. Initially, tests were performed but no diagnosis was determined. The illness began taking a new course—she developed an enlarged, malfunctioning heart. The best of medical minds were having difficulty diagnosing the problem. Finally, an analysis was done on her diet, since the illness appeared to be similar to Keshan disease, a disease of the heart seen in certain children in China. Keshan disease is due to a selenium deficiency, a mineral whose importance is discussed at length in Chapter Six. Indeed, testing did show that she was selenium deficient. A diagnosis of selenium-deficient cardiomyopathy was established, a disease which leads to the degeneration of the heart muscle. But even more important was the diet analysis. Her daily diet consisted of grits and sausage for breakfast, a hot dog with pork and beans for lunch, and pork and beans plus rice for dinner. Each of these meals contained a dose of nitrates. The only beverages she had were Kool-Aid and water. No wonder she was sick to her heart.

The real crime in this example is that food could be preserved by substances which are safe for human consumption. Herbs, spices, salt, vitamin C, and vitamin E are all proven food preservatives. More importantly, a natural herbal preservative is now available. Called Preservit-all™, it may be freely added to foods and beverages to safely extend shelf life. It is made from natural herb and spice extracts. Also, the oils of wild oregano and rosemary can be safely added to all types of foods to preserve them and halt microbial growth. Preservit-all™ and edible essential oils offer the additional benefit of improving flavor. In fact, they are culinary delights.

Consumers should demand that food be preserved only with compounds proven to be safe. Our food supply is highly corrupted, and this is getting worse every year. Since the food is contaminated with noxious food additives and deadly pesticides, along with thousands of other poisons, there is little chance that the human body can withstand this pressure. What's more, the majority of people have eaten processed foods, such as refined sugar, hydrogenated oils, and processed meats, throughout their lives. The quantity consumed varies greatly within the major effort must be made to avoid the intake of genetically engineered foods, which also contaminate the body. These foods contain foreign genetic materials, which cause toxic and/or allergic reactions. As compared to natural foods studies have proven that genetically engineered foods greatly increase the risks of allergic reactions. The potential damage is unknown, but it will likely be vast. Certainly, deaths have occurred from the intake of food additives. I personally know of several mysterious deaths that have occurred due to the ingestion of chemically-laced foods. When food additives were first introduced, toxic reactions were well documented. Unfortunately, today these reactions largely go unnoticed or undiagnosed. The combination of toxic additives plus genetically engineered components could prove devastating, potentially causing tens of thousands of illnesses and/or deaths.

Labeling of foods containing toxic additives, as well as genetically engineered components, must be mandatory. However, labeling alone is far from the answer. The growth of these crops must be prohibited. This is because genetically engineered crops contaminate surrounding natural crops. With time, all of the plant life on earth will become tainted. Write your congressman to demand that the growth of genetically engineered plants be halted as well as manditory labeling of such foods.

Much of the damage can be repaired by changing old habits, eating the most nutrient-dense, wholesome, health-giving foods and natural food supplements, and by taking special nutrients known as antioxidants, which are described in the next chapter.

CHAPTER SIX
Antioxidants to the Rescue

If you are plagued with an illness, such as diabetes, heart disease, high blood pressure, arthritis, lupus, lung disease, asthma, cancer, or any other disease of civilization, don't despair. There is hope, because natural substances known as *antioxidants* can come to the rescue.

Antioxidants can be defined just as the name indicates: they are anti (against) oxidation. Oxidation is a chemical reaction which normally occurs within the body. When oxidative reactions occur in excess, cell damage and even cellular death result. Antioxidants are useful, because they halt abnormal oxidative reactions before the damage occurs. Most Americans are deficient in this key group of nutrients. A deficiency of antioxidants greatly increases the risks for the onset of degenerative disease.

The rusting of a nail or piece of metal when exposed to the elements is an excellent example of the process of oxidation. When oxygen from the air reacts with the iron molecules, the nail or iron becomes rusty (oxidized). This is because oxygen from the air freely combines with iron, and the iron object eventually corrodes into oblivion. If left unprotected, a similar process can develop in the membranes (walls) of human cells, as well as the internal components of the cells, for instance, the genes. The fatty acids of the cell walls, the most vulnerable part of the cell, can actually become rancid as a result of the oxidative process.

Antioxidants shield the cells, as well as the genetic material, from damage due to a variety of noxious agents, for instance, toxic chemicals, heavy metals, radiation, chlorine, tobacco smoke, and stress. In particular, antioxidants protect us from reactions within our bodies which generate *free radicals*. Free radicals are molecules which provoke damage to human cells. Oxidation reactions are caused by free radicals.

Human beings are regularly bombarded with all manner of toxic chemicals. What's more, virtually everyone suffers from a significant amount of stress. Highly processed food creates additional stress upon the body. What's more, even normal healthy food can initiate stress if the individual eats excessively. As a result of all of these insults, each of us produces within our bodies tens of billions of free radicals every day. The ability of the body to quench or destroy free radicals before they cause tissue damage is dependent upon an adequate supply of antioxidants. Vitamin E, vitamin A, vitamin C, pantothenic acid, beta carotene, coenzyme Q-10, selenium, phenolic acids, and herbal flavonoids are examples of natural antioxidants which block free radical reactions. However, according to the latest research herbal antioxidants, particularly those found in rosemary, cumin, cinnamon, cloves, sage, and oregano, are infinitely more powerful in halting free radical damage than mere vitamins. Studies have determined that these spicy antioxidants are up to 10 times more effective at blocking oxidation (and, therefore, aging) than even the most powerful synthetic antioxidants known, i.e. butylated hydroxytoluene (BHT). Consuming these natural antioxidants provides tremendous protection against the ravages of aging and chemical toxicity.

Food Refinement: Its Effect on Antioxidants

The current American diet is an antioxidant depleted one. The refinement of food destroys approximately 90% of the naturally occurring antioxidants. What's more, many of these refined foods contain noxious substances, which deplete and destroy what few antioxidants there are left in the body. Margarine and refined vegetable oils are excellent examples. Both of these fats, which are common ingredients in processed packaged foods, rapidly deplete the body's reservoirs of antioxidants. In particular, vegetable oils induce the consumption of vitamin E and selenium. Anyone who consumes refined oils should take at least an extra 800 I.U. of vitamin E daily. For the vitamin E to be most effective as an antioxidant, it must be in the unbound state. These types of vitamin E molecules are known chemically as alpha-tocopherol or mixed tocopherols.

The Selenium Controversy

Selenium is a trace mineral of the utmost importance in human nutrition. It is one of the few minerals containing significant antioxidant properties. This is discussed in more detail in Chapter Eight. A debate exists about whether or not too much selenium is harmful. Thus, most nutritionists and doctors have been cautious in suggesting selenium supplements and have kept the dosages to a minimum. Yet, it is preferable for the individual to have higher amounts of selenium within the body than too little. This is documented by the fact that in regions of the world with near toxic levels of selenium in the soil or water, there is little or no cancer. Selenium may well be the single most important antioxidant for preventing cancer. The fact that Americans contract cancer in a ratio of one of every three individuals is a clear signal of epidemic selenium deficiency. If you live in states with selenium-depleted soils such as Wisconsin, Illinois, Indiana, Iowa, Michigan, Ohio, Maine, New York, New Jersey, Pennsylvania, and Florida, you need to take selenium supplements. What is the best dosage? That depends on how much selenium you are getting in your food and water (see Appendix A, chart #3). A good rule is to take at least 300 micrograms per day as a preventive measure. People living in low-selenium regions who are exposed to radiation, toxic chemicals, or excessive amounts of sunlight may need to increase this dosage.

Conditions Increasing the Need for Antioxidants

Certain circumstances dramatically increase the body's need for antioxidant protection. The following are a few of the more common ones.

I. Heavy Metal Pollution

Heavy metal pollution, that is the pollution of the atmosphere, land, water, and living creation with toxic heavy metals, is a massive problem and has reached epidemic proportions. Scientists have found unbelievably high levels of lead, mercury, aluminum, and cadmium within the soil and water. The result is increased levels of these toxic metals within our bodies. Even the Inuit living in the North Pole are affected. Scientists have discovered a 300% increase in mercury levels in the Inuits' hair over that of their ancestors 500 years ago. Even greater increases are seen with lead.

Metals that enter our systems cause the consumption of antioxidants. People at risk for metal poisoning include car mechanics, industrial workers, dentists, jewelers, painters, dialysis patients, road workers, battery manufacturers, auto industry workers, and artists. Also included are those who have lived in a home with lead pipes or who have used aluminum cookware and/or antacids over a prolonged period. Extra doses of antioxidants are needed to block the ill-effects of metal poisoning. In particular, certain minerals have been found to block the absorption of toxic metals, while aiding the body's ability to excrete them. Furthermore, certain herbs are powerful metal antidotes, because they contain substances which chelate, that is pull, the metals out of the body. Red sour grape (i.e. Resvitanol) is one of the most powerful metal antidotes. This is because it is rich in phenolic acids, such as malic, gallic, and tartaric acids, which are among the most effective natural metal chelators known. The following chart illustrates precisely which minerals, antioxidants, and herbs to take if you have a history of exposure:

1. Lead – Antioxidants/Minerals: take extra calcium, vitamin C, vitamin E, and selenium. Herbs: take Resvitanol, rosemary, and wild oregano.

2. Cadmium – Antioxidants/Minerals: take extra zinc (most important), vitamin C, and selenium. Herbs: take Resvitanol and wild oregano.

3. Mercury – Antioxidants/Minerals: take extra selenium (most important) and vitamin C. Herbs: take garlic, onion, oil of cilantro, and oil of cumin (the latter is a powerful liver cleanser/rebuilder and mercury is stored partially in the liver). Or, take Liva Clenz, a special combination of liver-purging edible spice oils, including oils of cumin and cilantro.

4. Aluminum – Antioxidants/Minerals: take extra selenium, vitamin C, and vitamin E. Calcium and magnesium also help by blocking aluminum absorption. Herbs: take red sour grape (Resvitanol) and wild rosemary.

5. Arsenic – Antioxidants/Minerals: take extra niacin, B_5, vitamin C, Nutri-Sense natural B vitamin drink mix, and selenium. Herbs: rosemary/sage herbal (such as Hercules Strength), oil of cumin, and oil of sage (the cumin and sage oils help purge toxic heavy metals from the liver so they can be eliminated from the body. Be sure to consume only the edible sage/cumin oils (see Appendix B).

6. Uranium/strontium – Antioxidants/Minerals: take extra selenium, vitamin C, and beta carotene. Herbs: aromatic juices of wild herbs, particularly Juice of Oregano; also, oil of rosemary and oil of cumin, or use Liva Clenz, a proprietary formula containing the oils of cumin, rosemary, cilantro, and sage.

II. Air Pollution

Air pollutants cause extensive lung damage. This means that Americans are suffering massive lung damage as a result of living in smog-infested regions, and this is especially true of those living in large cities. Researchers have proven that this damage is mediated by free radical reactions and that antioxidants halt these reactions. Vitamin E, beta carotene, vitamin C, folic acid, bioflavanoids, and selenium, as well as herbs, particularly rosemary, sage, oregano, black caraway, and fenugreek, are of particular value in protecting lung tissue from being damaged. Everyone living in smog-choked areas, such as Los Angeles, Chicago, Houston, and New York, should take at least 75,000 I.U. of beta carotene, 1200 I.U. of vitamin E, 500 mg of vitamin C, 400 mg of selenium, and 5 mg of folic acid. In addition, antioxidant herbs, particularly the edible oils of rosemary and sage, are highly protective. If you are constantly exposed to air pollutants, take three to five drops of edible oil of rosemary and oil of sage twice daily. These dosages will protect the internal organs, particularly the lungs, from the ill-effects of air pollutants. These oils are easy to take compared to pills. What's more, they are more cost effective as daily antioxidants for combating the toxicity of the modern world. A small amount, like three to five drops daily, provides the body with significant antioxidant protection, far more than would result from mere vitamins.

III. Radiation

Exposure to radioactivity greatly increases the need for antioxidants. Many of the health problems induced by radiation could be prevented by taking antioxidants, especially beta carotene, vitamin E, and selenium, along with the herbs rosemary, sage, cumin, and oregano. The effect is more powerful if the antioxidants are taken immediately before or after a radiation insult. Everyone on this planet is receiving increasing amounts of radiation, far more than our ancestors. Those acutely exposed to radiation from X rays, radiation leakage, ultraviolet rays, radiation treatments, etc. would benefit immensely by adding antioxidants to the diet.

It has also been discovered that radiation damage resulting from ultraviolet light can be blocked by certain B vitamins, particularly pantothenic acid, niacin, folic acid, and thiamine. Nutri-Sense is an excellent source of naturally occurring B vitamins and provides valuable amounts of thiamine, pantothenic acid, and niacin in an easy to absorb form. For folic acid, organic calves' or lamb's liver is the top source. Rosemary, sage, cumin, and oregano are the top anti-radiation herbs. In the aftermath of Chernobyl, herbalists successfully used these herbs to reverse radiation poisoning. I have personally seen before and after photographs of individuals with radiation poisoning, and the curative response was striking. In fact, the photographs of the villagers prove that the radiation-induced tumors were eradicated. What did the herbalists use? It was the aromatic juice of wild oregano. This juice/essence is now available as Juice of Oregano and Juice of Rosemary. To reverse radiation poisoning take Juice of Oregano and Juice of Rosemary, an ounce or two of each twice daily. Obviously, for severe radiation exposure, such as that occurring from a radiation leak, much more would be needed, such as five to 10 ounces daily.

Supplementing Your Diet

Flooding your blood with large amounts of protective antioxidants is an intelligent decision. This is because research has shown that the majority of health problems are related to too little antioxidant protection. For example, cancer patients have significantly lower blood levels of vitamins A, C, E, folic acid, beta carotene, and flavonoids than do normal people. These nutrients are rapidly consumed by the immune system in an attempt to battle the cancer. The same holds true for other degenerative diseases such as arthritis, emphysema, lupus, and heart disease. Most of us get too little antioxidant protection. It is not worth taking a chance, because, without consistent antioxidant protection degenerative diseases could strike at any time. Thus, it is necessary to take antioxidants in abundance.

It is likely that some individuals are concerned about getting too much of a good thing. This is difficult to do, since antioxidants are used up literally as fast as we consume them. This is because the intensity of the chemical reactions which cause disease is so great that the antioxidants are depleted almost as soon as you swallow them. Billions of molecules of vitamin E, beta carotene, and selenium are utilized every day by your liver alone to protect it from free radical damage. Without an adequate supply of these and other antioxidants, our tissues would age and degenerate very rapidly. In fact, this does occur in some extreme cases.

Stress can also induce premature aging. One reason it causes aging is that it provokes the loss of several important nutrients, including vitamins A, C, the B vitamins, zinc, magnesium, and selenium. The body's reservoirs of pantothenic acid (vitamin B_5) are rapidly diminished during stressful episodes. This vitamin has a potent antioxidant function. It is also needed for the synthesis of adrenal hormones. If the stress is prolonged and the levels of pantothenic acid become too low, a relatively serious problem can result: adrenal exhaustion. Without pantothenic acid, cells within the adrenal glands begin to die, a process known as *atrophy*. As a result, adrenal hormone production drops dramatically. People who are under stress should take high doses of pantothenic acid, as much as one to two grams daily. This is safe to take in high doses, but too much may cause loose stools, however this may, in fact, be of benefit to certain individuals. A superior way to treat the adrenal glands is to consume a natural source of adrenal hormones such as royal jelly. This is the food of the queen bee, and it is exceptionally rich in natural hormones, which are safe to consume. Royal Kick royal jelly is a premium grade royal jelly supplement, which is the richest naturally occurring source of pantothenic acid. Royal Kick is fortified with additional pantothenic acid, since researchers have shown that this combination exhibits exceptionally powerful activity. The royal jelly in this supplement is the highest grade possible, boasting nearly twice as much of the level of active ingredient as the commercially available types. Royal Kick is a significant agent, because it greatly strengthens the adrenal glands. Usually, the benefit is noticed quickly, like within a week or less. For adrenal exhaustion take a minimum of four to six capsules of Royal Kick every morning. Royal Kick is an ideal anti-stress formula, because both royal jelly and pantothenic acid are major stress fighters. To combat and reverse severe stress, take three capsules of Royal Kick, two or more times daily.

Beta Carotene to the Rescue

Beta carotene is an important factor in preventing cell and organ damage. In particular, it protects cells from the harmful effects of radiation. Beta carotene is found primarily in plants. Its function is to protect them from damage due to sunlight. Beta carotene plays a similar role in respect to human skin and is normally concentrated there in significant amounts. The value of this nutrient is so vast that an entire chapter could be devoted to it.

If you do not eat beta carotene-rich fruits and/or vegetables on a regular basis, it is likely that you are deficient in this important antioxidant. A prolonged deficiency could be risky. Beta carotene is of major importance in protecting the cell's nucleus from being damaged. In other words, it protects the genes from being harmed by toxic substances. Nuclear material, meaning the genes and chromosomes, is delicate and extremely vulnerable to harm by radioactive compounds, ultraviolet light, synthetic chemicals, heavy metals, and other noxious substances. In fact, the genes can readily be permanently damaged. This damage will likely occur when the immune system is malfunctioning. This is because the immune system is directly involved in the repair and replacement of nuclear material. Since beta carotene blocks this damage, a lack of it greatly increases the risks for cancer as well as infectious diseases.

The loss of the ozone layer is another reason for the high need for beta carotene. Ozone is known mainly for its harmful effects. Yet, it has a protective function as well. The ozone layer in the upper reaches of the atmosphere intercepts much of the potentially damaging ultraviolet waves from the sun. However, pollutants in the air, particularly substances known as *chlorofluorocarbons,* destroy the ozone molecules. This has led to a measurable decrease in the levels of ozone in the atmosphere. Every summer massive holes develop in the ozone layer, particularly at the poles. Thus, individuals living near the North and South poles, e.g. the Canadian provinces, Argentina, Southern Chile, South Seas, etc., are at a high risk of being exposed to toxic ultraviolet radiation levels. Because of a generalized depletion of the ozone layer, a greater amount of the potentially harmful ultraviolet waves are reaching every one of us now more than ever—enter beta carotene. If there is enough beta carotene in the skin, these waves are blocked before they can enter the body and cause damage.

This is why the consumption of beta carotene should be increased, and one of the best ways to do so is to consume large amounts of beta carotene-rich foods. People today receive significantly less beta carotene in the diet than did our ancestors, yet our needs are greater.

Food: The Best Source of Carotenes

Food is superior to supplements as a source of beta carotene. One reason is that food source beta carotene is relatively easy to absorb. Plus, foods contain a variety of other carotenes; substances besides beta carotene, such as lycopene, found in tomatoes and watermelon, as well as lutein, found in spinach, are also protective. Eating dried apricots is an easy way to get a daily dose of beta carotene. Purchase only the unsulfured variety, usually found in health food stores. Half a cantaloupe per day would also help, and for those who do not have to watch their carbohydrate intake, sweet potatoes are an exceptional source. For lycopene, a wedge of watermelon would suffice (this also provides a significant amount of beta carotene). Farm or garden-grown tomatoes are the richest source of lycopene. Natural lycopene (found in food) is superior to supplements.

The Body's Own Antioxidants

There are two basic categories of antioxidants: those found within food sources and those which are made within the body. Examples of the first type include vitamin E, beta carotene, lycopene, vitamin A, vitamin C, riboflavin, manganese, and selenium. The second type, those that can be synthesized in the body, includes coenzyme Q-10, glutathione, SOD (superoxide dismutase), catalase, and albumin. The human body is constantly working to produce adequate amounts of these antioxidants. However, before it can do so, it is necessary to supply it with the raw materials needed for synthesis. For example, the antioxidant enzyme SOD, which is found in every cell in the body, cannot be made without amino acids (from proteins) as well zinc, copper, and manganese. Glutathione synthesis is dependent upon the availability of proteins rich in the amino acids methionine and cysteine. This means that the diet must contain steady supplies primarily of animal proteins such as milk, eggs, fish, and meat, largely because these foods are richer than vegetable foods as a source of amino acids. These internal or "home-made" antioxidants are just as important as the dietary ones. The two work together to protect the body from all sorts of harmful chemical reactions.

Glutathione Inhibits Aging

Scientific studies are proving that glutathione inhibits the aging process. This protein/enzyme is the major antioxidant found within all animal cells. It is a universal antioxidant, that is it is found in every creature from insects to man. Every day our bodies synthesize untold millions of glutathione molecules. Volumes of research point to glutathione as being the number one anti-aging substance. This is best summarized by the following facts:

1. Levels of glutathione decline with age and are particularly low in those with premature aging.

2. People whose glutathione levels remain high are more free of diseases or sickness. In addition, tests show them to be biologically younger.

3. Animals fed substances needed for glutathione synthesis, such as methionine, cysteine, or selenium, lived longer than those that were not supplemented.

4. High glutathione levels are associated with a decreased risk of cancer, heart disease, diabetes, and other major killers.

The Liver—Our Body's Antioxidant Factory

The liver is the hub of all manufacturing activity. This is where antioxidants, such as SOD, catalase, coenzyme Q-10, and glutathione, are made. Thousands of other important substances are also produced in the liver. This organ is also the storehouse for most of the body's antioxidants. It is important to have a healthy liver in order to remain free of disease. If the liver fails to produce a sufficient quantity of antioxidants, disease and even death may result.

Don't Forget Your Daily Dose of Vitamin E

Vitamin E is not just for sexual vigor. It is one of the key antioxidants for protecting cell membranes. This is because the major constituent of cell membranes is fat. These fats include the essential fatty acids, cholesterol, and phospholipids (for instance, lecithin). Vitamin E itself is soluble in fat, which means it readily dissolves into cell membranes. By binding to the fatty acids of cell membranes, vitamin E directly stops the occurrence of reactions which would otherwise be damaging. Thus, it prevents these fatty substances from oxidizing. Such damage may lead to cell damage and/or death.

NASA and the Vitamin E Connection

A good example of cellular damage due to vitamin E deficiency is what happens to the red blood cells of astronauts. While in outer space, astronauts are exposed to dangerously high amounts of radiation from the sun. They have no earthly atmosphere to protect them from the sun's rays. The astronauts' red blood cells absorb some of this excess radiation, and the cell membranes break down. The result is tired, sick astronauts. The fatigue they experience is somewhat like that seen in anemic people. Researchers at NASA found that vitamin E stops this harmful reaction and, thus, they supplemented the astronauts' diet with the vitamin.

Vitamin E exhibits a variety of useful chemical functions. It aids in blood flow, hormone synthesis, and immune function, plus it is a major antioxidant for protecting human cells. Conditions in which vitamin E has proven helpful include some forms of anemia, low HDL cholesterol (the "good" cholesterol), heart disease, arthritis, acne, diabetes, infertility, fibrocystic breast disease, Raynaud's disease, lupus, leg cramps, and vasculitis (inflammation of the blood vessels). Vitamin E is not a miracle cure for these conditions, but if taken consistently in the proper form and dose, it often helps.

The Right Type of Vitamin E

There are many types of vitamin E available on the market. What is the right form? Certain brands claim to be all-natural. However, natural vitamin E is often chemically altered. This process is called *esterification*. This type of vitamin E is less potent as an antioxidant than the unprocessed vitamin E extract. Synthetic vitamin E is another type which is far less potent than the natural. What's more, few people realize that some products labeled as "natural vitamin E" contain as little as 10% natural E, the rest being synthetic. Unfortunately, this type of labeling is not illegal.

If you are confused about just how to procure the best vitamin E, here are some simple rules to follow when making your selection:

1. If your vitamin E is not producing results, it is likely that there is no active vitamin E in the product. In other words, the vitamin E you are using is probably a sham.

2. Any vitamin E product (400 I.U.) that costs less than $8.00 per bottle (for 60 capsules or more) is likely to be worthless. Pure natural vitamin E is rather expensive.

3. Vitamin E labeled as "dl" instead of "d" is synthetic and of little value. Man has not yet been able to duplicate natural E.

4. The only type of vitamin E with proven antioxidant activity is natural vitamin E extract. This extract is made primarily from soybean oil. The vitamin E is distilled out of the oil. If left unaltered, this extract is potent in antioxidant activity. Over 90% of the vitamin E on the market is esterified, i.e. chemically altered. Chemists bind the vitamin E molecule to substances known as acetate or succinate. Through this method the shelf life is greatly increased, while the antioxidant activity is diminished.

5. Read all labels. For antioxidant protection, select primarily products listing their vitamin E as being non-esterified. These unaltered vitamin E products are known as free tocopherols, mixed tocopherols, alpha tocopherol, etc. However, despite the chemical alteration, vitamin E succinate and acetate are of value especially for those with circulatory disease. Some products contain both vitamin E as succinate and/or acetate plus mixed tocopherols. This would also be acceptable.

6. Get as much vitamin E from food as possible. The top sources of vitamin E include rice bran, rice germ, wheat germ, oat bran, cold pressed oils, almonds, filberts, pecans, spinach, salmon, and sweet potatoes. Nutri-Sense, rich in rice bran and germ, may be taken daily as a natural vitamin E source. Crude pumpkinseed oil (Pumpkinol) is super-rich, containing about 10 I.U. per 2 tablespoons. Take it as a natural source of 100% unprocessed vitamin E. The vitamin E in Pumpkinol is the complete spectrum, including the potent antioxidant, gamma tocopherol.

Scientific Studies Prove the Worth of Antioxidants

There are untold thousands of scientific articles documenting various beneficial effects of antioxidants on health. Every week, hundreds of these articles are published. Antioxidants as a primary treatment and cure for degenerative disease is the trend of the future. Here are some examples from this wealth of scientific data:

1. The researchers Kikuchi and Koyama found that high-fat diets in rabbits caused the rabbits' red blood cells to become deformed due to free radical damage. However, when the rabbits were given vitamin E, the red blood cells stayed normal even though the high-fat diet was continued. Therefore, vitamin E acted as an antioxidant, protecting the red blood cell membranes from being damaged.

2. Drs. Manwaring and Csallany showed that organs which receive the highest amounts of oxygen such as the brain, lungs, and liver, are damaged by the oxygen if the organs are deficient in vitamin E. The addition of vitamin E protected the organs from this damage. Apparently, the liver was most sensitive to the oxygen-induced damage. This may be one reason the liver serves as the main depot for vitamin E storage.

3. Researchers Whitacre and Combs found that a deficiency of selenium leads to pancreatic damage. The outer membranes of the pancreatic cells become destroyed due to the ill effects of free radicals, which are toxic to the cell membranes. Damage to the pancreas is critical, as no food can be properly digested without it. You may recall that in every cell in the body there is an enzyme which protects cell membranes from free radical damage— glutathione peroxidase. Selenium is needed for this enzyme to work properly, and a deficiency of this mineral greatly diminishes glutathione peroxidase activity. In severe selenium deficiency the internal organs are left unprotected, and the cells may be readily damaged. In most instances supplementation with selenium rapidly reverses the damage. Other antioxidants which are highly protective against cancer include oregano, rosemary, and cumin. Juice of Oregano is the ideal spice tonic for cancer protection, and it works well with selenium. Take the two at the same time.

4. Sickle cell anemia is caused by free radical-induced damage to the cell walls of red blood cells. Rachmitewitz and colleagues proved that vitamin E at 400 I.U. per day resulted in a decrease in the number of sickled cells in patients with this disease. Apparently, vitamin E acts to prevent healthy red blood cells from turning into sickle cells. This is an impressive result, since sickle cell anemia has been regarded for years by the medical profession as being incurable.

5. The *Journal of the American Medical Association* reported recently that vitamin E supplements are effective in fibrocystic disease of the

breasts. The breasts are vulnerable to free radical damage, since free radicals love to attack polyunsaturated fats, and the breasts consist primarily of fatty tissue. Vitamin E apparently blocks this damage, although it would be more effective if combined with selenium. A report by Dr. Millner at the University of Pennsylvania shows that a common herb, rosemary, is even more powerful than vitamin E at protecting breast tissue. Merely adding rosemary to the feed of test animals halted the growth of malignant cells, saving many of the animals from fatal breast cancer. Oil of rosemary from a guaranteed wild source is even more powerful than the herb in providing dramatic protection against breast cancer. The edible type in olive oil can be safely taken internally.

6. Dr. Prasad found that the growth of melanoma tumor cells on animals was blocked by vitamin E. He suggested that fat soluble antioxidants, such as beta carotene and vitamin E, alter the physics of the cell membrane of cancer cells, leading to an inhibition of their growth.

7. Drs. Collip and Chen showed that selenium deficiency leads to heart damage in both children and adults and that, commonly, these age groups become selenium deficient. Much of this damage is corrected when selenium levels in the blood and tissues are increased.

8. Researchers Lloyd and Clayton have shown that both smoking and alcohol use induce a selenium deficiency. It is likely that the selenium is "used up" in an attempt to heal the tissue damage caused by cigarette smoke and/or alcohol.

9. Tiny arteries in the retina of the eye are vulnerable to damage from various noxious agents. Once these arteries are severely damaged, visual loss develops, and partial or complete blindness can result. This occurs in diseases such as diabetes and macular degeneration. The researcher Thornber and colleagues found that a high-sugar diet in animals damages the retinal arteries, leading to visual impairment and blindness. It is known that sugar causes this toxicity in humans as well. For example, sugar diabetes is the number one cause of blindness in America today. However, these researchers discovered that selenium protected the animals against damage to the retinal arteries even though the nutrient-poor, sugar-rich diet was continued. They also added chromium, which helps prevent sugar-induced damage to the eyes.

10. Dr. Prasad demonstrated that cancer-causing chemicals in the digestive tract are neutralized by vitamins C, E, and A.

11. Many researchers have shown that vitamin E decreases the incidence of breast tumors. Vitamin E is soluble in fat and will dissolve into breast tissue, protecting it from free radical-induced damage.

12. Recently, researchers have proven that high levels of beta carotene, folic acid, and B-12 diminish the odds for the development of lung cancer. Deficiencies of B-12 and, particularly, folic acid are common: virtually all smokers and drinkers are severely deficient. Both of these vitamins modify the rate at which cells reproduce, keeping the cells "under control," thus helping to prevent the onset of cancer.

13. Researchers Griffin and Lane showed that persons working around toxic chemicals known as hydrocarbons (oil and coal derivatives) had lower selenium and glutathione peroxidase levels than did the normal population. Both of these substances are required by the liver to detoxify hydrocarbons, which are often difficult to remove from the tissues. Certain antioxidant herbs stimulate the liver synthesis of glutathione, notably rosemary, sage, cumin, oregano, and black caraway.

14. Numerous researchers have determined that a lack of selenium and, thus, a lack of glutathione peroxidase, leads to skin damage and may even cause skin diseases. The skin's fatty acid coat is protected from damage by the sun, radiation, and/or free radicals by selenium, glutathione, vitamin E, and beta carotene. Treatment of diseases, such as eczema, psoriasis, vasculitis (inflammation of the blood vessels in the skin), age spots, and seborrheic dermatitis, with selenium and vitamin E leads to a beneficial effect in many cases. Other effective skin tonics include oil of rosemary, oil of myrtle, oil of lavender, and oil of bay berry.

15. Deficiencies of antioxidants cause damage to the blood vessels, particularly the arteries. This was illustrated in 1980 by Dr. Goto, who determined that damage to the inner lining of the arteries is often due to excess lipid peroxides circulating in the blood. Lipid peroxides, as described earlier in this chapter, are fats which are so toxic that they damage the fatty acids of healthy cell membranes throughout the body. High levels of these lipid peroxides are extremely damaging to the arteries, and, thus, heart attacks, hardening of the arteries, and even strokes may result. The lipid peroxides are rapidly abolished by the addition of prodigious quantities of antioxidants, particularly selenium, vitamin E, vitamin C, and beta carotene. Potent herbal antioxidants, such as rosemary, cumin, oregano, and sage, should also be added to the diet.

16. High vitamin E levels in the blood are associated with protection from heart disease, arterial damage, cataracts, cancer, and pollution induced cell damage. The blood levels necessary to achieve these protective effects are much higher than could result from consuming the RDA (Recommended Daily Allowance). A recent study showed that doses of vitamin E up to 60 times the RDA, i.e. 1000 I.U., are required to provide maximum protection from these and other free radical-induced diseases. Need there be any more debate? With the world as toxic as it is today, only a fool would believe that he/she will be protected merely by consuming only the RDA. By the standards described previously, the RDA for vitamin E (10-15 I.U.) is worthless.

17. Dr. H. Garewal of the University of Arizona recently showed that supplements of natural beta carotene caused pre-cancerous lesions in the mouth to disappear. When patients stopped taking the beta carotene, the lesions recurred. Research in Turkey and Greece indicates that oil of oregano also halts the growth of pre-cancerous lesions.

18. Researchers in the United States discovered that vitamin E is such a potent antioxidant that it not only prevented hardening of the arteries but also reversed it. They found that regular supplementation of vitamin E significantly reduced plaque deposits in the arteries, which means the vitamin worked better than cardiac surgery.

19. In Japan, researchers discovered that vitamin C offered significant antioxidant actions for protecting the heart and arteries. It is well known that the common surgical treatment for plugged arteries, known as angioplasty, frequently results in re-closure. This means that shortly after boring open the arteries with this procedure, the arteries refill with plaque and other obstructions. The closure is thought to be caused by oxidative damage to the arteries, which results from this traumatic procedure. The researchers found to their astonishment that a mere 500 mg of vitamin C prevents arteries from re-closing, meaning that this vitamin made the procedure much more effective and lasting.

20. In the Middle East researchers discovered that a Mediterranean spice, cumin, exhibits more powerful antioxidant effects than any vitamin or mineral. Using oil of cumin, they determined that a small amount, like a few drops per day, created massive antioxidant protection for the organs. In fact, oil of cumin raised the levels of glutathione, the body's number one antioxidant, by as much as

700%. That is an incredibly large increase, a fact which positions oil of cumin as being perhaps the premier preventive antioxidant. Such a protective agent would likely diminish the need for taking excessive amounts of commercial antioxidants such as vitamin E, vitamin C, glutathione pills, beta carotene, silymarin, etc.

Antioxidants are highly protective to the body. The following is a list of the beneficial actions of specific natural antioxidants.

Function	Antioxidant
1. Preservation of the elastic nature of skin	selenium, pantothenic acid, vitamin C, vitamin E
2. Increased ability of brain cells to use oxygen	glutathione, vitamin E, coenzyme Q-10, rosemary
3. Improved ability of cells to make energy	selenium, vitamin E, glutathione, coenzyme Q-10
4. Detoxification of ozone and radiation	beta carotene, selenium, glutathione, SOD, rosemary
5. Enhancement of the immune system	beta carotene, selenium, vitamin E, glutathione, vitamin C pantothenic acid, oregano
6. Improved blood flow to the heart	vitamin E, coenzyme Q-10, rosemary
7. Prevention of cancer	all antioxidants
8. Dissolving moles and brown spots	selenium, glutathione, oregano oil
9. Destruction of tumor cells	beta carotene, glutathione, selenium, oregano oil, rosemary oil

Herbal Antioxidants: The Anti-Aging Substances of the Future

Herbs, as well as spices, contain some of the most powerful antioxidants known. This is illustrated by the fact that various herbs and spices have been used since ancient times as preservatives. Many spices have been long known for their abilities to inhibit the spoiling of food. Furthermore, the ancient Egyptians used herbs and spices in mummification.

While the antioxidant potential of vitamins, minerals, and enzymes is critical, the value of the antioxidants in herbs and spices is even more profound. In fact, recent research proves that herbal and spice antioxidants are so powerful that they cause vitamin antioxidants to seem rather feeble.

It has been sort of in vogue to believe that synthetic chemicals are more powerful than natural ones. Recent research proves quite the opposite. For instance, Horwitt described how natural vitamin E is far stronger in biological activity than the synthetic. Incredibly, the same is true of natural herbal antioxidants. Rosemary is an excellent example. In Japan it was discovered that rosemary oil is a more powerful antioxidant than BHT, the synthetic chemical commonly used to preserve foods. Researchers found that rosemary oil is up to four times more effective than BHT and without the toxicity. Researchers in Europe found that an oil extract of the spice cumin was more powerful than any other antioxidant tested. Oil of cumin greatly increased the antioxidant levels in the liver, stomach, esophagus, and immune cells. Sage was found to be perhaps the most powerful herb/spice for protecting specifically fatty tissues from oxidizing. One study determined that sage oil was over 10 times more effective than synthetic antioxidants. Taintu describes how oregano, rosemary, and sage, as well as the essential oils of these herbs, effectively preserve food from oxidation, increasing shelf life by months. Spice and herbal oils may be combined specifically for preserving food and increasing shelf live. Preservit-all™ is such a combination and is ideal for preventing the spoilage of refrigerated foods. Simply add a few drops to any prepared food, and it will increase the shelf life considerably, while preventing microbial growth. Or, add a few drops to vegetables or on fruit for preserving freshness. Ancient civilizations emphasized the value of spices. The ancients valued spices like gold or jewels and developed hundreds of culinary and medicinal uses for them. Yet, perhaps most compelling was the value of spices/herbs in protecting food from spoilage, indicating their profound value as antioxidants.

CHAPTER SEVEN
The Number One Killer

Many advances have been made in the treatment of heart disease. Yet, despite these enormous efforts, cardiovascular disease remains the number one cause of death. There must be a reason.

In North America well over a million individuals die every year from heart disease. Other cultures, even some relatively modern ones, like the Japanese and French, do not have such a problem. Is it the lifestyle that makes the difference? In fact, diet is the primary difference between our culture and cultures where heart disease is rare. This may not come as a surprise. However, here are some examples for those who find this hard to believe.

The people of Crete, a Greek island in the Mediterranean, have a high-fat diet that is rich in natural, unprocessed foods. They enjoy good health and longevity. They are free of coronary artery disease. The incidence of stroke or high blood pressure is also minimal.

The Masai tribesmen of Africa eat large quantities of beef and drink whole milk regularly. What's more, butter is one of their staples. Yet, they develop coronary artery disease, high blood pressure, and atherosclerosis only after migrating to Westernized cities.

The Yemeni Jews, despite a diet rich in natural fat, including butter and lamb fat, were free of circulatory diseases and diabetes until they moved to Westernized cities. Now they suffer from these diseases in epidemic proportions.

The Inuit are free of coronary artery disease, heart attacks, strokes, and high blood pressure even though their diet is rich in foods such as seal and whale blubber. Those who now live on white bread, sugar, coffee, tea, and alcohol have developed a wide range of "modern" diseases.

Several societies in the Mediterranean are free of heart or circulatory disease, though their diets are up to 60% fat. The same is true for certain eastern European cultures.

Since the 1950s, an aggressive effort has been made by dieticians, the medical establishment, and the media to lay the blame on fats in our diet. Fats are only a part of the problem, although for the societies mentioned they pose no problem at all. What else, then, in our diet is to blame?

Sugar is More Dangerous than Fat

While fat can be natural, sugar is dangerous, because it is always unnatural. White sugar is a refined food and has no nutritional value. In fact, its consumption leads to the loss of nutrients.

Dr. Yudkin, a famous British researcher, has proven that the consumption of refined sugar deleteriously affects the circulatory system. He has shown that sugar causes a wide range of heart and arterial diseases. These harmful effects result whether the sugar is obvious (a teaspoon of sugar in your tea) or hidden (a doughnut, some ketchup, or a piece of bologna). Some people are particularly vulnerable to its ill-effects. Ultimately, an excessive intake of sugar compromises an individual's health by damaging the organs crucial for survival.

Sugar Stresses the Adrenal and Thyroid Glands

While you may not develop heart disease, the sugar you eat will disable other critical organs. Both the adrenal and thyroid glands must deal with the physiological upset that pure sugar causes in the body. Eventually, as a result of continuous sugar consumption, these delicate organs will burn themselves out. It so happens that most people with heart disease have malfunctioning thyroid and adrenal glands.

Some Fats are Bad

Unfortunately, many of the fats found in commercial foods are toxic to the circulatory system. These "bad fats" may be of either animal or vegetable origin. Primitive societies often have the luxury of consuming large amounts of the helpful or "good" fats. However, fat, by itself, is not the killer. It is the type of fat that is important. This is discussed in more depth in Chapter 12.

The American Diet—A Promoter of Heart Disease

What we eat is the number one factor predisposing us to heart disease. There are many elements within the diet that make us vulnerable.

The following questionnaire is useful to determine if your lifestyle is predisposing you to cardiovascular disease, a category which includes coronary heart disease, heart attack, stroke, and/or high blood pressure:

What are Your Risks? This Test Will Tell

Answer "yes" or "no" to the following questions. Add up the points to arrive at your score.

POINTS

1. Do you eat fatty or deep-fried foods? . . . . (5)

2. Do you regularly eat bakery goods such as doughnuts, cupcakes, pies, cookies, cakes, etc.? . . . . (5)

3. Do you eat cured meats such as bacon, hot dogs, bologna, sausage, ham, or corned beef? . . . . (5)

4. Do you regularly consume sugar added to foods, like coffee or tea, or in cereals, pop, candy, chocolate, etc.? . . . . (10)

5. Do you regularly drink alcoholic beverages? . . . . (10)

6. Do you smoke cigarettes? . . . . (10)

7. Were you previously a smoker or drinker? . . . . (5)

8. Do you have a family history of heart disease, high blood pressure, or stroke? . . . . (10)

9. Do you have a family history of elevated blood fats, cholesterol, or triglycerides? . . . . (10)

10. Are you considerably overweight (i.e. greater than 20 pounds)? (10)

11. Do you lead a sedentary life (i.e. little or no exercise)? . . . . . . (5)

12. Do you have elevated cholesterol and/or triglycerides? . . . . . . (20)

13. Do you have high blood pressure (above 140/90)? . . . . (25)

14. Have you recently had a stroke or heart attack? . . . . (50)

15. Do you have a diagnosis of heart disease, heart failure, enlarged heart, blood clots, or hardening of the arteries? . . . . (50)

16. Do you have symptoms of poor circulation such as memory loss, sluggish mental function, chest pain, shortness of breath, cold extremities, or leg pains/cramps? . . . . (15)

17. Do you regularly take birth control pills? . . . . (10)

18. Have you used drugs such as water pills, diet pills, marijuana, cocaine, or heroin for an extended period in the past, or do you currently use them? .... (5)

19. Do you drink coffee in excess of five cups a day? .... (5)

YOUR SCORE _____

10-35 Points Possible cardiovascular disease. Treatment would be preventive.

40-65 Points Probable cardiovascular disease. Treatment is needed. Failure to alter lifestyle and improve the diet could lead to significant disease. Stop the progression now before it is too late. Proper treatment at this stage could reverse much of the damage.

70-135 Points You have definite evidence of cardiovascular disease. Treatment is mandatory. The risk for further health complications is high. Failure to alter your lifestyle, diet, and nutrition could be life-threatening.

140-Above Danger—High Risk Stroke, heart attack, hypertensive crisis, or other cardiovascular complications could occur at any time. It is imperative that you alter your lifestyle and seek medical care immediately. However, do not expect the doctors to offer any miracle cure. The burden of cure rests with you. Aggressive changes in your dietary, nutritional, and exercise habits *could save your life.*

You can see from this test that a number of factors play a role in causing heart disease. The medical profession and news media have confounded the public on the subject of cholesterol, indicating that its excess in the diet causes heart disease. Yet, their view is wrong. I will now expose what I call the cholesterol hoax.

Cholesterol is Not the Culprit

Are my words controversial? Of course. Can I prove what I am saying? Absolutely. Cholesterol does not cause heart disease. The fact is cholesterol is an essential and normal substance made on a daily basis by the body. It has a variety of useful, in fact, lifesaving functions. Every cell in our bodies contains cholesterol. Without it, our cells would be vulnerable to disease, infection, and even cancer. How could such an important natural substance be deemed so harmful?

Cholesterol first got a bad reputation when it was found that many people with disease, not just heart disease, had high blood cholesterol. From this it was assumed that cholesterol was bad and that the cure would be the removal of cholesterol from the diet. This way of thinking is not much different than to assume that when the water level in a river is high, it is bad, and when it is low, it is good. No doubt, there is more danger of a flood if the water level is high, but that does not mean that the water itself is bad. The same is true of cholesterol. While its elevation is an indication of disturbed function and is associated with increased risk of certain diseases, including heart disease, it is likely that it is the function of the body that is bad, not the cholesterol.

In other words the cholesterol is elevated for a reason. Its elevation may be serving a useful function. This is because cholesterol itself is an antioxidant. It is made in the liver according to the body's needs. A cholesterol level that is too low is just as dangerous as a level that is too high. There is thorough proof that an extremely low cholesterol is associated with a breakdown in the immune system and cancer. There is evidence that drugs which artificially lower cholesterol cause a number of cancers. To reiterate, every cell and organ in the body needs an adequate amount of cholesterol to remain free of disease. In particular, the immune cells need a steady supply of this valuable nutrient. Eventually, it will be proven that the regular intake of cholesterol molecules as naturally found in foods is highly protective of health and cannot cause harm. If your cholesterol level is too high or low, the following charts may be of interest to you.

Causes of High Cholesterol Levels

1. Excess dietary sugar

2. Excess dietary starch

3. Excess hydrogenated or processed fats (lard, shortening, cottonseed oil, palm oil, margarine, etc.)

4. Liver dysfunction

5. Amino acid deficiency

6. Essential fatty acid deficiency

7. Deficiency of natural antioxidants such as vitamin E, selenium, and beta carotene

8. Increased tissue damage due to infection, radiation, or oxidative activity (free radicals, etc.)

9. Fiber deficiency

10. Vitamin C deficiency

11. Carnitine deficiency

12. Biotin deficiency

13. Food allergies

14. Alcoholism

Causes of Low Cholesterol Levels (below 150)

1. Immune decline

2. Chronic hepatitis

3. Cholesterol-lowering drugs

4. Essential fatty acid deficiency

5. Liver infection or disease

6. Manganese deficiency

7. Adrenal stress

8. Street drugs (cocaine, marijuana etc.)

9. Excessive exercise (especially in females)

10. Low-fat diets

11. Vegetarian or macrobiotic diets

12. Psychological stress

13. Cancer

As you can see, eliminating eggs from the diet is not the answer. If you have a cholesterol problem, a superior approach is to determine why imbalances in your chemistry exist. You can also see that causing the cholesterol to drop too low is not wise.

Where Does Cholesterol Come From?

Most of the cholesterol found in the blood is made within our own bodies. The liver synthesizes more cholesterol each day than can possibly be absorbed from the diet. Under normal circumstances, the equivalent of 10 or more eggs worth is manufactured daily. This cholesterol is used to seal off damaged tissues, arterial walls, and cell membranes. It is also utilized in the synthesis of adrenal hormones. In addition, cholesterol is a vital component of nerve and brain tissue. Few individuals realize that you can actually have a cholesterol deficiency and that this deficiency can damage the heart. The heart cannot function adequately unless the nerves which control it are healthy—a state dependent on an adequate supply of cholesterol and other nerve nourishing substances.

How Diet Influences Cholesterol Levels

Diet is another source of cholesterol. However, there is no need to specifically avoid foods high in cholesterol. Most foods naturally rich in cholesterol, such as eggs, fresh meats, liver, and butterfat, fail to cause a significant increase in blood cholesterol levels. This fact may astonish many individuals. However, it shouldn't shock anyone, because if you think about it, it makes a lot of sense. At the beginning of this chapter a number of examples were given of societies whose diets are high in unprocessed fats, and yet, these societies have low mortality from heart disease. These people also have normal cholesterol levels despite eating a variety of cholesterol-rich foods. There are several reasons for this effect:

1. Cholesterol-rich foods contain certain natural substances which lower blood cholesterol and assist the body in the metabolism of fats. This includes compounds such as lecithin, essential fatty acids, manganese, B vitamins, and carnitine.

2. When cholesterol is eaten, the body recognizes this and, by a sophisticated mechanism, reduces or curtails cholesterol synthesis in the liver.

3. Most cholesterol-rich foods (butter, eggs, organ meats, shellfish) are also rich in a variety of other nutrients. Often, these foods are listed within one of the categories of the wholesome basic food groups. Eliminating them usually results in their replacement by less nutritious foods (i.e. Egg Beaters vs. real eggs).

4. Most of the foreign diets which are high in fat and cholesterol are also low in refined sugars and starches. In contrast, the American diet is high in fats as well as refined sugars and starches. Cholesterol levels increase if the diet is high in either sugars or starches, since the liver makes cholesterol from the breakdown products of sugar.

Sugar Raises Cholesterol Levels

Now you have it. The truth is whatever *causes* an abnormal elevation in blood cholesterol is harmful. Refined carbohydrates of all types lead to an elevation of blood fats. These include white sugar, brown sugar, malt, corn syrup, corn starch, maltodextrin, dextrose, glucose, white flour, and white rice. Hundreds of case histories and numerous research studies have proven that these depleted foods cause an elevation in cholesterol and/or triglycerides by a phenomenon I call *glucose overload.*

How Does Sugar End Up as a Fat?

All the aforementioned carbohydrates are broken down by the body into a single common substance: glucose. Starch is nothing more than a chain of glucose molecules. These chains are broken apart by digestive enzymes. Sugar consists of single molecules (glucose, dextrose, etc.) or double molecules such as white sugar (sucrose). Sucrose is broken down by digestive enzymes into glucose and fructose. This is where the phenomenon of glucose overload becomes important.

When you consume more glucose (or fructose) than you can burn as energy, the body has no choice but to process it into stored energy: fat. This connection is best illustrated by the following case history:

Mr. Jacobs, a retiring executive, came to me for one reason; he was scared to death of undergoing bypass surgery. There was reason for him to be concerned: he was constantly plagued with angina. He underwent two coronary angioplasties, operations where the cardiologist tries to open clogged coronary arteries with a plastic catheter. Both of these procedures had failed. He was placed on medications and given the standard heart-saver diet used by hospitals and their dieticians.

I attempted to find out why Mr. Jacobs had this problem. Although he never had a heart attack, he was a mild diabetic and was grossly overweight. He was a sugar addict supreme, reveling in all sorts of candies and sweets. Even though he didn't drink or smoke, he followed a sugar-rich diet which was likely the cause of his heart troubles.

Testing showed that Mr. Jacobs was actually allergic to sugar. Whenever he ate sugar or other refined carbohydrates, his triglycerides skyrocketed to as high as 1,000. Due to his extreme addiction to sugar, Mr. Jacobs was a tough nut to crack. Yet, being a businessman, he was accustomed to discipline. Mr. Jacobs was placed on a diet free of sugars and starches. Instead, he was instructed to eat foods such as vegetables, meats, whole fat milk products, and low-sugar fruits. Needless to say, his triglycerides came down to normal in no time. He dropped 25 pounds, his heart pain decreased, and he is now able to exercise and take long walks, though prior to his therapy he was relatively debilitated.

Had these problems been discovered and addressed earlier, the risky coronary angioplasties could have been avoided.

Regarding bypass surgery, I do not think Mr. Jacobs would have lived through it. Currently, having kept to his diet, Mr. Jacobs has lost nearly 50 pounds and is walking over five miles a day—without any angina. Needless to say, he is indeed happily retired.

Triglycerides

For the heart patient this term is the companion evil to cholesterol. A triglyceride is a fat formed from three (therefore the "tri") fatty acids attached to a molecule known as glycerol. Most of the triglycerides found in the body do not come directly from dietary fats per se; they are made in the liver from any excess sugar which hasn't been burned. As has been stated, glucose and many other sugars originate from processed foods. These sugars can also come from whole foods which naturally contain carbohydrates. This includes the natural sugars in milk, the starch of a baked potato, or the sugar in a bunch of grapes. In a vulnerable person any of these foods could lead to elevated triglycerides.

Most Americans get an excess of starch and/or sugar in their diets. Unless you are a marathon athlete or a college wrestler, it is likely that you are not burning up the sugar you eat fast enough. The extra sugar will enter the liver and will then be synthesized into fat. While this extra fat may not be a problem for a healthy person, it is deadly to the individual afflicted with heart disease.

These extra fats may not make it to the front of your abdomen or the outside of your hips. Unfortunately, they are often deposited in organs of crucial function: the liver, arteries, brain, and heart.

The liver is the factory responsible for making important molecules known as *carrier proteins*. These proteins are responsible for carrying minerals, vitamins, and fatty acids such as cholesterol or triglycerides in the blood. The well known HDL ("good") and LDL ("bad") cholesterol are carrier proteins made in the liver. A malfunctioning liver cannot make sufficient quantities of HDL cholesterol, and a liver infiltrated with fat is not able to work up to speed. The less HDL cholesterol you have, the more likely it is that fats will be deposited into your arteries.

In the worst scenario fats plug up the arteries in the heart, leading to angina, sudden death, or heart attack. However, more likely causes of heart problems follow in the next few pages.

Heart Disease is Often a Biochemical Disorder

Dr. Cooley, the noted cardiovascular surgeon from Texas, stated that no more than 20% of all heart attacks are due to occluded coronary arteries. Thus, blood clots and fat deposits play only a partial role. What, then, accounts for the other 80%? Likely causes are biochemical and nutritional imbalances within the heart itself or in organs which support cardiac functions. Medical authorities have long associated disorders of the thyroid gland with heart disease. Emotional and psychic stress, with their powerful effects upon the brain and nervous system, play a major role as well.

The health of the liver has an enormous bearing upon diseases of circulation. As stated previously, the liver synthesizes HDL and LDL cholesterol. These are also known as lipoproteins, since they consist primarily of protein and fats, i.e. lipids. Much of the fatty acid metabolism in the body is controlled by the liver. It synthesizes carnitine and taurine, nutrients of critical importance to the heart.

Carnitine—Fat Burner

Individuals trying to lose weight have always searched for that miracle pill that could help them effortlessly burn excess fat. Little did they know that nature makes its own fat burner: carnitine. This is an amino acid found in certain foods. It is also synthesized in the body, primarily in the liver. Carnitine transports fats into cells so they can be used for their primary purpose—as a source of fuel. Fats cannot be properly combusted without adequate amounts of carnitine.

Hearts Love Fat

You may have a lovely heart, but did you know that your heart loves fat? In fact, according to Guyton's textbook of human physiology fat is the primary fuel used by the heart. It specializes in the oxidation of fats into energy. The reason the heart prefers fats is that they are a more efficient form of energy. The heart needs to be efficient in its energy production more so than any other organ. After all, our hearts never sleep—if your heart stopped to take a breather, you would be dead. The heart pumps 13,000 pints of fluid throughout the body each day. With this huge workload, it needs to have the most effective energy conservation mechanism possible. Fats *are* the most productive source, providing over twice the amount of energy per gram as do sugars, starches, or proteins. Here again, the health of the heart depends upon a properly functioning liver—enter carnitine. Carnitine binds to the fatty acids and carries them into the heart's muscle cells. Once reaching the mitochondria, tiny factory-like organs located within the cells, carnitine releases the fatty acids. The mitochondria, which are found within the heart cells in great numbers, then burn the fats into energy. This energy is used to keep the heart pumping. Remember, the heart is the only organ in the body that *never gets to rest.*

Those who promote a low-fat, high-carbohydrate diet for heart disease never take the above-mentioned facts into account. They neglect a most fundamental part of normal human physiology—that heart tissue prefers to utilize fat above all other dietary sources of caloric energy. The fact is strict avoidance of fats is catastrophic to the heart muscle. This muscle will degenerate unless it is supplied with fatty acid-rich foods on a regular basis. Ironically, heart-nourishing fats are found in the very foods prohibited for heart patients. In other words, the prohibited fat-rich foods, such as eggs, meats, and whole milk products, provide fuel fats desperately required by the heart. What's more, foods rich in fat, such as meats, chicken, eggs, avocados, whole milk products, and nuts, contain carnitine and other nutrients which help the body metabolize the fats which they naturally contain. This is another principle that the anti-natural fat dieticians and nutritionists fail to grasp.

Carnitine is made in the liver from two amino acids: lysine and methionine. These amino acids are in the category known as "essential" amino acids. This means that the body cannot make them. Thus, you must get them in the diet. Without sufficient lysine or methionine, a carnitine deficiency will result. Vitamin C is also needed for the carnitine synthesis reaction to proceed.

Sugar: The Poor Man's Food

From this you can see that the heart is dependent upon fats, proteins (amino acids), and vitamins. It does not need even a pinch of sugar. Sugar damages the heart in the following ways:

1. It depletes valuable minerals from the body, minerals helpful to cardiac function.

2. It takes up calories in the diet where heart-nourishing calories are needed.

3. It disrupts protein metabolism and interferes with carnitine synthesis.

4. It destroys B vitamins needed by the heart such as thiamine, biotin, pyridoxine, and niacin.

5. It leads to the production of excess quantities of triglycerides and other fats, which are ultimately deposited in the arteries. Its use can lead to the development of high blood pressure, which places added stress on the heart.

6. It causes hardening of the arteries. The once flexible tubes become rigid. This forces the heart to work exceptionally hard, leading to heart muscle strain and/or damage.

Dietary Sources of Carnitine

There are numerous consequences of carnitine deficiency. In essence, fats can build up throughout the arteries and within the cells, since, without this key nutrient, they cannot be fully metabolized. The liver produces some carnitine on a daily basis. Vegetarians with high cholesterol and triglycerides are assuredly carnitine deficient, since there are essentially no vegetable sources. Meat products constitute the major sources. Here is a comprehensive listing of carnitine-rich foods:

Animal Products	**Plant Sources**
Lamb meat and fat (the richest known source)	Avocado (the richest vegetable source)
Beef	Brewer's yeast
Liver, heart, and other organ meats	Wheat germ
Whole milk	Peanuts
Cream	Peanut butter
Chicken or turkey breast	Cauliflower
Fatty fish	Cabbage

In addition, carnitine supplements may be useful. Research has shown that supplemental carnitine is particularly valuable for lowering triglyceride levels. Other conditions responding favorably include mitral valve prolapse, high blood pressure, heart failure, obesity, and coronary artery disease. Some cases of cardiac arrhythmia also respond to carnitine supplementation. Carnitine can also help raise HDL cholesterol levels, while lowering total cholesterol.

Despite their obvious fat content, carnitine-rich foods should be added freely to the diet. Carnitine losses from food due to cooking can be considerable. If meat is cooked excessively, losses of carnitine are extensive. Broiled meats lose their carnitine in the juices; do pour the juices from the bottom of the pan over your meats. Make gravies with these juices, and do not throw them out for fear of their fat content. Be sure to use whole grain flour instead of white flour as a gravy thickener.

Avocado is a great source of carnitine, since it is usually eaten uncooked. What little carnitine is found in cauliflower and cabbage is lost in cooking unless they are steamed or eaten raw.

Lamb Fat—A New Heart Saver?

Eat your lamb chops nice and juicy and don't trim off any of the fat; that lamb fat is loaded with carnitine. For centuries people in eastern Europe, Palestine, Turkey, and Greece made use of every part of their lambs, fat included. They rendered this fat and kept it for use in cooking. Heart disease was nonexistent despite their eating pure fat.

Of course, there is no need to start eating pure animal fat of any kind. However, you can eat your fill of lamb without trimming the visible fat. It tastes better that way. Try to eat lamb chops and steaks medium-rare. Remember, well done meat loses much of its carnitine. Be sure to also consume the juices from the cooking process, since this is where much of the carnitine is found.

Lard: The Heart's Doom

Lard is bad for the heart. It is a processed fat and is added relatively freely to the food supply. Many deep frying fats contain lard. Whenever you see the word "shortening" on a label, you can be assured it contains lard. Lard is harmful in part because it easily becomes rancid. It also contains a high fraction of polyunsaturated fats, which are quite toxic.

Lard has no nutritional value. It should be avoided entirely.

Protein is Good for the Heart

If you are plagued with heart disease, high blood pressure, or hardening of the arteries, you probably need more protein. While this may be contrary to what doctors say, the fact is the heart is made of protein and it direly needs protein to survive. We have been told that we get too much protein. To a degree this may be true. Yet, the average individual is not eating enough high-quality protein. Let me explain.

If 40% to 80% of the diet is in the form of deep-fried fat, greasy foods, chips, snacks, flour, sugar, and sweets, then something has to be displaced. These foods have to replace something. That something usually is high-quality foods such as proteins, vegetables, nuts, and fruits.

How often do you make these high-quality proteins a regular part of the diet?

- fish, fresh or frozen
- eggs, whole milk, or cheese (i.e. hard or cottage)
- fermented whole milk products
- chicken (baked or broiled)
- beef or lamb
- bee pollen, sunflower seeds, or pumpkin seeds
- fresh nut meats and nut butters

If you are losing portions of these excellent protein foods, you may have become deficient in certain components of proteins needed to maintain cardiovascular fitness, mainly carnitine. This amino acid is made from lysine and methionine, which are found primarily in high-quality protein foods such as those listed previously.

Animal proteins are the primary source for both of these amino acids, especially methionine. Both lysine and methionine are rare in plants. Exceptions include soybeans, oatmeal, and lentils, which are a good source of lysine. Unless the diet is carefully constructed, vegetarians routinely develop lysine and methionine deficiencies. The deficiency is of serious concern, as it may lead to cirrhosis of the liver, which is irreversible. Thus, carnitine deficiency is relatively common in vegetarians, since this substance is made from these amino acids.

Taurine: Another Unique Amino Acid

Taurine is another important protein-derived nutrient. Like carnitine, it is synthesized by the liver. However, in contrast to carnitine, dietary sources of taurine fail to supply worthwhile amounts. The human body depends almost entirely on the liver's ability to synthesize it from another amino acid: cysteine. Fortunately, cysteine is found in a wide variety of foods, particularly animal proteins.

The heart and blood vessels need taurine. Just as carnitine carries fats, taurine carries minerals into the cells. Minerals can be lost from the body in many ways. For example, sugar causes the loss of potassium and magnesium in the urine. Taurine helps prevent the loss of these valuable lifesaving minerals by binding them tightly within the cells.

Sudden Death and Taurine Deficiency

This is a story you have probably heard before. An aspiring executive of a major corporation dies of sudden cardiac standstill, leaving behind his wife and children. Was it preventable? It probably was, and taurine may well be a major player in this scene. Patients admitted to the hospital with acute chest pains had significantly higher concentrations of taurine in their blood than did normal people. You are probably wondering how a taurine deficiency could be represented by an increase in blood levels. It is because taurine is deficient within the cells. When the body is under stress, taurine is lost from the cells into the bloodstream and eventually is excreted into the urine. What's more the high amount of taurine means the body is using it to fight stress. Most cases of sudden death or heart attack occur during stressful events. Once taurine is depleted, valuable minerals, such as calcium, potassium, and magnesium, are easily washed out of cells. Without these minerals, the nerves of the heart become irritable and unstable. Thus, a fatal cardiac arrhythmia can result. Do you remember the deaths that occurred when dieters were following the liquid protein diet? Many of the fatalities were due to cardiac arrhythmia, which resulted in sudden death. These formulas were composed of incomplete proteins and contained no taurine. It is likely that the lack of taurine led to potassium deficiency and that this was the primary cause of these unfortunate deaths. To test yourself for taurine deficiency use the Web site, **NutritionTest.com.**

Medical Uses for Taurine

Taurine keeps the nerve and muscle cells of the heart calm. It helps the cells of the body hold onto the minerals they so desperately need. It is no surprise, then, that taurine has been found useful in the treatment of a variety of diseases, including:

1. High blood pressure
2. Congestive heart failure
3. Heart rhythm disturbances
4. Atherosclerosis
5. Epilepsy
6. Gallbladder disease
7. Alzheimer's disease

Sources of Taurine

Goat's and cow's milk, as well as cheese, contain some taurine. However, the only significant source is mother's milk, which contains ten times the amount found in cow's milk. It is likely that with the baby-boomer explosion statistics will show in 20 to 30 years that breast fed babies will have a far lower incidence of heart disease or high blood pressure than those fed formula or cow's milk.

Many excellent taurine supplements are available. In addition, cardiac patients should take riboflavin and pyridoxine, since the liver needs them to synthesize taurine. In addition, vitamin B_{12}, magnesium, and zinc are needed for taurine to be properly metabolized. Be sure to also consume enough high quality protein foods, because amino acids are needed for the internal synthesis of taurine.

Watch Out for the Mineral Thieves

Simple sugars and refined starches, such as white flour and rice, cause the loss of cardio-protective minerals, while high quality foods, such as proteins, fruits, and vegetables, help you retain them. A list of substances which deplete heart nourishing minerals from the body includes:

- white sugar
- corn syrup
- white flour
- coffee
- distilled water

- iced tea
- soft drinks
- some forms of fiber (if taken in excess)
- diuretics

Diuretics May Wash Your Life Away

Are you taking water pills for your heart trouble? Water pills, known by the medical term *diuretics,* can be very dangerous. Tens of thousands of fatalities in the elderly are due to the side effects of these drugs. The reason they are so dangerous is that they wash out valuable nutrients such as potassium, magnesium, chloride, sodium, and zinc. If tissue levels of any of these minerals become too low, sudden death or stroke can occur. Nature has provided many diuretics, which can remove excess fluid without adverse effects. Taurine was mentioned as a useful treatment for congestive heart failure, a condition wherein fluids overload the heart and lungs. Potassium itself is a diuretic, as is magnesium. Many herbs stimulate the kidneys to eliminate water. A partial list includes alfalfa, uva ursi, parsley, wild cranberries, and wild strawberry leaves. Watermelon is an excellent diuretic, and chlorophyll, which is found in dark green leafy vegetables, has a gentle but effective stimulating action on the kidneys. Parsley is perhaps the most powerful diuretic of the dark greens. It is also one of the best natural sources of magnesium and potassium. So, if you suffer from fluid retention, eat plenty of watermelon and parsley on a regular basis. For a natural tea with diuretic actions use WildPower Tea. This tea is made from an old Native American remedy—wild strawberry leaves. A natural and safe diuretic, wild strawberry leaves aid in fluid loss without depleting minerals. In fact, wild strawberry leaves aid in mineral nutrition, because they are a top source of potassium (see Appendix B). Gene's wild powerdrops are another natural diuretic formula. The purple powerdrops are made with wild cranberries, which makes them an ideal heart and kidney tonic. Take 5 to 10 drops of this pleasant tasting and extremely effective tonic twice daily. To order see the Web site, WildernessHerbs.com or call 1-800-243-5242.

Heart Medications and the Symptoms they Create

No reasonable cardiologist or internist will tell you that medicines cure heart disease. At most, medications help relieve some of the symptoms. There are several types of heart medicines, the major categories being beta blockers, calcium-channel blockers, anti-arrhythmics, digitalis compounds, vasodilators, anti-clotting agents, and diuretics. Few doctors have the time to tell you about the side effects these medicines create. The following is a list of the more common symptoms and toxicities caused by their use:

Symptoms
1. indigestion
2. dizziness
3. fatigue
4. headache
5. impotence
6. depression
7. palpitations
8. constipation or diarrhea
9. numbness or pain in the nerves
10. breathing difficulty
11. hair loss

Toxicities
1. bone marrow damage
2. blockage of the nerves in the heart
3. liver damage or inflammation
4. kidney damage
5. sudden death (from cardiac arrhythmia)

It is totally bizarre that heart medications cause damage to the very organ they are being used to treat. Unfortunately, fatal heart attacks have been caused by a variety of prescription as well as non-prescription drugs.

Causes of Heart Disease

Their are numerous factors predisposing individuals to heart attack, heart failure, stroke, and high blood pressure, some of which have already been discussed. Let's review some of these factors in more detail.

I. Fat and Sugar Intake

The theory that fats in the diet are the primary factor in causing heart disease is just that. This idea was started by a researcher named Ancel Keys. In 1953 he noted that certain cultures whose diets were high in fat also had a high incidence of heart disease. Thereafter, his theory became accepted as fact. There is some truth to the theory, but only on this basis: Americans and other people who have a high incidence of heart disease eat massive quantities of *refined fats*. Thus, it is not the fat itself but how it is processed or refined that makes it damaging. That brings us to the topic of sugar. It is proven that sugar intake is related to the increased incidence of a wide range of circulatory diseases.

Dr. Yudkin, former professor of Nutrition and Dietetics at Queen Elizabeth College of London University and now Emeritus Dean of

Nutrition, first noticed that many of the same countries who had a high intake of fat had a higher intake of sugar. When looking at fat alone, Yudkin found no evidence that people who had high intakes of saturated fats from foods naturally rich in fats, such as milk, cheese, eggs, or meat, had any greater incidence of heart disease than those who did not eat these foods. However, what he did find was that high intakes of sugar had an obvious relationship to the occurrence of heart disease. What follows are some glaring statistics:

Deaths from Heart Attacks or Heart Failure Per 100,000 People

Per capita sugar consumption	Deaths
20 lbs. of sugar per year	60 deaths
120 lbs. of sugar per year	300 deaths
150 lbs. of sugar per year	750 deaths

Note the dramatic increase in fatalities as sugar intake increases. The most vulnerable group appears to be men, aged 40 to 65, whose sugar intake is high. Apparently, the younger individuals can withstand the extra sugar, and the older ones have survived despite their sugar intake. Thus, if the sugar is going to destroy you, it will do so right in the prime of your life.

You might ask, "Is taking the sugar bowl away the answer?" Partially, it is, but hidden sugar is even a more sinister culprit. Most of the per capita consumption comes from sugar which is blended into the food supply. There are, of course, more obvious sources of hidden sugar such as a candy bar or a can of pop. So many foods in the supermarket contain sugar that it would take a book twice this size to list them. There is an easier way—just read the label. If it contains any of these sugar or starch derivatives, don't buy it:

Sugar Additives	Starch Additives
cane sugar	barley malt
corn syrup	malt syrup
dextrose	corn starch
fructose	dextrin
glucose	maltodextrin
levulose	
maple syrup	
molasses	
sucrose	
sugar	

Are refined sugars and starches really the villain? Yes, but they are not the only ones.

II. Iron, Iron, Everywhere

The food processors probably believe they are doing us a favor by "fortifying" our food. After destroying up to 95% of the nutrients in the foods, they fortify them with only a few of the ones that were originally removed. One of these few is iron. Why are foods, such as white flour and rice, cereals, as well as various other grain products, fortified with iron? These foods do contain small quantities of naturally bound iron, though much of it is lost during their refinement. Perhaps the food processors are themselves aghast at the devastation they wreak on the foodstuffs and feel they must do something in return. Cost effectiveness is the more likely motive. Thus, they fortify the food with iron in the form of iron sulfate (a by-product of industry and manufacturing) and add a few B vitamins. While no complaint can be registered against the B vitamins, the added iron may pose a problem: there is an increased risk for heart disease and cancer when there is excess iron within the body.

Iron Overload: Its Effects upon Vitamin E

Iron is found naturally in water and soil. Certain foods are rich in iron, but they are rich in natural iron. Natural iron exists in a chemical form that is harmless to the body. However, the iron added to food is no different than that found in iron filings—and it is a chemical form that causes toxicity. We can see how this works in nature versus how it works with iron additives by the following example. Foods naturally rich in iron often contain significant amounts of vitamin E. This natural iron does no harm to the molecules of vitamin E. However, the iron used in food fortification destroys vitamin E, both in the food to which it is added and within the body. Here again, humanity is unable to duplicate nature. Natural processes within iron-rich plants, such as spinach and parsley, render the iron harmless once it is absorbed from the soil. Not so with inorganic iron, which is highly reactive within the body.

Vitamin E, Inorganic Iron, and Your Heart

Vitamin E is a key nutrient for maintaining a healthy heart. It helps keep blood vessels open by preventing excessive blood clotting. As an antioxidant it protects the muscle and nerve cells of the heart from damage due to toxic compounds (such as inorganic iron). Vitamin E improves the pumping power of the heart and keeps it from becoming easily fatigued. Furthermore, it improves the ability of the blood to carry oxygen to the cells. This makes it clear that as far as diseases of circulation are concerned it is imperative that you retain whatever vitamin E you have in your body and not destroy it. Most people don't even get the RDA of vitamin E through their diets. The tiny amount they do consume is quickly destroyed by any inorganic iron there might be in the food. Thus, in many individuals there is little or no vitamin E available in the body to protect it against heart and circulatory diseases.

Foods Containing Added Iron

All foods containing wheat flour also contain added iron. The exception is stone-ground wheat flour or products made thereof. A partial list of foods fortified with synthetic iron includes:

- breads
- muffins
- pastries
- cake mixes
- cookies
- pies
- doughnuts
- malted milk
- pudding
- pasta
- crackers
- noodles
- pancake mixes
- creamed soups
- frozen dinners
- gravies
- pretzels

In addition, most breakfast cereals are fortified with iron. This includes virtually all cereals made with wheat, rice, corn, or barley. Cereals that are not fortified include Shredded Wheat, oatmeal, oat bran, rice bran, Triple Bran, Red River, Nutri-Sense, and some granolas. The latter are known as whole grain cereals.

If you are eating large amounts of any of the foods in the above list, the added iron is probably destroying most of the vitamin E in your body. Extra doses of vitamin E are needed.

In addition, iron in excess is stored and deposited within the body. It can end up in the liver, heart, bloodstream, red and white cells, and even in the skin. Once within the tissues it interacts with harmful compounds called free radicals to cause tissue damage. The heart is particularly vulnerable to the ill-effects of iron excess.

A certain amount of iron is necessary, particularly for menstruating females. In fact, blood loss is the only way nature can reduce iron stores in the body. This is why excess iron is so dangerous to men. Whatever extra iron they get through the diet (or from vitamins containing iron) ends up building up within the body. This extra iron is thought to be the major reason women who menstruate have a much lower incidence of heart disease as do men of the same age. This is further proven by the fact that after menopause, women become susceptible to cardiovascular disease. Women who use birth control pills are also at risk. Since menstruation is significantly reduced, their iron stores increase and so do their risks for heart attack, high blood pressure, and stroke.

The best way to tell if you have iron overload is to have a blood test which measures levels of a compound known as *ferritin.* Ferritin is a storage form of iron found circulating in the bloodstream. It consists of iron bound to protein molecules. Most medical laboratories can measure it. Levels above 90 mean there is too much iron stored in the body. Remember, if blood levels are high, the tissues themselves are overloaded. Red blood cells use iron in the synthesis of hemoglobin. Once that has been achieved, the excess iron is dumped into areas where it is not needed. It can then act as a catalyst for free radical reactions, which are dangerous to the cells and their membranes. It is thought that these reactions eventually damage the cells of the heart and arteries, leading to cardiovascular disease.

If you are not anemic, or if you have a proven case of iron overload (verified by a high ferritin level), you should avoid the following:

- white flour fortified with iron
- foods containing white flour
- multiple vitamins with iron
- excess quantities of red meat
- foods containing blood (e.g. blood sausage)
- white rice fortified with iron
- cereals fortified with iron

In addition, get rid of some blood. I don't care how you do it—whether you give it to the blood bank or have your doctor dispose of it. If you have too much iron and you are a male or post-menopausal female, blood-letting is the safest cure. This is far from an old wives' tale re-enacted. I have listed at the back of this book several scientific articles which provide proof for what I say.

How Often Should I Get My Blood Removed?

That depends on how much extra iron you have in your body. The removal of one pint every six months would do for most, although it may be necessary to draw it as often as once per month. This, of course, must be done under a doctor's care.

Once the excess iron has been removed, the result will be superior health. This is because with less iron in the body, there will be a significant reduction in the number of free radical reactions. Minimizing the number of these reactions is important. If free radicals get into the cell nucleus and are allowed to reproduce unchecked, they can damage the genetic material. If the genes or chromosomes are damaged, a wide range of serious problems can result ranging from mutations to cancer.

III. Thyroid Disorders

Both hypo (too little) and hyper (too much) thyroidism can lead to circulatory diseases. Hardening of the arteries and high blood pressure are commonly related to hypothyroidism, while cardiac arrhythmia is often caused by hyperthyroidism. A fatal type of cardiac arrhythmia can also occur in severe cases of hypothyroidism. This is due to an extreme deficiency of potassium within the nerve cells of the heart. In these cases the hypothyroid condition, if left untreated, leads to a gradual loss of the body's potassium stores.

In hypothyroidism there is often an elevation of cholesterol and triglycerides. This is due to a decreased rate at which food is metabolized. Thus, many hypothyroid patients are overweight. The combination of obesity plus hypothyroidism significantly increases the risks for the development of cardiovascular diseases.

Certain foods contain chemicals which block the production of thyroid hormone, particularly raw soybeans, cabbage, broccoli, rutabaga, cauliflower, kale, Brussels sprouts, watercress, carrots, carrot juice, turnips, and peanuts. Cooking partially inactivates the interfering chemical, known medically as *goitrogens*. Thus, in most instances it is wise to eat these foods cooked. Raw peanuts or soybeans should never be eaten. Fortunately, peanut butter and soybean products are heated to a high enough degree that the goitrogens are destroyed. If you eat the suspect foods frequently, it is a good idea to supplement the diet with extra iodine, since goitrogens block iodine absorption by the thyroid gland.

IV. Alcohol Consumption

Alcohol causes heart disease. It directly damages the arterial walls, causing hardening of the arteries, and traumatizes the heart muscle itself. Alcohol disrupts liver function and often causes permanent liver damage. A properly functioning liver is absolutely essential for the maintenance of a healthy cardiovascular system. Alcohol also causes direct damage to the heart and causes a disease of its own: alcoholic cardiomyopathy.

It is interesting to note that over the last several years certain scientific researchers have published data claiming that alcohol has a positive benefit on cardiac function. They base these claims largely on the fact that alcohol causes a rise in HDL-cholesterol. The researchers have gone so far as to presume that a drink or two of alcohol per day could prevent heart disease and extend life span. However, these researchers do not take into account that certain people who consume alcohol develop a condition in which the heart muscle degenerates, which is known as cardiomyopathy. Alcohol depletes thiamine and other B vitamins from within heart tissue. If the level of thiamine within the nerves of the heart becomes too low, the muscle fibers which are nourished by the nerves begin to degenerate. Cardiomyopathy has been successfully treated with a nutrient known as coenzyme Q-10. Treatment with selenium has also been shown to help. Thiamine may also be effective. Abstinence from alcoholic beverages is a must.

If you have high blood pressure and you drink one or more alcoholic beverages per day, guess what? The alcohol is probably causing your blood pressure elevation. The cure is abstinence, combined with dietary changes and nutritional supplements (see Chapter 11).

V. Cigarette Smoking

Everyone is aware that cigarettes are bad for you. Smoking chokes the supply of oxygen to the lungs, blood, and heart. Less well-known is the fact that cigarette smoke destroys vitamins C, E, folic acid, and vitamin A, which are key nutrients for maintaining healthy circulation. In addition, smoking generates harmful free radicals. Your risk for having a heart attack is far greater if you smoke—you know it and your insurance company knows it.

It has been proven that secondhand smoke, the type you get from being around smokers, is also a killer. If you are around smoke consistently, your risk for having a heart attack can increase as much as two-fold, even if you don't directly puff.

What Can I Eat?

By now, many of you are probably thinking that I have taken away all the "good things" of life, right? Wrong! I have only steered you away from the harmful ones. You can eat, snack, and indulge until you are full—providing you eat foods that are good for you. Now that your mouth is watering, here is a list of some healthy snacks. In addition, I have provided numerous recipes plus "Two Weeks of Eating Right" in the latter portion of this book.

Snacks for the Cardiovascular Patient

The following snacks are high in vitamins, minerals, and fiber. There is no need to snack on foods containing added sugars, starches, chemicals, and toxic oils. Notice the emphasis on low-sugar foods, which are the ideal snack for cardiovascular patients.

Sliced Vegetables

carrots	green peppers	zucchini
celery	red peppers	radishes
cucumbers	pickles	turnips

Sliced Meats

roast beef	chicken
roast lamb	turkey

Fruits

cantaloupe	honeydew	grapefruit
strawberries	watermelon	papaya
kiwi	guava	

Nuts and Seeds

almonds	pecans	pumpkin seeds
Brazil nuts	pine nuts	sunflower seeds
filberts	pistachios	walnuts

Other

boiled or poached eggs (preferably farm fresh)
feta cheese
farmer's or Swiss cheese (contains no dyes)
herring (unsweetened)
olives
sardines
shrimp
wild rice
wild game

Nutritional Supplements For the Heart Disease Patient
Fish Oils—Too Good to be True?

The proof is overwhelming. Eating two or more servings of fish per week decreases the risk of developing heart disease. Eating fish regularly is a good idea. However, in order to dramatically decrease the risks, take supplemental fish oil. Reputable medical journals all over the world have reported that fish oil supplements protect the heart, decrease blood fats, diminish blood clots, and improve circulation. Be sure to attempt to find the finest fish oil supplements available.

Perhaps the most important benefit of fish oils for heart patients is decreased risk of sudden death due to blood clots. In the proper dosage fish oils act as a blood thinner. Drugs, such as aspirin, Heparin, and Coumadin, also thin the blood, but they are far more dangerous. If taken properly using high quality products, fish oils are entirely safe. They are nature's blood thinners par excellence.

If you are taking fish oils regularly, you must increase your dose of vitamin E. This is because fish oils become rancid easily unless there is plenty of vitamin E around to protect them.

Eating fatty fish on a regular basis is another way to get these important oils. Be sure to buy the wild varieties of fish versus farmed raised. Wild fish is significantly richer in essential fatty acids than farm raised, as the latter are fed an entirely different diet than the type eaten in the wild.

Vitamins

Most vitamins play an important role in assisting cardiac function. Vitamins A, C, D, E, thiamine, niacin, B_5, and B_6 appear to be most critical. Thiamine deficiency causes shortness of breath and arrhythmia. A lack of it even predisposes to angina.

Vitamin B_5 (pantothenic acid) is extremely important, since it is needed to keep the adrenal glands healthy. Without it, these glands fail to produce sufficient quantities of key adrenal hormones which keep the heart pumping strong. Cardiac patients should take at least 500 mgs of vitamin B_5 daily, although dosages as high as 5,000 mg are entirely safe. For a superior adrenal boost use a premium grade royal jelly such as Royal Kick. Such a supplement has a major impact on preserving the integrity of cardiac function by strengthening the adrenal glands. If you suffer from a heart disability, take Royal Kick, two to six capsules every morning with breakfast. Since Royal Kick is fortified, this dosage provides the 50-plus steroids naturally contained in royal jelly plus over 500 mg of pantothenic acid. Thus, you receive precisely the adrenal boost you require from one simple supplement. The point is strong adrenals lead to a strong—and protected—heart.

Minerals

Minerals are critically important to cardiac function, because they play a major role in assisting cardiovascular function. Heart-nourishing minerals include calcium, magnesium, zinc, silicon, manganese, copper, potassium, and chromium. Cardiac patients should receive healthy doses of all these minerals. Magnesium, chromium, and manganese are particularly important, since cardiac patients are almost always deficient in them. Chromium plays a special role, since without it blood fats cannot be properly metabolized. A drawback of most chromium supplements is that very little chromium is absorbed into the bloodstream. This is even true of brewer's yeast, particularly if the individual is allergic to yeasts. However, recently a new type of natural chromium has become available. It is a type of chromium found naturally in wilderness grapes. Known as Resvitanol, it is made strictly from sun-dried mountainous grapes and is naturally rich in chromium. Incredibly, a heaping teaspoon of this powder (equal to 12 capsules) contains nearly 100% of the daily requirement. Impressive results have been observed in the reduction of blood fat levels, as well as blood pressure, with Resvitanol. One study resulted in dramatic improvement: six individuals with stubborn high blood pressure had a normalization of blood pressure from taking only 6 capsules daily. What's more, they were able to halt their medications. Other excellent sources of naturally occurring chromium include rice bran/rice germ (use Nutri-Sense), oat bran, nuts, seeds, beans, and organ meats.

Radishes, Nuts, and Mushrooms for a Healthy Heart

What these foods have in common that is of value to the cardiac patient is that they are all rich sources of the mineral selenium. Selenium helps prevent damage to the heart's muscle. Without it, muscles throughout the body tend to degenerate. The heart, being a muscle, is no exception.

Recently, scientists in the Netherlands discovered that heart attack patients have significantly lower selenium levels than controls. What's more, these levels were low for up to a year prior to the heart attack. These results indicate that the loss of selenium from the body leads to gradual but serious heart damage.

Selenium probably exerts its protective effects through preventing damage to the heart from those nasty free radicals (see Chapter Six). In other words, selenium keeps the heart from being poisoned by the body's own metabolic toxins. Other selenium-rich foods are listed in Appendix A in Part III of this book.

The Healing Powers of Edible Essential Oils

It has been long known that toxins cause tremendous damage to the heart muscle and arterial walls. Substances which neutralize and/or destroy toxins preserve heart and arterial health. Recently, it was determined that infection also damages the cardiovascular system and that, in fact, certain chronic infections may largely cause heart ailments. During my internship I first realized the role of infection and toxicity when attending heart surgery. The surgery in question was a cleaning out of the carotid arteries of the neck. What shocked me was what I saw inside the arteries: toxic sludge. That sludge certainly harbored germs. This sludge is found in the arteries of virtually all North Americans. There is an answer to this dilemma: edible essential oils. This is because such oils offer the rare benefit of a dual action: they are both anti-toxic and antiseptic. Plus, they act as solvents and, thus, greatly aid in cleansing the arteries. Cardio-Clenz, a liquid edible essential oil formula, is powered by wild and high mountain herbal/spice extracts. It contains oils of oregano, juniper, celery seed, and more, all of which are completely edible and safe. Crude unprocessed and edible essential oils are ideal for heart health. They help detoxify poisons, support immunity, destroy germs, and strengthen the arteries. The value of this is emphasized by the findings of recent research which proves a connection between infection and heart or arterial disease. Herpes viruses, staph, strep, and the bacteria chlamydia have been determined to infect the heart and arteries.

Use Cardio-Clenz to detoxify the entire cardiovascular system. It is a completely natural heart/artery tonic for the heart and arteries. Its cleansing actions include the removal of toxic metals, noxious germs, and arterial sludge. To cleanse the cardiovascular system from the inside out take 5 to 10 drops twice daily under the tongue or in juice/water.

Conclusion

Erroneous diet is the biggest factor increasing the individual's risk for heart disease. Exposure to toxic chemicals and metals, as well as alcohol consumption, also play a major role. Cigarette smoking, as well as the passive inhalation of smoke, directly damages the heart and arteries, perhaps irreparably. However, statistically, sugar is the number one cardiac poison. Nutritional deficiencies are always involved in heart and arterial diseases. What's more, the latest research indicates that infections also play a significant role. If you can avoid the poisonous substances, reduce your dependency upon medications, boost your immune system and cleanse it of germs, eliminate the refined sugar, and vastly improve your diet/nutritional status, you can have a healthy heart and excellent circulation. Then you too can succeed in the quest for excellent cardiovascular health.

CHAPTER EIGHT
The Number Two Killer

Cancer is a disease which must be prevented. With one of every three Americans getting cancer at some point during their lifetimes, the reasons are obvious. Once cancer becomes established, it is difficult to eradicate. Usually, monumental efforts are required to reverse it. What's more, these efforts often fail. Thus, the only logical solution is to completely prevent it from developing.

There are numerous reasons cancer is so prevalent today. Here are some of the more critical ones.

Preventing Cancer: The Importance of a
Healthy Digestive Tract

What we eat and drink has a greater bearing on the incidence of cancer than any other factor. We have discussed the time bombs, and it is crucial that you avoid these. In other words, to avoid cancer it is imperative to halt the consumption of cancer-causing foods. Yet, it is also what we don't eat that accelerates the risks: enter the importance of fiber.

Fiber: A Missing Link in Cancer Prevention

There has been a dramatic decrease in the amount of fiber in the diets of Americans over the last century. Low-fiber diets are clearly associated with an increased risk of digestive cancers, especially colon and rectal cancer. Breast cancer is also more common in women who have a history of constipation as a result of low-fiber diets. Fiber greatly enhances colonic function by increasing the strength of the contractions of the muscles in the colon wall. Fiber decreases the time that stool and wastes remain in the body. With low-fiber diets, fecal matter remains in the colon for extended periods. Normally, food should be digested and its residues eliminated within 24 to 36 hours. However, low-fiber diets may result in wastes staying within the intestines for days or even weeks. It is only logical that waste products remaining in the body for that long will lead to tissue damage. The colon and rectum usually bear the brunt of this damage, although other organs, such as the liver, pancreas, breasts, and skin, are also negatively affected.

It has been discovered that wastes can leak from the bowel into the bloodstream. These wastes then contaminate the organs and/or tissues in the body. The point is the appropriate amount of fiber is required so that the body can eliminate the wastes efficiently.

Thus, fiber is of great importance to health by accelerating the removal of wastes from the body. The normal elimination of wastes results in improved digestion, and overall health will be dramatically enhanced. What's more, the risks for developing cancer will be greatly diminished. This is because the health of the immune system is dependent to a large degree upon the ability of the body to remove wastes. The immune system itself has several direct connections to the small intestine and colon. Both of these digestive organs are lined with untold millions of white blood cells. In addition, the gut contains many immune organs, such as the appendix and lymphatic glands, which serve protective functions. In fact, over one half of the entire immune system is positioned within or near the intestines. If these immune organs are diseased as a result of waste contamination, the body's ability to ward off cancer is severely compromised.

The intestines love fiber. Fiber massages the intestinal walls, improving muscle tone and increasing local circulation. It maximizes the removal of poisons and intestinal wastes. While it is better to have too much fiber than too little, it is possible to consume it to excess. For instance, an excess of fiber can cause mineral/vitamin deficiency by actually removing food and nutrients from the body too quickly. Be sure to consume fiber in a "reasonable" amount. The best fibers are those found naturally in foods such as whole grains, vegetables, and fruit. It is virtually impossible to overdose on fiber by merely eating it in food. Some fibers are more gentle on the body than others. The best fibers are those which can be partially digested such as that found in vegetables, fruit, squash, wild rice, and brown rice.

No matter what condition you might have, increase your intake of roughage and fiber. Your life may depend upon it.

The Role of Friendly Bacteria

Although fiber is a major factor for intestinal health, there are others of equal importance. A healthy amount of helpful intestinal microbes is necessary for optimal colonic function. In fact, most of the weight of each bowel movement consists of bacteria and other microbes. There are a greater number of bacteria in the intestines than all the cells in the human body. This underscores the importance of intestinal microbes such as Lactobacillus acidophilus, plantarum, bulgaricus, and bifidus. These bacteria are beneficial, since they perform several useful functions. They aid digestion, synthesize vitamins, decompose carcinogens, and add to the bulk of the stool. If the numbers of these bacteria drop too low, they may be overtaken by potentially harmful ones. Antibiotics are the number one factor causing a decline in the quantity of useful intestinal bacteria. Since most people either take antibiotics medicinally or get them via the food chain, taking an acidophilus supplement is highly recommended.

Food may contain natural helpful bacteria, that is fermented food. To improve the health of the bowel, as well as the rest of the body, increase the intake of acidophilus/bifidus rich foods. The best dietary sources of these organisms include fermented products, especially yogurt, quark, sauerkraut, and acidophilus milk. The regular consumption of fermented milk products and/or Lactobacillus supplements is crucial for preventing cancer. However, the regular consumption of fermented food is perhaps the most reliable means of the achieving the Lactobacillus Cure.

Your Thoughts Can Affect Your Digestion

It is important to have a healthy mental outlook. Digestive and intestinal disorders can have much of their origin in our minds. Stress has a profoundly negative effect upon the activity of the digestive glands. Anger, grief, depression, anxiety, and worry disrupt digestion and, thus, alter body chemistry.

Certain chemicals can be released from the brain, which have a direct effect on the muscular and skin cells lining the intestinal walls. These potent substances may cause irritation and inflammation, which leads to nausea, stomach pain, indigestion, and colitis. If prolonged, negative thoughts greatly increase the susceptibility to cancer. Peace of mind is a prerequisite for digestion and health to be at its best.

Top Sources of Fiber

There are many sources of fiber for use as dietary supplements. Try to eat a large amount of fresh vegetables and fruit daily. The best way to get fiber is to eat fresh raw or lightly cooked vegetables, as well as fresh fruit, particularly watermelon, strawberries, kiwi, papaya, pears, and apples. Fiber supplements of exceptional value include:

- alfalfa (leaves and seeds)
- chlorella
- ground flaxseed
- kelp
- oat bran
- psyllium husks
- rice bran
- wheat bran (assuming you are not allergic to wheat)
- Nutri-Sense (rice bran/polish plus flax)

Whenever fiber intake increases, the need for fluid increases dramatically. Fiber absorbs water. In fact, it can absorb so much that it can actually dehydrate the intestines. This is evidenced by the fact that a high fiber intake without a corresponding increase in fluid intake may lead to bound stools (constipation). Anyone who takes a fiber supplement must drink at least six 12 oz. glasses of water per day. This is in addition to any other drinks taken such as warm drinks, milk, juice, etc. Otherwise, you could get more constipated than you were in the first place. Fiber is activated by water. Use the two as a team for the best effect.

Nutri-Sense is an excellent source of fiber. The type of fiber it contains is primarily soluble fiber, which is the safest and most nutritious type. Soluble fiber is a cancer-fighter, because it not only helps maintain proper elimination, but it also is a useful source of fuel. Nutri-Sense is an ideal fiber/protein supplement, and it is well tolerated by the majority of individuals. It provides soluble types of fiber, which are the most useful types for stimulating the growth of the Lactobacilli.

It is important to realize that the healthy bacteria, that is the Lactobacillus, thrive if they are provided with the correct environment. Of greatest importance is the fact that they must be provided with the proper food for survival. Lactobacillus use soluble fiber as a source of energy. It is the Lactobacillus which are the main preventive agents for blocking the development of digestive cancer. Plus, they increase the bulk of the stool, greatly aiding elimination. To enhance the growth of these microbes, take Nutri-Sense, three tablespoons in juice or water daily.

Diseases Caused by a Lack of Fiber

Since the advent of food processing, that is the use of manufacturing procedures which deplete the food of nutrients, there has been a rise in the incidence of degenerative diseases. In Chapter Two the negative effect of food processing on vitamin/mineral content was discussed. Yet, fiber is also a nutrient, and food processing removes most of it. The following is a list of diseases resulting from low fiber intake:

1. arthritis
2. cancer
3. cholesterol elevations
4. diabetes
5. diverticulitis
6. duodenal ulcer
7. gallbladder disease
8. gastric ulcer
9. heart disease
10. hemorrhoids
11. high blood pressure
12. hypoglycemia
13. inflammatory bowel
14. obesity
15. triglyceride elevation
16. venous disease (varicose veins and blood clots)

Constipation, although not a disease in itself, is due primarily to a lack of fiber. It is one of the most common health maladies in America today. Most cases of constipation are cured simply by adding additional fiber to the diet. However, be sure to increase water intake simultaneously. Dehydration is a major cause of constipation. For stubborn cases where fiber alone fails to resolve the problem, a variety of remedies are listed on page 271. Food allergy may also cause constipation. The primary culprits include wheat, rye, corn, barley, cheese, sugar, nuts, white flour, and the various processed foods made with these ingredients.

Certain foods greatly activate the intestines, improving digestion and promoting elimination. A partial list includes:

- figs
- dates (fresh)
- oregano
- cabbage (raw)
- sauerkraut
- watermelon
- grapes (fresh)
- cucumbers (fresh)
- parsley (raw)
- beets with tops (fresh)
- ground flaxseed
- turnips with tops (fresh)
- horseradish
- onions (raw)
- garlic
- radishes
- Jerusalem artichokes
- pears (fresh)

Gene's Powerdrops™ is a high quality herbal/dietary supplement for activating the intestines. Made from wild vegetables, herbs, and berries, this juice is extremely potent. Only small amounts are needed, like 5 to 10 drops once or twice daily. Take it as an intestinal tonic for a safe means of stimulating digestion and eliminating poisons. This is the original and only wild, raw greens and berry extract available. Its impact is far greater than mere commercial or organic vegetables or fruit. To order call 800-243-5242. Note: the item is rare, so shortages are possible.

Cancer Begins in the Mouth

Oral hygiene should be considered important by the dentist and physician alike. Unfortunately, many doctors fail to emphasize how critical proper dental hygiene really is.

The health of the oral cavity, the gums, and the teeth are directly related to one's susceptibility to cancer. The healthier and stronger the gums and dentition are—the more free of disease they are—the less vulnerable an individual will be to the development of cancer. There are several reasons. Cancer is directly related to the health of the immune system. Infected teeth and gums cause great stress upon immunity, and certain infections in the mouth can actually depress the immune system throughout the body. Chronic infections in the gums or roots of the teeth are directly related to the cause of certain cancers. In these instances the chronic infections poison the immune system's central defenses. In essence, the immune system becomes paralyzed. Because of this, cancer can more easily gain a foothold. Furthermore, a healthy oral cavity prevents the spread of infection, acting as a guardian for the rest of the body. When its structural components, such as the gums and enamel, degenerate, whether due to nutritional deficiency, poor diet, excess sugar, or other stressors, existing infections within the mouth can spread to infect other tissues. If the oral cavity becomes damaged by disease or trauma, i.e. invasive dentistry, various microorganisms contracted through the environment may enter the bloodstream, causing systemic disease. Remember, billions of microorganisms of all types live in the mouth—bacteria, fungi, yeasts, and viruses—many of which can cause disease. Even a slight imbalance within them can lead to ill health.

Over 95% of Americans have gum disease, and most have had one or more cavities. Many factors play a role in creating this. Refined sugar, white flour, soft drinks, pastries and/or candy, if consumed regularly, will assuredly cause gum disease. The consumption of excess quantities of soft drinks is associated with erosion of the enamel. This leads to infections of the teeth themselves, known more commonly as cavities. Deficiencies of calcium, vitamin D, vitamin C, bioflavonoids, zinc, coenzyme Q-10 and folic acid are associated with gum disease. Regarding vitamin D, sunlight is required since it dramatically stimulates the synthesis of this vitamin within the skin. Vitamin D is essential for the formation of strong enamel. Getting plenty of vitamin D through sunlight exposure as well as through supplements and food is perhaps the best defense against dental disease.

Folic acid and coenzyme Q-10 are critically important for gum integrity. Researchers have determined that a deficiency of these nutrients leads to receding gums, which is a breakdown of gum tissue. When this damage occurs, the gums are readily infected. Thus, to keep the gums healthy, a regular intake of folic acid and coenzyme-10 is advised.

Supplementation with coenzyme Q-10 and folic acid has proven in scientific studies to prevent gum disease and in some cases can even reverse the damage.

Your Water May Be Constipating You

Constipation is truly the plague of modern civilization. Up to one half of all Americans have it. There is plenty of proof that those who are chronically constipated are highly susceptible to cancer. However, few people realize that certain types of water can cause constipation – particularly chlorinated drinking water. Chlorine compounds in tap water kill the helpful intestinal bacteria, leading to the overgrowth of harmful bacteria, yeasts, or even parasites. In addition, despite chlorination, tap water may itself harbor parasites and/or their cysts. If you are easily constipated, you might be reacting to the water you drink.

The alternative certainly isn't to stop drinking water. The simplest solution is to purify the water at its source. This subject is discussed at length later in this chapter. I do not recommend drinking distilled water, as it increases the excretion of valuable minerals. This includes cancer-protective minerals such as calcium, silicon, zinc, and selenium.

Toxic Chemicals and Cancer

Toxic chemicals play a major role in the genesis of cancer. These chemicals are found within the food, water, air, and soil. Some are added directly to food when it is processed. For example, the preservative BHT is added to corn oil. Another example is food dyes, which are added to everything from Kool-Aid to pickles. Others are absorbed directly from the soil into the food or are found as residues on the food when crops are sprayed. Still other chemicals are ingested through drinking water. Our fresh water supplies are quickly becoming a toxic nightmare. They are laced with poisons and carcinogens, the result of industrial wastes, agricultural runoff, pesticides, herbicides, and radioactive chemicals, which seep into ground water stores. Unfortunately, these wastes are accumulating faster than they can ever be removed. Even the highest, most remote mountains are contaminated. Humankind should work aggressively to halt the use of earth-destructive chemicals.

Our Grain is Contaminated—The Aflatoxin Story

Natural chemicals can also contaminate the environment. Molds which grow on stored grain release several potent chemicals. Aflatoxin is one example. This poison is 100 times more potent in causing cancer than PCBs. PCBs are highly toxic synthetic chemicals made from the residues of coal and oil production.

Aflatoxin is the most powerful carcinogen known. The grain crop of 1988, especially the corn, was heavily contaminated with aflatoxin. Stored corn, already weakened by the drought, became infested with a fungus, which released aflatoxin in minute quantities. However, enough of the chemical got into the food chain through corn and cattle products to increase all of our cancer risks. For example, in Texas millions of pounds of milk were dumped due to aflatoxin contamination, and it doesn't take much. Millionths of a gram can initiate precancerous or cancerous changes. This serious health threat was thoroughly exposed in *The Wall Street Journal* (February 23, 1989).

Unfortunately, government surveillance of aflatoxin contamination of grain, milk, or meat is inadequate despite laws in existence to protect the public from it. Dr. David Wilson of the University of Georgia was quoted by the Journal as stating that neither government nor industry are capable of dealing with the problem. Mr. R. Leonard of the Community Nutrition Institute in Washington, D.C. says there will be an increase in cancers for decades after the aflatoxin exposure. This emphasizes the importance of the grain- and corn-free dietary guidelines found within this book. Risks can also be greatly decreased by taking antioxidants, particularly the highly powerful antioxidant spice oils, as outlined in Chapter Six. People whose diets consist primarily of grains, such as wheat, rye, and oats, or who eat large amounts of corn products probably have increased amounts of aflatoxin in their livers as well as in other tissues. For those who are concerned that they were or are being exposed, take daily doses of vitamin E (1000 I.U.), beta carotene (50,000 I.U.), and selenium (400 to 600 mcg.). In addition, a scientific study published in 1989 describes how oregano, particularly the oil of wild Mediterranean oregano, completely halted the production of aflatoxin, reversing its toxic effects. It is believed that spice oils, such as oregano, sage, cumin, and rosemary oils, block the ability of aflatoxin to induce cancer. If taking oregano oil, the amount of vitamin E and beta carotene may be reduced.

Oreganol brand wild oregano is exceptionally high grade and is the ideal type to consume. It contains the P-73 wild oregano compound which is the subject of modern research. Research at Georgetown University determined that the P-73 oregano oil dramatically improved the immune health of laboratory animals infected with fungus as well as the bacteria, staph. Animals given P-73 thrived, while those who didn't died. The Oreganol P-73 wild oregano contains a variety of active ingredients, including the potent antiseptic carvacrol. Scientific studies prove that wild oregano oil completely halts the formation of aflatoxin and various other fungal toxins. Take the Oreganol oil of wild oregano, 2 or more drops twice daily. Add a few drops to any suspect food.

Furthermore, avoid the consumption of large amounts of commercial grains, especially corn, and limit the consumption of commercial milk, consuming instead organic milk.

Avoid low carvacrol (55% or less) types of wild oregano. Note: the oil of oregano made by North American Herb & Spice is 100% wild high mountain Mediterranean source.

Unfortunately, for many people there is no way to escape having some intake of aflatoxin. The food sources are numerous, and it is difficult, if not impossible, to avoid them all. In these cases, reliance must be placed on helping the body detoxify aflatoxin through the antioxidant program outlined previously and by taking substances known as *liver protectors.*

Liver Protectors—The Answer to Toxic Scares

The aflatoxin problem is not the first toxic scare to surface in the last 20 years. Chernobyl, Bhopal, Three Mile Island, Love Canal, and the U.S.A. dioxin contamination are just a few examples. Each time one of these disasters is revealed, we are told of the potential or actual damage to human health. Yet, do you ever remember being told that you can do something about it—that if these toxins reach you through food, air, or water you can protect yourself? To a large degree you can, through liver protectors. In the case of aflatoxin poisoning, protection and treatment of the liver is of utmost importance, since aflatoxin exerts its primary toxicity on liver cells and, thus, greatly increases the risks for liver cancer.

Why Protect the Liver?

It is of critical importance to protect the liver, because it is the primary organ responsible for processing and removing toxic compounds. Well over 90% of the detoxification processes for substances such as aflatoxin, dioxin, pesticides, and hydrocarbons occur in the liver. These chemicals damage the liver and/or cause liver cancer, which is becoming increasingly more common in the U.S. every year. So, it is important to provide the liver cells significant protection. The liver contains billions of cells, and these cells are in dire need of protection. The following are the liver protectors which can be used to boost your anti-toxic defenses.

Protector:
BEET JUICE WITH TOPS (fresh-squeezed)
Comment

Fresh beets and beet tops contain special substances which protect liver cells from damage. They also help heal liver cells once they are injured. Beets also contain a substance which stimulates the flow of bile, thus reducing liver congestion. Hepatitis, whether caused by viruses or chemicals, often responds to beet juice. However, to gain these benefits you have to drink at least a quart or more per day.

Protector:
CHLORELLA

Comment

This is an excellent protector, since it helps pull poisons out of the liver. This may be due in part to its high chlorophyll content. Chlorella also minimizes the toxin load on the liver by aggressively binding to a variety of harmful substances, including cadmium, lead, mercury, pesticides, herbicides, and chlorinated hydrocarbons (PCBs THMs, TCEs, etc.). It is likely that chlorella will remove aflatoxin as well.

Protector:
LIPOIC ACID

Comment

Lipoic acid actually seals off and stops damage to liver cells which have been exposed to toxic substances. It is the treatment of choice for certain types of mushroom poisoning, conditions which would otherwise be fatal. It is useful in the treatment of most types of chemical hepatitis.

Protector:
BIOTIN

Comment

Whenever liver damage occurs, the liver cells swell and become infiltrated with fat. In order for these cells to recover quickly from toxic insults, it is necessary to metabolize or dissolve this fat out of the cells. Biotin accomplishes this well. Its primary role as a B vitamin is to modulate fat metabolism, in other words it helps the liver burn excess fat. At least 5 to 10 milligrams per day of biotin are needed to accomplish this.

Protector:
ROSEMARY OIL AND HERB

Comment

Rosemary extracts, as well as the pure herb, have been proven in many research studies to induce a dramatic, protective effect on the liver. Improvement of the liver's ability to remove poisons, synthesize valuable enzymes, and produce bile, as well as tissue healing after chemical exposure, has been documented. One study showed that a significant rise in liver content of glutathione—as much as 400% above normal—occurred following therapy with rosemary extract. Glutathione peroxidase (GP), as described in Chapter Six, is the cells' front line of defense, and the liver cells are no exception. In fact, the liver contains more GP that any other organ in the body. A good guideline is that whenever the liver is stressed, its GP levels drop. The most valuable agents which raise GP levels are the antioxidants of the aromatic herbal family such as rosemary.

An excellent wild and time-tested rosemary is produced by North American Herb & Spice Co. under the name Oil of Rosemary. For potent liver protection take five drops of this edible oil of rosemary in juice or water twice daily. Or, take a rosemary/sage herbal, such as Hercules Strength, two capsules twice daily.

Protector:
BIFIDOBACTERIA

Comment

The existence of harmful bacteria within the intestines is bad news for the liver. This is because the liver receives 80% of all blood flow from the intestines. No doubt, this blood carries vitamins, minerals, sugars, amino acids, and other nutrients to the liver, where some of these substances are utilized. Yet, this blood also delivers all sorts of by-products resulting from bacterial fermentation within the intestines. If allowed to multiply in excess, noxious bacteria will release substances which compromise the liver's ability to function. What's more, the harmful bacteria can enter the blood stream and flow into the liver. The liver has the capacity to kill bacteria, since 30% of its weight is made up of cells somewhat similar to white blood cells *(Kuppfer cells)*, which function to filter out foreign invaders. Even so, the added burden of these bacteria and the toxins they produce places tremendous stress upon the liver. This may be why people who regularly eat fermented milk products live such a long and healthy life, since these food products contain prodigious quantities of friendly bacteria (Lactobacillus bifidus, plantarum, and acidophilus). These friendly bacteria act to "crowd out" the harmful ones, reducing their overall number and, thus, diminishing the toxic load on the liver. Bifidobacteria are also useful for inactivating cancer-causing chemicals found within the bowel before they travel to the liver. A healthy liver means a long and healthy life.

In addition to consuming fermented milk products friendly bacteria may be taken in supplemental form. Best results are achieved if both Lactobacillus bifidus and acidophilus are taken.

Protector:
LECITHIN

Comment

For years it has been known that choline and other components of lecithin improve liver function. Lecithin is used by the liver to make bile and other fatty substances such as triglycerides. Perhaps more importantly, lecithin contains choline, which has been shown to protect liver cells from chemically-induced damage. In animals given cancer-causing chemicals a deficiency of choline induced cancerous changes in their livers. When choline was added to the diet, these changes were blocked. Choline works best when consumed with a diet rich in high quality proteins such as eggs, fatty fish, nuts, and meats. For a natural choline-rich food supplement excellent for liver health, take Nutri-Sense, three tablespoons daily.

Protector:
CUMIN OIL AND HERB

Comment

Cumin is an herb from the celery family which has a medical history as ancient as humanity itself. Recently, scientific research has shown that this aromatic spice protects the liver in particular from chemically induced damage. Everyone living in the U.S.A. is receiving a daily dose of toxic chemicals. Less than 200 years ago there was no such thing as a synthetic chemical. Now we are being bombarded by tens of thousands of them. The production of pesticides alone exceeds several billion pounds per year. Even a trace of pesticides is toxic to our bodies, and most of us are being exposed to massive amounts.

Today, Americans are experiencing a significant degree of liver toxicity or damage as a result of these ubiquitous chemicals. A name can be coined for this condition: the Toxic American Liver Syndrome. Every day the liver must attempt to rid the body of a host of chemical poisons absorbed from the water, air, and food. For example, every minute it must deal with pesticides and herbicides from the food, chlorinated compounds, and heavy metals from the water, and ozone and chloroform as well as other noxious gases from the air. This is why cumin is so valuable. It protects liver cells from free radical damage, acting as an antioxidant. In fact, its antioxidant activity, in terms of protecting the liver, greatly exceeds that offered by vitamin antioxidants such as beta carotene, vitamin C, and E.

The liver-healing effects of cumin can be quite dramatic. This pungent spice also greatly aids the liver's ability to produce bile, which is desperately needed for fat digestion. Plus, bile is the means for the liver to rid itself of toxic chemicals. The fact is cumin, particularly oil of cumin, is perhaps the most effective bile stimulant known. Oil of cumin should be in your protector pharmacy *just in case*. Note: a special liver detoxification formula is now available. Known as Liva-Clenz, it contains a proprietary combination of bile-stimulating and liver-enhancing edible essential oils, including oils of cumin, coriander, cilantro, and rosemary. As a liver tonic take 5 drops twice daily. Natural darkening, i.e. a rich brown coloration, of stools is a normal consequence.

Hydrogenated Fats and Polyunsaturated Oils

Refined fats play a greater role in cancer causation than perhaps any other factor. A definite increase in cancer risk is seen with the consumption of processed fats and oils, particularly that of refined vegetable oils. Deep frying oils, most of which are hydrogenated, greatly contribute to this risk. In fact, the current American dietary practice of consuming refined fats and oils plays a greater role in causing cancer than any other single dietary factor. High quality cold-pressed oils and extra virgin olive oil have not been correlated with increased risk. In fact, they may help decrease the risk.

Iron Overload—A Cancer Promoter?

There is a great deal of proof that there is such a thing as too much iron. This condition is known as *iron overload*, and it afflicts tens of millions of North Americans. It has been discovered that an excessive amount of iron increases the risk for the development of all types of cancer. Richard G. Stevens, Ph.D., the top researcher in the field, found that as little as a 3% rise in blood iron levels above the norm increased cancer risks in men by as much as 40%. This is an astonishing finding. Higher levels of iron further exaggerate the risks. Women did not show such a pattern. This is because their blood iron levels are consistently lower due to menstruation. However, the few women who did have excess levels of iron also had a higher rate of cancer.

Women who are of menstruating age but have no periods, as well as women who take the pill, can also develop iron overload. Women who have very light periods are also losing a smaller amount of iron, and so their iron levels may be high.

I have consistently seen that cancer victims have excess iron in their blood. This finding has been confirmed by many cancer researchers. Yet, until recently no one has discussed why excess iron predisposes to cancer.

Iron Overload Depresses the Immune System

Iron in excess is bad for health, because it helps initiate a breakdown of the immune system. The presence of iron greatly enhances the rate at which the cells' most critical components – the genetic material – becomes damaged. Iron somehow interacts with certain toxic molecules (remember the free radicals) to generate destructive chemical reactions. These reactions damage both the cell and its nucleus. Once the genes are repeatedly traumatized, the cells can become cancerous. This is the same destructive process that occurs within the body from a nuclear bomb or if there is a meltdown (as in Chernobyl).

Potentially dangerous chemical reactions are occurring within our bodies every day. Plus, we may become poisoned from the environment, i.e. radiation and toxic chemical exposure, which aggravates the internal toxicity. Here is where iron is the demon. If levels are excessive, the iron interacts with free radicals to, in essence, poison us. The cells of the immune system are particularly vulnerable. White blood cells divide rapidly; millions of them are made every hour. When they attack a microbe or detoxify a poison, hundreds of chemical reactions occur. In essence, they give off their own form of radiation. In the presence of iron these reactions can backfire and actually kill the white cell. Having too much iron inside the body is potentially catastrophic. It makes what are normal physiologic processes go haywire. The iron-mediated reactions may accelerate to such a degree as to go out of control. All sorts of cellular damage results. You can imagine the problems that will occur if immune cells are destroyed at a rate faster than they are made. Most certainly the body will be left completely vulnerable for all sorts of infections or even cancer.

Contaminated Water: A Major Factor in Cancer Causation

Unfortunately, our most valuable resource is being destroyed—our fresh water supply. Every well, river, and lake in the U.S. is polluted. In fact, the fresh water supplies throughout the world are now tainted with toxic chemicals, heavy metals, and other contaminants. Even the ice caps and icebergs contain measurable amounts of these poisons. Your cancer risks are directly related to the degree to which your drinking water is polluted. In some regions the water is so toxic that the individual would be better off not to drink any water at all. Recent research indicates that cancer risks from drinking chlorinated/polluted water may be as high as 300%. Of course, each of us needs a certain amount of fluids. Water is essential to life. I am not suggesting that you totally curtail your fluid intake. What I am suggesting is that you do something to upgrade the water you drink.

What You Bathe in may be Harmful to your Health

You get more pollutants in your system through the water you drink than by direct contact, right? WRONG! Most people today are skimping on drinking tap water. Do you know anyone who has cut down on the number of baths or showers they are taking? You absorb more water through a bath or a 15 minute shower than it is likely you would drink in one day. Most people do not drink more than a quart of water per day. Immediately after taking a shower or bath, an individual can gain as much as three pounds. However, it is unlikely that there is any noticeable weight gain because the water evaporates very rapidly. But the toxic chemicals remain.

Let's look at this another way. For every 50 pounds of body weight, up to one pound of water and impurities are absorbed during a typical bath or shower. Thus, a person weighing 140 pounds would absorb over a quart of bath or shower water! The more you weigh, the more you will absorb. How is all of this water absorbed? Through the skin. The skin is like a sponge. It is the largest organ of the body and has an unbelievably large surface area. This is due to the innumerable tiny crevices and folds found in the skin. If spread out, it would cover an area the size of a tennis court or greater. Toxins from the water or environment can easily penetrate it. This poses a problem. When toxins enter our bodies through the digestive tract, they are confronted by cells of the immune system, which decompose and detoxify them. If toxins get past the immune cells, the liver siphons them out of the blood and attempts to eliminate them However, direct absorption through the skin of harmful substances, such as pesticides, herbicides, hydrocarbons, and heavy metals, is often more damaging to our delicate immune systems than other means of exposure. A number of research studies have proven that the absorption of toxic chemicals through the skin is far more dangerous than a similar exposure through drinking water. Direct absorption through the skin of toxic substances can and has caused ill health and even death.

There is another danger in tap water: pharmaceutical drugs. Residues of drugs are found in virtually all public water supplies.

Researchers are finding increasingly high levels of potent drugs, including estrogenic and psychotropic agents, in public water. Even more ominous is the finding of residues of genetically engineered drugs, which is evidence of the existence of bizarre germ residues in public water. These drug residues and genetically engineered germs negatively affect health. The residues must be removed, otherwise it is virtually certain that epidemics of toxic reactions and/or germ infestations will strike. In fact, the epidemic is current. For instance, children are prematurely developing breasts and pubic hair, and men are developing breasts. Drug residues are the likely cause. However, the municipalities are failing to resolve this. It is up to you to take action to protect and/or cleanse your water.

Purifying Your Water: What are the Options?

Many of you are now so concerned that you may stop drinking tap water entirely. I do not advise this. You need fluids daily to keep from dehydrating and to maintain proper kidney function. A better alternative is to drink tap water after removing impurities. Water purification is a huge, multi-million dollar industry. Companies large and small have jumped on the bandwagon. These next few pages will help you sort out fact from fiction so you can make the best choice possible in your attempt to improve the quality of the water your drink, shower, wash and/or bathe in.

Distillation

In this process water is heated to the point where it becomes steam. The steam, along with other vapors, including potentially toxic ones, goes through tubes where it condenses back into water. For example, chlorine in the water readily vaporizes into highly toxic chlorine gas when water is heated. Some toxic vapors remain in the water even after it is distilled. What is left behind is particulate matter, including impurities and all the minerals naturally contained in water.

Distillation is expensive and wasteful. A great deal of energy is consumed in the process. However, that is the least of the waste. Look at what is left behind. Yes, many impurities are removed, but so are the life-giving minerals such as calcium, magnesium, zinc, and selenium. It is bad enough that the food is depleted of these minerals. If you deplete the water too, you can really get into trouble. It is a fact that hard water rich in these and other minerals has an anti-cancer effect. We need all the cancer protection we can get. For this reason I strongly recommend against drinking distilled water.

Reverse Osmosis

Reverse osmosis water purifiers are wasteful in a different way. It typically takes six to eight gallons of water to make one gallon of purified water. That's right! Eight gallons go down the drain. The limited resources of fresh water cannot withstand such waste. Fresh water makes up only 3% of the total water on the earth. Fully 2% of this is locked up in glacial ice at the North and South Poles, and in icebergs. In fact, less than 1% of all the water in the world is available for human use. Can you imagine the problems that could result if everyone used such wasteful methods?

In reverse osmosis water is forced through a very fine membrane that is designed to remove minerals from the water. For example, reverse osmosis purifiers are often used in conjunction with salt-based water softeners to remove the sodium, which the softeners put into the water. If these systems are not properly maintained by regular changing of the membranes, they can actually result in putting sodium or other contaminants back into the water (from the unclean membrane). Only about 10-25% of the water is actually forced through the membrane producing demineralized water. The rest of the water is wasted. In 1990 *Consumer Reports* magazine found that most of the RO units wasted at least 13 gallons of water per day. Models that constantly run a small amount of water to the drain waste nearly 40 gallons a day.

All types of reverse osmosis units remove the valuable minerals such as calcium, potassium, and magnesium. The following is an example of the ill effects which occur from drinking water treated with reverse osmosis:

Mrs. J. was plagued with a history of repeatedly injuring her muscles and ligaments. At the slightest strain, such as picking up a bag of groceries or opening a jar lid, she would injure herself. I suspected magnesium deficiency, since its lack leads to the muscles being easily injured and torn. Mrs. J. had one of the lowest blood magnesium levels I had ever seen. Not to my surprise, she had been religiously drinking reverse osmosis water for over four years. This habit was the likely the cause of her systemic magnesium deficiency.

Water Softeners

In the United States water softening is a multi-billion dollar business. You probably either know someone who uses a softener or have at least seen one. They are distinctive, as one prominent feature is a large container to hold the salt which is used in the softening process. Water softeners work on an ion exchange basis. Water is directed through resin beads, which are charged with the salt. As the water flows through the resin beads, calcium and magnesium ions are removed from the water and replaced with twice as many sodium ions. This produces so-called "soft" water. Calcium and magnesium are important minerals for cardiovascular health, while sodium intake, primarily from heavily processed foods, is associated with some types of heart problems.

Water softeners need to recharge these resin beads regularly. This recharging process, called regeneration, flushes large quantities of salt water through the resin beads to clean off the calcium and magnesium that has built up and to reseed the beads with sodium. Regeneration typically occurs every three or four days depending on water use. In addition to wasting a considerable amount of water through this process, it is also injurious to the environment. Numerous municipalities have banned salt-based softeners due to the severe environmental problems caused by the high quantities of salt introduced into the sewer system. For example, it makes it very expensive to reclaim that water to use for other purposes. Salt damages sewer lines and kills plants and even trees. The use of softened water is highly correlated with an increased incidence of cancer, heart attacks, and strokes. Don't waste your water or health by drinking softened water.

Bottled Water

Now you probably suspect what I am leading up to. Bottled water from the French Alps, right? Wrong! I believe that the only truly natural way to drink water is to drink running water. Stagnant water of any type, whether it is bottled under the most sterile conditions or if it is in a fetid pond, is not water as nature intended it. Running water, which undergoes all the natural processes, is the best way to go. Water that originates as rain or snow, percolating from the ground—filtering through the many layers of rock and soil from which it absorbs and carries minerals: this is ideal. I realize that the ideal is not always possible, and in this respect, some of the higher quality bottled waters are acceptable. But how do you know which ones are truly high grade?

"Bottled Water Fizzles Out"
So says the Water Quality Association

In 1987 this respected organization tested bottle water found on the shelves of New York City's supermarkets. They found that 96% of the bottled water tested worse for chemicals and bacteria than did water from the tap! This proves my point. Bottled water is becoming a huge and highly competitive industry. Not everyone is as careful as you might think, and though that sealed bottle of water might look pure, it is likely laced with all kinds of contaminants, and possibly even bacteria and parasites.

Tap Water Purifiers: The Logical Solution

I would not take you through this journey without providing you with some answers. Tap water is far from perfect. It contains both useful and harmful elements. However, the harmful elements can be removed effectively. This is through in-house water filtration and purification units. This is especially important for those who bathe or shower frequently.

The finest purifiers are those which remove toxic substances, including the chlorine and toxic hydrocarbons, while retaining the health-giving minerals. It is important to retain as much calcium, magnesium, silicon, and selenium in the water as possible. These minerals exert powerful protection against heart disease, arthritis, cancer, as well as other illnesses. In addition, once dissolved in water, these minerals are readily absorbed by the body. This is because water acts as a solvent, causing the minerals to be ionized. Once in this state, the minerals are readily absorbed by the body. A recent (2001) German study proved that the trace minerals in tap or spring water are nutritionally highly significant. The development of osteoporosis in women was inhibited by mineral water intake.

Due to the importance of skin absorption, the ideal alternative for water filtration systems is a whole house water system. There are significant differences among systems marketed as "whole house." An effective sophisticated system is manufactured by LifeSource Water Systems in Pasadena, California. This system is filled with high-grade granular- activated carbon, an effective medium for removing the chlorine, bad odors, and bad tastes often found in tap water. In May, 1994, The Environmental Protection Agency published a study entitled, "Is Your Drinking Water Safe?" which noted that amendments to the 1974 Safe Drinking Water act require that "granular activated carbon (GAC) filtration, an effective but expensive technology, be considered the best available technology for controlling synthetic organic chemicals."

One feature of this unit that is particularly important is its automatic back-washing. Back-washing is a vital step for filtration, as it serves to clean, refresh, and resettle the filtration bed. As water flows into the filter, the granular-activated carbon compresses and channels. When water channels, it goes over the same surface areas which then gradually become less effective. The back-washing creates turbulence within the carbon, cleaning, refreshing and resettling it. This ensures effective filtration over a much longer time by eliminating the channeling that would otherwise occur.

The LifeSource Water System even includes a feature for lessening hard water problems. Rather than employing the ion exchange process which depletes water of vital minerals, like calcium and magnesium, while substituting sodium, the unit physically conditions water to reduce hard water problems while maintaining the healthy minerals. Thus, no sodium is added. The extra sodium from the softened water contributes to kidney disease and high blood pressure.

The LifeSource system cleanses the water without adding noxious ingredients. No chemicals, salts, or residues are added to the water through this process. After treatment with this system, the water noticeably improves in taste and is odor free. Home owners should contact LifeSource Water Systems about their whole house water treatment units. It would be difficult to compare the value of such a unit for your home versus, for example, a new set of kitchen cabinets, TV, or some new furniture. To me, there is no comparison between these. Health is not an exchangeable commodity. There is no way to put a dollar figure on it. For more information about the water treatment systems which are available contact:

Lifesource Water Systems
523 S. Fair Oaks Avenue
Pasadena, CA 91105
(800) 992-3997

Unfortunately, apartment dwellers and renters are not usually able to install household purifiers. However, they can still adequately clean up their water. Many countertop models are available on the market. It is easy to get confused in this area due to the wide selection available and the variations in price. When looking at countertop and under-the-sink units, consider the following:

1) To be safe and effective it is important to be able to change the filters frequently. Some counter top units require that the whole unit be replaced rather than simply the filter. This means more expense. The natural tendency would be to replace the unit less frequently if it means a greater expense. Get a unit with a standard size replaceable filter that you can buy at a variety of sources. Don't rely on only one potential source for replacement filters. For typical use, change the filters every six months.

2) The ideal is loose granular carbon, which can be back-washed. Unfortunately, the vast majority of countertop and under-the-sink units use compressed carbon block. The problem with compressed carbon block is that there is no way to clean, refresh, and resettle the carbon to ensure continuous effective filtration. As the water flows over carbon block and toxins are taken out of the water, the surface area begins to saturate with the toxins. It becomes steadily less effective as a filtering medium. Buy carbon block filters rated at 1 micron or less. **Change the filters frequently**.

3) Activated carbon purifies water much like nature does through

topsoil or sand. Water within deep wells or aquafers gets purified by percolating through thousands of acres of topsoil, silt, rock, and sand. The purifying of the water through this process is related to surface area contact. The longer the contact, the more is absorbed. Activated carbon has a tremendous surface area for contacting and holding on to pollutants such as chlorinated hydrocarbons, pesticides, herbicides, PCBs, THMs, TCE, benzene, gasoline, drug residues, and many similar compounds. One pound of carbon has the same water filtration capacity in terms of surface area as 112 acres of topsoil.

The key to taking advantage of this tremendous filtration capacity is that the water must have ample contact time with the carbon. Thus, if the water runs through the carbon too fast, as is the case with most water treatment units, fewer poisons will be removed. Quality whole house water filtration systems, like the LifeSource system described previously, are designed to maximize contact time.

Pure water means better health. Every river, lake, stream, and well in this country is contaminated. With one out of three Americans developing cancer at some point in life, it is life-threatening not to purify your water. It makes little sense to "go all out" and eat pure, wholesome foods while drinking water which is full of toxic substances. Our water is contaminated with everything from parasites and pesticides to gasoline. Don't be fooled. The water in this country is getting worse by the day. Soon, water will be the most precious commodity on this earth. What you drink and bathe in is every bit as important as what you eat. When seeking preventive health care, try to cover as many bases as possible. Proper dental hygiene, pure water, clean air, and nutritious foods are important. Reducing or eliminating any contact with water-borne toxic chemicals is a major step in the right direction.

The Role of Stress

Do you know anyone whose cancer developed after a period of severe mental stress? In fact, this is what most commonly happens. In these cases the genetic tendency for cancer already exists. Usually, the cancer arises because the severe emotional and/or psychological stress stimulates its growth. Stress has an extremely negative effect upon the nervous system. The nervous system controls the function of the immune system. Stress or negative emotions, such as anger, guilt, or depression, is transmitted from the brain through the spinal cord. The nerves send aberrant messages into the internal organs, resulting in the release of poisonous and immunosuppressive chemicals. The immune system of the majority of individuals is already compromised by toxic chemicals, heavy metals, poor diet, and nutritional deficiency, and, thus, it will readily collapse under severe stress. Even a relatively brief episode of stress, if severe enough, can precipitate the onset of cancer. This is illustrated by a specific case. A father was very close to his daughters. The youngest girl, his "baby," developed a monstrous disease: multiple sclerosis. Soon afterward, the father was stricken with kidney cancer and died promptly. It may be argued that there already was an underlying cancerous tumor and the stress merely served to hasten its development. This may indeed be true. Yet, many of these individuals have been sensitive to the ill effects of stress possibly for a lifetime. The role played by stress in the causation of cancer is so great that it would not be an exaggeration to state that 80% or more of all cancers have their immediate origins in some form of mental pressure or strain. Grief, distress, fear, worry, and anger have disastrous effects upon the body's functions. Researchers have discovered that these emotions cause the release of chemicals from the brain called neuropeptides. These potent compounds have a profound immune suppressive actions. Scientists have traced a pathway from the brain to the immune cells, proving that negative emotions can stop the immune cells dead in their tracks. This results in part from the release of chemicals from the nerve endings, which poison the immune cells. When this happens, harmful microbes or cancers cells can invade any tissue in the body. The point is to be careful of what thoughts you allow yourself to entertain. As described by Judy Kay Gray, M.S., if you suspect that negative thought patterns are circulating in your mind, patterns which are having a detrimental effect upon your health, it is possible to change them. By changing your thoughts from negative (minus) to positive (plus), your health will change for the better. Disease indicates the need for change. No one can change the situation better than you. For some, this may be the best cancer prevention of all.

Nutritional Deficiencies and Cancer
Selenium Deficiency

This mineral is a key factor in cancer prevention. Regions with the highest soil and water concentrations of selenium have the lowest cancer incidence. The Great Lakes region (Wisconsin, Illinois, Indiana, Michigan, and Ohio) has one of the highest cancer rates in the world. As you may have presumed, this region has virtually no selenium in its soil. Many coastal states also have selenium-deficient soil, particularly those in the northeastern and northwestern regions.

Selenium activates an enzyme in the body known as glutathione peroxidase. The function of this enzyme is to protect cell membranes, genetic material, and the immune system from damage due to toxic chemicals, heavy metals, radiation, and stress. Without selenium, this enzyme becomes powerless to protect us.

When selenium or glutathione deficient cells are bombarded with cancer causing substances, their genetic material goes haywire. This is the beginning of cancer. This is because the genes control the rate at which cells reproduce. A tumor is essentially cellular reproduction gone out of control. Selenium may well be the most important cancer-protective nutrient known. To thoroughly evaluate your selenium and glutathione status use the Web site NutritionTest.com.

Beta Carotene

This nutrient is instrumental in preventing cancer, especially cancers of the skin and mucous membranes. Recent research is proving that beta carotene actually helps the body destroy tumor cells. The activity of special antitumor cells known as macrophages is greatly increased by supplemental and/or dietary beta carotene. In addition, beta carotene itself is directly toxic to certain tumors. Beta carotene is found primarily in vegetables, tubers (root plants), and fruits. Rich food sources include:

alfalfa leaves	green onions
apricots	kale
asparagus	mustard greens
avocados	parsley
beet tops	persimmons
broccoli	pimentos
butter	pumpkin
cantaloupe	red peppers
carrots	romaine lettuce
chard, Swiss	spinach
chili peppers	sweet potatoes
chlorella	tomatoes
collards	turnip greens
dandelion greens	turnips
endive	watercress
escarole	winter squash
yellow squash	

National Cancer Institute and Beta Carotene

The NCI, as well as the American Cancer Society, recommends that diets include foods rich in beta carotene. They know that the evidence is clear: diets enriched with foods, such as those just mentioned, prevent cancer. Take heed of this and include prodigious quantities of these foods in your diet. A good rule is to snack on beta carotene-rich vegetables every day in addition to including them with your meals.

How Beta Carotene Works

Beta carotene exerts its protective effects in a number of ways. It directly protects cells from the damaging ions induced by radiation. People receiving X rays should greatly increase their beta carotene consumption. Computer operators should also increase their intake. Beta carotene also enhances the body's ability to utilize oxygen at the cellular level. If the oxygen concentration within the cells is high enough, cancer cannot develop.

The loss of the earth's ozone layer is allowing a greater amount of radioactive particles to penetrate the atmosphere than ever before. These extra ions are also penetrating our bodies. Once these ions enter the body, they cause damaging reactions which can destroy the nuclear material (genes and chromosomes) within the cells. Beta carotene blocks these reactions. By increasing the consumption of beta carotene-rich foods, it is possible to minimize damage to the body caused by the sun's radioactive waves. Use only natural sources of beta carotene. Synthetic beta carotene has not been proven to be protective.

Vitamin E

Cancer patients are often deficient in vitamin E. Does this mean cancer is caused by vitamin E deficiency or that it can be cured by it? There is no evidence to prove this yet. All it means is that vitamin E helps protect the body against cancerous degeneration. Vitamin E in doses up to 1200 I.U. has a stimulating action on immune function. White blood cells which contain adequate quantities of vitamin E are able to survive longer and are more effective in killing foreign invaders, including cancer cells. It also boosts immunity by conserving other antioxidants such as glutathione, selenium, and coenzyme Q-10.

Vitamin C

This vitamin offers its most potent anti-cancer actions when it is consumed in fresh fruits and vegetables. There has been much discussion regarding the beneficial effects of vitamin C supplements upon cancer. No doubt, vitamin C is a critical nutrient for assisting immune function. Even so, there is no firm evidence that supplements of synthetic vitamin C, whether powder or pills, have any curative or antitumor action in respect to existing tumors. On the other hand, studies have shown that regular consumption of vitamin C-rich foods, such as fresh citrus fruits and dark green leafy vegetables, greatly diminishes the incidence of cancer. This protective effect may not be from the vitamin C per se but from a combined action of vitamin C, bioflavonoids, pigments, citrus oils, chlorophyll, and other naturally occurring components in the whole fruit/vegetable, including the fiber. A natural vitamin C supplement called Flavin-C is available. The ingredients include acerola cherries, rose hips, immature orange, and immature tangerine, all of which are top natural sources of vitamin C and bioflavonoids. It was Dr. Szent Gyorgi, the Hungarian Nobel Prize winner, who proved that unprocessed natural vitamin C is far more effective in disease reversal than the synthetic vitamin. Note: beta carotene, vitamin C, and bioflavonoid status can all be evaluated through taking the tests on the Web site, NutritionTest.com. The cost is approximately $1.00 per test.

Fish Oils

Fish may well be brain food. Did you know it is also immune food? Fish oils have significant anti-tumor action. They exert this effect primarily by preventing the spread of cancer into the tissues. Fish oils may also help block the formation of tumors. What's more, they greatly aid the white blood cells, stimulating their ability to kill cancer cells as well as germs.

The chemical name for fish oils is *eicosapentaenoic acid* (EPA) and *docosahexaenoic acid* (DHA). Their actions may be due in part to the dramatic improvement in circulation they cause. Fish oils decrease the sludging of blood, acting as a natural blood thinner. Cancer often spreads to other tissues through the blood. Cancer cells metastasize by attaching to platelets, which transport these invaders from their primary site to more distant sites throughout the body. By decreasing the stickiness of platelets, fish oils help stop this from happening. They also help dramatically improve the circulation. This leads to an increase in the oxygen content of the blood. Cancer cells grow best when the tissue oxygen concentration is low.

It has also been discovered that fish oils directly enhance the function of white blood cells, making them more effective in fighting infection and destroying malignant cells. A word of caution: only high quality fish oils exert this protective effect. The best source is eating fish rich in EPA and DHA, although fish oil supplements are also helpful. EPA/DHA-rich fish include salmon, tuna, whitefish, sardines, bluefish, trout, mackerel, halibut, and herring.

Foods that Improve the Odds

Diet has a major influence upon cancer risk. What you eat has a direct impact upon the integrity of the immune system. If the immune system is damaged by poor diet, the risk for the development of cancer greatly rises. What you drink makes a difference too. Pure water, fresh juice, and pure milk aid the body. Alcoholic beverages, sugar-laden drinks, and stimulants harm it.

Fruits and vegetables offer the highest degree of protection against cancer. However, herbs and spices are also potent anti-cancer substances. Cultures which have a high intake of fresh fruits and vegetables, as well as herbs and spices like garlic, oregano, basil, and rosemary, have a significantly lower cancer incidence. In some societies with extraordinarily high intakes of anti-tumor plants, cancer is literally non-existent. Let's examine some of the reasons.

The Wonder of Fruits

Fruit is good for you for a number of reasons. First, they are highly digestible. The digestive organs put out far less energy to digest fresh fruit than to process, for instance, a piece of bread or a slice of roast beef. Fruit is loaded with anti-cancer substances. A word of caution: only fresh fruit provides these benefits. Fruit which is picked unripe, stored, fumigated, and waxed, or which is laden with pesticides or herbicides, is not likely to have cancer-protective benefits. Unfortunately, the majority of our fresh fruit is in this sorry condition. Thus, the following information holds true only if the fruit is fresh and free of contamination.

Protective Effects

Certain types of fruit exhibit protective effects against cancer. For example, people living in citrus-growing regions, such as Florida and California, eat large quantities of fresh citrus fruits and, thus, have a reduced incidence of intestinal and stomach cancer. Citrus fruit is a rich source of two key nutrients: vitamin C and bioflavonoids. Both inactivate toxic or cancer-causing chemicals. They also protect our bodies from the harmful effects of these chemicals. Researchers have shown that a diet high in fresh citrus fruit leads to a reduction in the amount of cancer-causing chemicals, known as *mutagens,* in the feces. Note that these anti-mutagenic effects results from *naturally occurring* vitamin C and bioflavonoids. The majority of individuals are unable to eat fresh citrus fruit on a daily basis. As an alternative, take Flavin-C, two or three capsules twice daily.

In addition, bioflavonoids and vitamin C help keep the cellular cement in place. The cells in our body are bound to each other by connective tissue which is, in essence, microscopic ligaments. Vitamin C is required for the synthesis of these connective tissues, and bioflavonoids plug the gaps, acting as a sort of cellular glue. Vitamin C is needed on a continuous basis to keep the bonds tight and prevent the glue from breaking down. In this way vitamin C and bioflavonoids help prevent the invasion and spread of cancer. The tighter the "fit" of the cells, the more difficult it is for tumors to grow, invade, or metastasize.

Scurvy is an extreme example of a breakdown in the cellular cement. In this condition the tissues of the body literally disintegrate, as if they are becoming "unglued." This vitamin C and bioflavonoid deficiency disease is occurring with increasing frequency in North America and not just in alcoholics or the elderly. A recent report indicated that as a result of excessive consumption of processed foods up to 60% of teenagers are severely vitamin C deficient.

If the vitamin C and bioflavonoid deficiency becomes extreme and prolonged, the gaps between cells and within cell membranes become so extensive that the body becomes invaded by all sorts of toxins, infections, and tumors. Cancer itself may be a form of a scurvy-like disease due to the degeneration of the connective tissues.

People who crave fruit or sour substances are likely deficient in vitamin C. Those who crave the rinds of citrus fruits or who love to suck on lemons or limes usually have a deficiency of bioflavonoids. As a child, I always craved sour foods (unfortunately, some candies, like Sweet Tarts, are sour tasting, so I craved and ate those also). Food sources rich in both vitamin C and bioflavonoids include:

Vitamin C

black currants	lamb's quarter
broccoli	mustard greens
Brussels sprouts	papaya
cantaloupe	parsley
citrus fruit	pimento
elderberries	potatoes
green, yellow, and red peppers	red cabbage
guava	spinach
hot peppers	strawberries (vine ripened)
juices (unsweetened citrus,	tomatoes
tomato, vegetable, papaya,	turnip greens
guava, etc.)	watercress
kale	
kiwi fruit	

Note: Crude unsweetened black currant juice (Currant-C™) is an ideal means of consuming large amounts of natural vitamin C. So is Potent-C, a crude natural vitamin C supplement made from wild rose hips. The Potent-C contains 40 mg of crude natural vitamin C per teaspoon.

Bioflavonoids

alfalfa
apricots
blackberries
black currants
blueberries
broccoli
buckwheat
cantaloupe
cherries
citrus pulp
citrus rind
elderberries
grapes
green and red peppers

herbal teas (especially those
    containing rose hips)
plums
pure raw vinegars
raspberries
red onions
strawberries
tangerines, especially tangerine juice

Here are some excellent, simple ways to get your daily dose of bioflavonoids:

1. Douse your salad with raw vinegar. Doctor Bronner's grape vinegar or raw apple cider vinegar are excellent choices. Other good brands are found in specialty shops, health food stores, and some supermarkets. The more crude the vinegar is, the richer it is as a source of bioflavonoids.

2. Drink one or more cups daily of herbal tea containing rose hips or other flower buds. Or, for an aromatic bioflavonoid treat consume Essence of Orange Blossom or Rose Petals as a bioflavonoid-rich tea and tonic. Simply add a tablespoon of either of these refreshing, nourishing essences to hot water, and drink as a tea.

3. Drink fresh-squeezed tangerine, grapefruit, or orange juice every day. Tangerine is an exceptionally good source.

4. Use bioflavonoid-rich sauces/chutneys, such as those made from tart fruit like mango, papaya, or pomegranate, with any meat dish. Pomegranate Syrup is an extremely tart, tasty bioflavonoid food. In the Mediterranean it is a frequent addition to protein/fat dishes such as any dish containing meat or cheese. Use it with eggs, cheese, beef, lamb, and chicken dishes, and for a wonderful taste add it to stir fry (see Appendix B). With its deep red color it is obvious that this sauce is super-rich in bioflavonoids. Also, mix this syrup with

cold water to make a refreshing, nutritious drink.

5. Drink crude unsweetened black currant juice (i.e. Currant-C™). Black currants are the top juice source of both vitamin C and bioflavonoids, far exceeding citrus juice. Gene's powerdrops ™ is an extract of wild currants and various other wild berries. A potent natural source of bioflavonoids, it is available both in a dropper bottle and in gelatin capsules. Only a small quantity of this concentrate is needed, like 10 to 20 drops daily or 1 or 2 gelcaps. This is a rare nutritional supplement, because the berries are picked wild. It is the ideal way of procuring a daily dose of natural unprocessed bioflavonoids.

Bioflavonoids can help as a part of your cancer protection regimen. They are also useful in treating and preventing the following conditions:

- anemia
- bleeding gums
- blood clots
- bruising
- diabetes
- glaucoma
- heavy menstrual bleeding
- uterine fibroids
- hemorrhoids
- miscarriage
- urinary bleeding (if not due to a tumor)
- varicose veins

Vitamin C in Fruit Inactivates Carcinogens

Foods rich in vitamin C preserve the health of the tissues. Just how vitamin C acts as a natural preservative is best illustrated by some common observations. When a food is cut open, it rapidly loses its vitamin C content. As the vitamin C disappears the food becomes susceptible to oxidation, which is represented by loss of taste as well as color changes. A good example of this reaction is what happens to a banana and potato when they are peeled—they turn brown. This is the process of oxidation in action. It results from rapid loss of vitamin C into the air. If we become severely deficient in vitamin C, a similar process occurs within our bodies.

Toxins and carcinogens, that is cancer-causing chemicals, cause our tissues to oxidize, and vitamin C prevents this reaction from occurring. In addition, this vitamin can actually help the body destroy harmful chemicals. Meats preserved with nitrates are a good example. As described in Chapter Five nitrates are chemicals used in the production of processed and cured meats. Examples of foods processed with nitrates include hot dogs, bologna, bacon, sausage, ham, pastrami, and corned beef. Nitrates are responsible for the bright reddish color of these meats. Thus, nitrates are used both for preservation and consumer appeal. However, the very thing manufacturers use to cure these meats acts as a powerful cancer-initiating substance after it is ingested. You can visualize the harmful effects of nitrates actually "curing" your innards. Here is where vitamin C enters the picture. Substantial doses block the toxicity of nitrates and stop them from producing their most harmful effect—cancer. Today, food processors are taking advantage of vitamin C's powers, because they add it as a preservative to many cured meats.

Cured meats are associated with a significant increase in the incidence of cancer of the esophagus, intestines, pancreas, and stomach. Ironically, vitamins C and E, as meat preservatives, are just as effective as are nitrates but without the toxicity. Spices, such as sage, rosemary, cloves, and oregano, are also excellent meat preservatives. Perhaps the toxic nitrates will one day be replaced by natural substances which are entirely safe for human consumption.

Fruit in the Grocery Store
May Not Be as Fresh as it Appears

The problem with food presented in the grocery store is that looks can be deceiving. Sometimes you can tell that the fruit is picked green; note the major difference in color, texture, and shape of commercial tomatoes versus the tomatoes grown in a garden. A similar measurable difference occurs in the nutrient content as well. When a fruit is allowed to ripen naturally on a tree or vine, the nutrient content increases dramatically. This is due to the interaction between sunlight and the fruit. During the ripening process, sunlight is needed to induce chemical reactions within the fruit, resulting in an increased concentration of nutrients. This increased nutrient content is the major reason fruit ripened on the tree or vine tastes so much better than artificially ripened fruit. On the other hand, prolonged storage, gas-induced ripening, waxing, and fumigation all lead to the loss of delicate nutrients such as riboflavin, folic acid, vitamin C, magnesium, potassium, chromium, manganese, vitamin E, and beta carotene.

Oranges Without Vitamin C, Anyone?

In some instances eating a "fresh" orange from the supermarket provides no more vitamin C than eating a plastic one. At the Rockefeller Institute Dr. Michael Colgan determined that some oranges found on supermarket shelves actually scored zero in vitamin C content. This is a universal dilemma in America. This is because the majority of fruit available is not totally fresh and certainly is not sun ripened. Fruit in season which is ripened on the vine by the sun is more reliable in its nutrient content than winter fruit. Certainly, if you have access to organically grown fruit, this is the best option. Do not be entirely discouraged about the options available. Many fruits retain their vitamin C content despite the litany of abuse they receive. A partial list of such fruits includes:

avocado	lemons	strawberries
cranberries	limes	papaya
kiwi fruit	melons	pineapple (fresh)

Vegetables

Vegetables may be the premier food category for the prevention of cancer. There are many reasons for this protective effect. The fact that most vegetables are rich in the most effective anti-cancer nutrients known is of major importance. These are flavonoids, indoles, sulfones, carotenes, ascorbic acid, chlorophyll, and fiber.

Vegetables are a low-stress food. In other words, they are relatively easy to digest. Very little effort or energy is required by the digestive tract to process them. Proteins, on the other hand, require a great deal more energy to be broken down into an absorbable form. Even so, protein is of critical importance, because it is required as the building block of all cells.

Since vegetables are readily digested and are gentle upon the body, they are one of the most valuable foods in the fight against cancer. Digestion consumes up to 60% of the energy used by the body on a daily basis. If you have cancer, eat plenty of vegetables to help you conserve bodily energy for the most important use: the destruction of the cancer. Focus especially on those vegetables proven to block cancer, particularly broccoli, cauliflower, cabbage, kale, watercress, radishes, turnips, turnip greens, arugula, beets, Brussels sprouts, and spinach.

Raw Versus Cooked Vegetables

Contrary to what some health advocates advise, not all vegetables need to be eaten raw. Sometimes steaming vegetables, sautéing lightly in butter or olive oil, or even simmering them in a small amount of water, can be superior to eating them raw. If broccoli, cauliflower, and Brussels sprouts are lightly cooked, they provide far more nutrition than if they are eaten raw. This becomes readily apparent by seeing how much more vibrant and intense their colors appear once they are gently steamed or sautéed. Thus, for certain vegetables cooking serves to activate the nutrients (by breaking down the fiber), making them easier to digest and assimilate.

Some vegetables appear to have a more potent cancer-preventive effect than others. A good example is the vegetables of the cabbage family—the *cruciferous* vegetables. This family includes cabbage, Brussels sprouts, cauliflower, broccoli, mustard greens, brown mustard, watercress, kale, and kohlrabi. Research has shown that these vegetables contain natural chemicals which block the formation of tumors in a variety of organs, including the breasts, liver, lungs, stomach, colon, and rectum. The fact is numerous scientific studies document how cruciferous plants contain substances which can even stop the spread of cancer once it is established.

Cabbage exerts a highly protective action against diseases of the stomach, including stomach cancer. Along with the other cruciferous vegetables, cabbage protects against the occurrence of breast cancer.

It is amazing that the cruciferous vegetables are so powerful in preventing and combating cancer. God was indeed generous in providing them for our use. We do not yet know all the reasons they are so effective. They contain their own unique group of chemicals, known as indoles and sulfones, which are potent cancer fighters. Cruciferous vegetables also contain a wide variety of flavonoids; there are dozens of different flavonoids in vegetables such as broccoli, kale, watercress, Brussels sprouts, arugula, and kale. In addition, cruciferous plants are rich in antioxidants such as vitamin C, selenium, vitamin E, flavonoids, and beta carotene. Regardless of the reason the research is indisputable. Add cruciferous vegetables to the diet freely and in large quantities—a piece of advice for peace of mind.

A Little Chlorophyll With Your Vegetables, Anyone?

Chlorophyll is found in all types of vegetation. It serves as the blood of the plant. Just as animal blood is red (hemoglobin is the plant's molecular equivalent to chlorophyll), the blood of plants is green. Chlorophyll exerts powerful anti-cancer protection. It helps prevent the accumulation of potential cancer-causing compounds by inactivating them and transporting them out of the system. In addition, it is a rich source of naturally occurring magnesium, needed by all cells in the body for their proper health. Chlorophyll-rich vegetables include parsley, watercress, alfalfa, spinach, broccoli, kale, collards, and other dark greens. Seaweed, chlorella, and spirulina, that is the edible algaes, are also top sources. Chlorophyll is a valuable anti-cancer compound. Include chlorophyll-rich foods and supplements in the diet on a regular basis in order to combat or prevent cancer.

Strike Gold With Yellow and Orange Vegetables

Vegetables and tubers with a deep yellow or orange color are among the richest sources of beta carotene in the world. These include pumpkin, squash, carrots, and sweet potato. Their bright yellow and orange colors are due to the high concentration of carotene pigments.

Pumpkin soup is one of the best ways to achieve the beta carotene value. Squash and sweet potatoes may also be pureed for making cream soups. You can also enrich any of your favorite soups in beta carotene by adding diced pumpkin, squash, or carrots. Sweet potatoes, if you can handle the high starch content, are an excellent snack or dinner addition. Use them as a side dish instead of baked potatoes.

Special Vegetables for Special People

You are a very special person. Your body has a right to be cared for. Cancer is an invasion of your inner privacy. It can be an invasion of your rights. A good example of this is cancer in a teenager resulting from exposure to the estrogenic drug, DES, while in the womb. DES and many other cancer-causing chemicals have been used extensively in the food chain. Another example is the development of cancer from exposure to toxic chemicals such as asbestos, chlorinated hydrocarbons, mercury, etc., in the workplace. Sadly, this happens to millions of individuals every year. Thousands of other chemicals are being used in our foods even though they haven't been shown to be safe. On the contrary, many of them have been proven to be harmful. Eating copious amounts of vegetables listed in the following special category can be instrumental in preventing chemical-induced cancer:

broccoli	Brussels sprouts
cabbage	carrots
cauliflower	cucumber
garlic	kale
kohlrabi	mustard greens
onions	parsley
pumpkin	red peppers
squash	turnip greens
watercress	zucchini

The Anti-Cancer Powers of Aromatics: Spices to the Rescue

Columbus traversed the globe, reaching the New World for one reason: to gather spices. Yet, modern society has failed to comprehend the enormous value of these substances for the human body. During the Middle Ages and even prior, such as in ancient Rome, spices were essentially worth their weight in gold, not just because they tasted good but because they were used as medicines. Now modern research has discovered the reasons. Aromatic spices are among the most powerful medicinal plants known, far more powerful than many of the herbs currently in vogue. Many individuals think of echinacea and goldenseal as powerful immune boosters, but few people realize that wild oregano is up to 50 times more powerful and that even the most powerful types of echinacea are rather impotent in comparison. Research in Poland proved that of some 40 herbs only wild oregano dramatically stimulated immunity.

Pycnogenol and vitamin E are regarded as powerful antioxidants. Yet, did you know that they cannot compare to the antioxidant and preservative powers of two simple spices: rosemary and sage. Perhaps it is time to re-evaluate our understanding of just what is a powerful herb. Could it be that the spice kitchen is where the strongest immune-boosting and disease fighting capacities exist? The latest research certainly points in that direction. According to research published in 1998 by Cornell University spices are among the most protective substances against disease known. The following is a list of the most powerful disease and cancer-fighting spices and their benefits:

Medicinal Spice	Beneficial Function
Cinnamon	Kills germs; stimulates white blood cells
Cloves	Potent germicide and excellent antioxidant
Allspice	Listed by Cornell University as one of the top four germ-killing spices; strong antioxidant
Sage	Extremely effective preservative and antioxidant; possesses anti-cancer properties
Rosemary	Anti-cancer, especially against breast cancer in test tube and animal research. Top quality antioxidant
Cumin	Dramatically stimulates anti-cancer enzymes, notably glutathione; anti-parasitic and anti-fungal
Oregano	Kills cancer cells outright in test tubes; the most powerful spicy germ killer; valuable antioxidant; also, rich in anti-cancer flavonoids; Note: the anti-cancer effects were proven in the test tube using only wild oil of oregano P73. Do not use Spanish thyme or Thymus capitus.

Garlic: Nature's Anti-Cancer Substance

A perusal of cancer-preventive foods and herbs would be incomplete without a discussion about garlic. This herb has been used extensively as a remedy for a wide range of ailments for untold centuries. Current research indicates that garlic boosts immunity, kills germs, improves circulation, lowers cholesterol, and combats cancer. Garlic contains a number of compounds which improve immune function. These compounds are known as sulfated amino acids, and there are dozens of them in garlic. It is also an excellent source of selenium, which is the top anti-cancer mineral. Here is a list of some of garlic's immune-enhancing properties, as discovered by researchers recently:

1. Inhibits the growth of tumor cells in test tubes

2. Prevents chemically induced stomach and colon cancer

3. Prevents skin cancer induced by the chemical dimethyl benzanthracene

4. Causes the destruction of bladder tumors in animals (by injecting garlic extract directly into the tumor)

5. Increases the activity of white blood cells, improving their ability to destroy tumor cells

6. Helps increase the production of antibodies by B-lymphocytes

7. Increases the activity of white blood cells in the human body known as *killer cells*, whose function is to destroy cancer cells

8. Improves the function of the skin's immune system

9. Increases body stores of the antioxidants glutathione and selenium

10. Destroys harmful microorganisms which depress the immune system

Incredibly, garlic offers an enormous amount of benefits—perhaps more than any other plant—and research is beginning to tell us why it is so valuable. Garlic is one of the richest dietary sources of selenium, a mineral critical in maintaining immune defenses. Selenium is the most powerful anti-cancer mineral known. Garlic is also rich in glutathione and other sulfur-containing compounds. These compounds benefit the immune system in a variety of ways. In addition, garlic is directly toxic to cancerous cells as well as to certain microbes such as fungi, yeasts, and viruses.

Garlic provides benefits whether it is eaten raw or cooked or if it is taken in a supplemental form. However, it is not a good idea to eat excessive quantities of raw garlic. A clove or two a day or every other day is usually sufficient. Larger amounts can be consumed if the garlic is cooked or if it is taken in the form of an extract. While garlic may not be a total cure for cancer, it is one of the most important foods to consume for preventing it. When possible, purchase fresh or organically grown garlic instead of garlic powder or paste. Commercial garlic is irradiated, a process which destroys some of its useful properties, so always opt for organically grown garlic if available.

Summary

One out of every three households has or will be stricken by cancer. Those who have experienced the physical and mental trauma that it causes understand the following facts:

1. that cancer, once it develops, is difficult to treat and cure

2. that cancer often leads to a slow, painful death

3. that often, much mental and emotional trauma strikes both the cancer victim and his/her loved ones

4. that at this time, there are no known cures in modern medicine for cancer

These facts make it obvious that there is only one simple solution — prevent cancer from developing. This can be readily accomplished. It is being accomplished in numerous civilizations besides ours, where people eat wholesome foods rich in protective and immune-enhancing nutrients. Although Americans have the added burden of living in a toxic, polluted environment, they also have the luxury of being able to consume a plethora of protective nutrients by taking nutritional supplements and by having a wide variety of nutritious foods available.

CHAPTER NINE
What About Food Allergies?

Wholesome foods are good for you, right? Indeed, they are, as long as you are not allergic to them. While processed foods are the ones most likely to cause allergic intolerance, even totally natural foods may be the culprits. Throughout this book you have been told that eating right means consuming certain natural, unprocessed foods. However, this fails to account for the fact many individuals are allergic to several perfectly wholesome foods, which otherwise should be a part of a healthy diet. In fact, the right diet cannot be designed without knowing precisely what are an individual's food allergies, since each person's set of allergies are unique. In other words, even totally natural foods could make you ill if you are allergic to them.

Your Unique Set of Food Allergies

No one knows exactly why each individual has his/her own distinct set of allergies. Sometimes the reasons can be determined. A common cause is the excessive consumption of a specific food for a prolonged period of time. Eventually, the individual develops an allergy to that food. Other allergies may develop early in life and can persist to a degree into adulthood. Some food allergies can even be inherited. Prolonged drug therapy may damage an individual's immune system, increasing the vulnerability to food allergies. However, no one knows for sure why one person is allergic, say to wheat, while another is allergic to oats or beans.

Regardless of the cause, numerous common symptoms are likely due to food allergies. Even in the absence of noticeable symptoms, it is likely that you are allergic to several foods, especially if you are chronically ill. In addition, many diseases can be aggravated by continual exposure to such foods.

The Great Mimicker

Food allergies are probably the most prevalent cause of symptoms which mimic other diseases. A partial list of the symptoms they cause includes:

abdominal pain
anxiety
arrhythmia
back pain
bedwetting
bloating
burning eyes
burping
canker sores
chest pain (non-cardiac)
chills
chronic cough
colitis
confusion
cracked eyelids
cracked skin
crying spells
diarrhea
dizziness
earaches
ear discharge
eczema
eye discharge
fainting spells
fatigue
fever blisters
flatulence (gas)
flu-like symptoms
fluid retention
food cravings
gagging
headaches
hives

hoarseness
hunger pains
hyperactivity
indigestion
itchy ears
itchy mouth
itchy skin
irritability
joint aches
memory loss
mood swings
muscle aches
muscle twitching
neck pain
palpitations
ringing in ears
runny nose
salt cravings
shortness of breath
sleepiness
sneezing spells
sore throat
stomach pain
sweats
swollen ankles (or feet)
swollen eyelids
swollen fingers
urinary frequency
urinary urgency
violent behavior
weight gain
vaginal discharge

If you have five or more of these symptoms, it is possible that you have food allergies. If you have 10 or more, food allergies are likely the cause of some of your symptoms. People who have 20 or more of these symptoms usually have multiple food allergies, and certain illnesses can result if these allergenic foods are not eliminated.

Allergies *Can* Predispose to Disease

Did you know that certain diseases can be caused or aggravated by the foods you eat? Intolerance to eggs, for example, could lead to a gallbladder attack. Sensitivity to pork or pork products can cause arthritis. Cheese or milk allergy may provoke sinus attacks or migraines. Citrus fruit, especially oranges, may irritate the bladder and predispose to bladder infections. Intolerance to refined sugars, such as cane sugar or molasses, can provoke joint pain, lower back pain, or arthritis. On a more serious level wheat allergy predisposes individuals to colon and/or breast cancer as well as lymphoma. Allergy to aspirin or foods containing natural aspirin can cause or worsen asthma. Mold allergy often results in lung irritation, which could lead to bronchitis or even pneumonia. Here is a partial list of diseases or conditions having a food allergy component:

- Alzheimer's disease
- Arthritis
- Asthma
- Breast cancer
- Bronchitis
- Colon cancer
- Diabetes
- Diverticulitis
- Eczema
- Hardening of the arteries
- Heart disease
- High blood pressure
- Hypoglycemia
- Lupus
- Obesity
- Osteoarthritis
- Pancreatitis
- Parkinson's disease
- Peptic ulcer
- Psoriasis
- Psychosis
- Rectal cancer
- Rheumatoid arthritis
- Schizophrenia
- Stomach cancer
- Ulcerative colitis

A Time When Butter Is Not Better

Here is an important concept: butter is better than margarine because butter is natural and margarine is synthetic. While this is true, there is a quirk. Butter is not better if you are allergic to it. In this case, neither butter nor margarine can be recommended. Instead, whip a mixture of extra virgin olive oil, Austrian cold-pressed pumpkinseed oil, and flaxseed oil as a replacement spread. Or, make a blend of olive oil and coconut fat as a spread and for cooking. Or, make a blend of butter and Austrian pumpkinseed oil (i.e., Pumpkinol) as a spread or for cooking, if you are not allergic to butter.

Food Allergy Testing

The Food Intolerance Test performed by Nutritional Testing Laboratories is an excellent test for determining food allergies. This test has an accuracy of 78%, far greater than scratch (30%) or Rast (5-10%) testing. It is easy to perform, requiring only a single tube of blood. Over 200 foods and food additives are tested. It is true that no allergy test is 100% accurate. Yet, the value of this test is so great that I rarely begin dietary recommendations without it. You can imagine why. Think how awful a patient would feel and how embarrassed I would be if I recommended eating whole wheat bread in the event of a severe wheat allergy. Do not expect such monumental results from ELISA or RAST testing, which are less accurate and thorough than the food intolerance method.

Once your food intolerances have been determined, take the following course of action:

1. Avoid all foods you are allergenic to for at least 90 days.

2. Stay off of all foods to which you are known to have had severe allergic reactions during your childhood. These may not show up in the test, since it is likely that you have diligently avoided eating them.

3. Re-introduce the allergenic foods one at a time and keep track of the symptoms they produce. If you are symptom free, you may add the food into the diet. A word of caution: moderation should be used in regard to your food allergies. Overconsumption of any food can result in food intolerance.

4. Certain foods to which you are severely allergic may need to be avoided forever. This is particularly true if you have significant health problems.

Why *You* Should Have a Food Allergy Test

The above gives further credence to my belief that in the case of the chronically ill individual, it is difficult to design a proper diet without knowing what the food allergies are.

I have a wheat allergy. Whenever I eat it, I tire easily. If I have a large enough dose, I fall asleep at my desk. One of my patients knows when I have eaten a piece of bread with lunch. I have an observable loss in my ability to concentrate so much so that she would say, "You've eaten wheat today." Wheat is really the only food I crave. However, I never made the connection until I had a Food Intolerance Test performed on myself. The only other reliable way to find out would have been to stay away from wheat for a month or two, and then re-introduce it. Most of us are not that disciplined.

You too would benefit immensely if you discovered exactly what your allergies are. You have only one chance to live life to its fullest. You deserve the finest health care. Medicine today is geared to give you the best. Don't skimp when it comes to your health.

Fortunately, your doctor, providing he/she is open-minded and willing to help, can order this test. You do not have to see me to have it done. All he/she needs to do is order a special tube from the lab and draw one tube of blood. It is advised that you fast overnight. The blood can then be shipped from any state in the U.S. directly to the lab where the test is performed. Within days you will receive the results. Once you know your allergies, you can better apply the principles of this book to eat right, stay healthy, and remain young. For ordering information and prices you or your doctor can contact:

Biotrition (Nutritional Testing Laboratories)
1701 Golf Rd., Tower 2 – Suite 606
Rolling Meadows, IL 60008
Phone: (847) 640-1377

Discovering your food allergies is an integral component toward the effort to achieve better health. Give yourself that special treat – it will be well worth it.

CHAPTER 10
What Your Allergies Mean

This chapter describes the importance of discovering precisely what are each individual's food intolerances. The information is of the greatest value once it is determined exactly what foods you are allergic to. However, even if you don't get your allergies tested this information is invaluable for helping to construct an optimal diet.

There are several categories of potentially allergenic foods and food additives. These categories may be divided as follows:

- Protein-rich foods
- Sugars
- Fruits
- Vegetables
- Grains
- Nuts and seeds
- Spices
- Natural chemicals
- Synthetic chemicals
- Fats and oils

Protein-Rich Foods

Allergists know that of all food components, protein is the most likely one to cause allergic reactions. This is because protein becomes an easy target for immune reactions. In other words, the white blood cells of our bodies readily attack it. White blood cells have a biological means to recognize protein quickly. Furthermore, these cells are geared to attack and digest any potentially offensive protein.

The body may recognize naturally occurring proteins as poisons, which results in an immune response against those proteins. The protein-immune reaction leads to a wide range of symptoms, including rash, digestive disturbances, joint pain, muscular pain, urinary irritation, and even back pain. Examples of protein allergy include intolerance to seafood, fish, pork, beef, milk, chicken, cheese, wheat gluten, rice protein, and soybeans.

Food allergy tests should include testing for all of the common high protein foods, including meats, fish, shellfish, poultry, eggs, beans, grains, and milk. If the individual is allergic to numerous high protein foods, this may signal a deficiency of substances required for the digestion of protein, notably the digestive enzymes and stomach acid. The digestive enzymes are needed to completely digest the proteins. Incompletely digested proteins are much more likely to cause allergic reactions than thoroughly digested food/protein. This is because poorly digested proteins may be recognized by the immune system as foreign, and, thus, it will attack them. Allergy to proteins may also warn of vitamin B_6 and zinc deficiency, since these nutrients are required for optimal activity of the digestive enzymes. Multiple protein allergy also indicates a lack of stomach acid. All protein digestion begins in the stomach, a process which is dependent upon adequate amounts of stomach acid.

Incompletely digested proteins can be absorbed intact, causing an immediate allergic response. In this instance, immune cells in the blood attack the circulating food proteins as if they are foreign invaders. Allergy to foods rich in protein can result in rather severe reactions, including asthma attacks, joint pain, hives, swollen throat, and even allergic shock. Individuals who react this violently may be sensitive to the actual protein particles or to some other ingredient such as the iodine in shrimp.

Sugars

Sugar, that is refined sugar, is the bugaboo of modern humanity. Refined sugar depletes nutrients and disrupts the hormonal system. It also suppresses immune function. Eventually, as a result of continuous consumption of refined sugar, the immune system begins to recognize it as a toxin. In other words, it becomes sensitized to the sugar. As a result, allergic intolerance to various sugars may develop.

Allergic intolerance to sugars is manifested by reactions to cane and beet sugar, molasses, maple syrup, malt syrup, sorghum, and even honey. Most reactions to honey are to the heated and refined varieties.

It is important to realize that reactions to sugars may be subtle; in other words, usually there are no obvious symptoms. Common sugar-induced symptoms include fatigue, apathy, depression, irritability, joint pain, panic attacks, anxiety, hyperactivity, heartburn, headaches, and constipation. No one regards these as being allergic reactions, yet they are.

The existence of multiple sugar allergies is a warning of poor adrenal gland function. The adrenal glands are a primary organ for processing sugars and starches as a source of fuel. They also regulate blood sugar levels. In other words, they are intricately involved in sugar metabolism. The frequent consumption of highly refined sugars, such as cane sugar and corn syrup, places enormous stress upon the adrenal glands.

When an intolerance develops, the immune system reacts to sugar as if it were a poison. Sugar depresses immune function. It disrupts hormonal balance. It depletes nutrients. Ultimately, it becomes a physiological poison. It not only poisons the body, but it also irreparably harms the brain, causing a wide range of mental symptoms, including depression, agitation, mood swings, and even violent tendencies.

Sugar sensitivity/allergy is exceedingly common, occurring in perhaps as many as one in three Americans. It is seen in a variety of conditions, including yeast infection, hypoglycemia, diabetes, PMS, obesity, hyperactivity, high blood pressure, heart disease, arthritis, fibromyalgia, attention deficit disorder, and psychological disorders to name a few. With the exception of food dyes, it is the most common allergic intolerance occurring in children. Children who crave sugar are often allergic to it. The same is true of adults.

Case history:
Mental confusion, depression, and memory loss eliminated

Mr. F., a 36-year-old male, was in severe distress when he came to see me. He was losing his memory, fighting depression, and had feelings of mental confusion and agitation. Immediately, I noticed he was unusually nervous and agitated. When I shook hands with him, his hands were cold and clammy, this being a sign of severe adrenal distress. Upon discussing his condition with him, I discovered that his diet as a child was high in refined sugar, which he craved. He ate significant amounts of sugar on a daily basis, and his consumption easily equaled the average American amount of about 150 pounds per year.

A Food Intolerance Test was performed, which revealed that Mr. F. had severe sugar allergies, indicating a high reactivity to white sugar, molasses, and malt syrup. He was placed on a diet very low in sugar and was even restricted in the amount of natural sugar (fruit, bread, etc.) he could consume. Improvement was rapid, with the depression and confusion ceasing within two weeks. The improvement in memory took a bit longer, but it was restored to normal within four months. Today, Mr. F. is a happy man, and due an improved sense of well-being he is pursuing the jobs and goals which he had always desired, proving that mental illnesses *are not always in your head.*

Fortunately, Mr. F. discovered this preventive and curative approach before the psychiatrists got to him. However, the majority of individuals never get the chance to try nutritional cures for their mental symptoms. Millions of individuals suffering with chronic depression, mood imbalances, psychosis, mania, and anxiety could be cured by a nutritional approach *without the use of mind-altering drugs*. The nutritionally oriented practitioner must take the attitude of finding out *why* these mental symptoms exist and not just automatically assume they are psychiatric in nature.

Case history:
Alzheimer's-like disease with nearly total memory loss dramatically improved

Joe, a pleasant 65-year-old retired painter, had one major problem – his memory was nonexistent. In fact, he was an hour and a half late for his first appointment, as he could not remember where he put the directions his wife had given him *even though he had her written directions with him while he was coming over in the car*. Despite the seemingly incurable diagnosis of Alzheimer's disease, it was evident after examining him that diet played a major role in his illness. Thus, he was tested for food allergies. Routine blood chemistries were also performed. It was determined that he was extremely allergic to sugar. Furthermore, his blood sugar was abnormally high. Upon further history elicited from his wife it was found that his sugar levels had been elevated for years but that no one had treated him for it. All the while, refined sugar continued to be a major part of his diet.

Although all of this is astonishing, what was even more compelling was his dramatic improvement. After three weeks on the treatment program of avoidance of allergenic foods, low carbohydrate diet, and nutritional supplements, he was able to *drive to the clinic unassisted and without directions*. He continues to experience lapses of memory whenever he cheats on his diet or goes without his supplements. The stricter he is in avoiding sugar and his other allergenic foods, the better is his memory.

As discussed in both of these case histories proper treatment for the mental patient involves a combination of dietary guidance plus the elimination of any allergies. In addition, nutritional supplements assist in resolving the symptoms and may aid in the cure of the disease. The following is a rather comprehensive list of natural substances, vitamins, and minerals which have proven helpful in mental disorders:

Amino Acids

gamma aminobutyric acid (GABA)
glutamic acid
taurine
tryptophan

glutamine
phenylalanine
tyrosine
5-HTP

Vitamins

B_{12}
folic acid
niacinamide
niacin
pantothenic acid
riboflavin
biotin

thiamine
pyridoxine (B_6)
para-amino benzoic
acid
vitamin C
vitamin E

Minerals

calcium
chromium
magnesium
molybdenum
potassium
zinc

chloride
iodine
manganese
natural lithium
sodium

Herbs

St. John's wort (wild, high-mountain type is superior)
gingko biloba
wild sage

wild rosemary
valerian root

Other Substances

crude liver extract
fish oils (EPA/ DHA)
lecithin
choline

essential fatty acids
flaxseed oil
inositol

How Nutrients Affect Brain Chemistry

There are several mechanisms by which nutrients improve brain function. The most important of these are listed below:

1. **By increasing the production within the brain of natural chemicals known as *neurotransmitters***

    Just as the name suggests these substances help the neurons, that is the brain cells, transmit messages throughout the brain. Neurotransmitters also are responsible for sending messages through the spinal cord, which then transmits them to the internal organs. Thus, a deficiency of nutrients within the brain can affect tissues or organs anywhere in the body. Vitamin B_6 is an excellent example. Even if a mild deficiency exists—you may remember from Chapter Two that nearly seven of ten Americans are deficient—a decrease in neurotransmitter synthesis will occur. Without adequate levels of neurotransmitters, the entire nervous system can become disabled. This presents a two-fold problem for allergy patients. They may develop mental symptoms, plus their defenses for fighting allergic reactions are weakened. The nerves control the function of every organ, tissue, and cell in the body. Even the immune system is controlled by them. Thus, for long-term treatment of allergies it is advised that any nutritional deficiencies affecting the brain be identified and corrected. In these cases, diagnostic testing for nutritional deficiency may be necessary. Written tests are another valuable resource for evaluating "mental" deficiencies. (See Dr. Cass Ingram's *Self-Test Nutrition Guide.*)

2. **By improving circulation within the brain**

    Without proper blood flow, the brain cannot get the nutrients it needs. Yes, vitamins and minerals are important to the brain, but even more critical are fuel and oxygen. For fuel, the brain relies on glucose, and oxygen is needed to help burn it into energy. The brain uses 20% of the oxygen produced in the body. Even a mild reduction in blood flow leads to an oxygen deficit, which then causes symptoms such as memory loss, mental fatigue, confusion, and/or irritability.

    Certain natural substances, such as herbs, vitamins, minerals, and flavonoids, increase blood flow to the brain. Blood flow enhancers include gingko biloba, rosemary, riboflavin, niacin, pyridoxine, magnesium, resveratrol (found in dried grape products), and fish oils. Certainly, the function of the nervous system will improve dramatically if the nutrients which enhance blood flow are consumed on a regular basis.

3. **By reducing or eliminating the transmission of abnormal nerve signals within the brain**

In some individuals the neurons generate all kinds of garbled, disordered messages. These messages actually accumulate and impede the brain's ability to send the internal organs appropriate signals. Certain nutrients and/or herbal extracts effectively block the production of the aberrant messages, giving the brain cells time to normalize. If the brain suffers from toxic insults, such as may occur from exposure to noxious chemicals or poor diet, the function of the nerves is further disrupted. Herbs which help block disruptive brain signals include St. John's wort, rosemary, neroli orange extract, cumin, and sage. These herbs are edible and are entirely safe for human consumption. Both rosemary and sage are fat soluble antioxidants, meaning they are highly specific for blocking toxicity of the fatty organs such as the brain and liver. A rosemary/sage herbal called *Hercules Strength* is available. For combating mental disorders, take two capsules three times daily. For neroli orange there is a high quality natural extract known as *Essence of Orange Blossoms*. Made from the essential oil-rich bitter orange blossom petals from neroli orange trees, this is admired as a delicate beverage in the Mediterranean. In fact, people living in the Mediterranean call the hot beverage made with it "white coffee." It receives this name because it is famous for giving a natural mental boost without caffeine. To balance mood add one tablespoon to juice or hot water (as a tea) twice daily after meals.

Fruits

Almost everyone is aware that citrus fruit commonly causes allergic reactions. This is true for the majority of citrus fruit, although allergies to grapefruit and tangerines are somewhat rare. Perhaps most common are allergic reactions to lemons and limes. This may be caused by a reaction to the potent essential oils contained in the rind of these fruits. In addition, the chemicals used on them, such as pesticides, fungicides, such as those made from cyanide, and dyes, are toxic to the immune system. These chemicals are concentrated mainly in the rind.

Fruits rich in salicylates are another category of potentially allergenic fruits. Salicylates are powerful chemicals in the same family as aspirin. They are found in relatively large amounts in several fruits, including apples, apricots, grapes, oranges, blackberries, raspberries, boysenberries, gooseberries, cherries, strawberries, tomatoes, peaches, plums, prunes, nectarines, and currants. Almonds also contain a high amount, and 15 almonds have as much aspirin-like pain killing power as is found in a single aspirin. Asthmatics are often reactive to salycilate-containing foods.

Some fruits rarely cause allergy. A partial list includes:

- apricots
- cantaloupe
- guava
- mango
- pears

- avocado
- figs
- kiwi fruit
- papaya
- watermelon

Case history:
Childhood asthma cured in a 9-year-old boy

Johnny suffered from asthma attacks about once per week. His mother had tried everything from drugs to dietary changes. When I first saw him he was taking several asthma medications.

A Food Intolerance Test showed that Johnny was highly allergic to salicylates. These chemicals, whether in drugs or in foods, have been shown by scientific research to provoke asthma attacks. Thus, Johnny's mother was instructed to carefully remove all salicylate-containing foods and medicines from his diet. This resulted in a gradual but complete cure of his asthma. In addition, he was told to eliminate refined sugar, flour, and processed vegetable oils, and his diet was supplemented with B complex vitamins and essential fatty acids. Processed vegetable oils, especially brominated oils found in soft drinks, are a major cause of asthma attacks.

Vegetables

Vegetables are certainly as natural as a food can be. Yet, ironically, it is possible to develop an allergy to certain vegetables. Vegetables most likely to cause allergic intolerance include corn, peas, string beans, carrots, and celery.

Normally, vegetables are regarded to be totally digestible and non-fattening. Yet, certain individuals may develop bloating, fluid retention, and/or weight gain from eating vegetables. Do you happen to be eating mostly vegetables and/or salads and you still are not losing weight? An allergy to lettuce or any number of salad vegetables could be the culprit.

Lettuce allergy causes weight gain

Mrs. T. had a history of a persistent weight problem despite dieting. Even on a minimal calorie diet she gained weight. Food intolerance testing determined that, among other things, she was allergic to lettuce and endive, which she ate daily while dieting. After removing these allergic offenders, she rapidly lost 15 pounds.

That Child May Be Snubbing His Nose for a Reason

There may be good reason a child refuses to eat certain vegetables such as peas or asparagus. Instinctively, he/she may be aware that the food doesn't agree with his/her system. Forcing the child to eat allergy causing foods only exacerbates the problem. Unfortunately, allergy testing in children is often inconclusive. This is because the immune system of young children is immature. Thus, the immune system fails to respond in a measurable degree. Food allergies can be more accurately determined in children ages 10 and above. By this time the immune system has matured sufficiently so that the allergic foods can be measured.

Vegetable allergies can be related to conditions under which the vegetables are grown. Celery that is exposed to excess amounts of ultraviolet light may contain toxins known as *furocumarins*, which can cause a relatively severe allergic reaction. Alfalfa sprouts contain a potent chemical which can be toxic to the immune system. Corn, especially if stored in elevators, often becomes contaminated with toxins secreted by molds, including aflatoxin. The immune system often reacts violently to contaminated corn or its by-products such as corn syrup, corn starch, corn oil, dextrin, or corn flour. Genetically engineered corn contains chemicals previously unknown to the human body. Thus, allergic reactions to genetically engineered corn may be far more violent than those to non-GE corn.

Pesticide and herbicide contamination of fresh vegetables is rampant. Unfortunately, the majority of fresh vegetables contain residues of these toxic chemicals. The residues are primarily on the skin, so they can be somewhat removed by washing. Even so, enough pesticide or herbicide molecules can get into the internal parts of the plant to cause an allergic reaction. The best way to solve this is to buy only organically grown vegetables. However, this is not always feasible, and most supermarkets do not carry organic produce. Currently, several major supermarket chains have begun carrying a limited supply of organically grown fruits and vegetables. Also, surfactants may be available in supermarkets. These are biodegradable soap-like compounds, which help remove pesticide residues from vegetables. Ask for them in your supermarket or health store.

Despite the problems of contamination, fresh vegetables are still an excellent food. Overall, they contain far less contaminants than do processed or canned ones, plus the majority of the contaminants can be removed by careful washing or peeling. Yet, by far the ideal choice is organic vegetables, which should always be purchased in preference to the commercial vegetables. Because of the plethora of health benefits they provide and their added nutritional density, it is wise to include as many fresh, chemical-free vegetables in the diet as possible.

Grains

Grain intolerance may well be the most common allergy. Individuals with grain allergies usually react to the protein portion of grains. In the case of wheat this protein is known as *gluten*. Gluten intolerance can induce a variety of disturbances, including intestinal inflammation, malabsorption of vitamins and minerals, blood sugar imbalances, back/muscular pain, and mental disorders. Even certain diseases, such as intestinal cancer, fibromyalgia, colitis, malabsorptive syndrome, and lupus, may be caused by wheat allergy. Gluten-containing grains include wheat, rye, buckwheat, barley, and oats. Headaches are commonly caused by grain allergies, as is illustrated in the following case history.

Case history:
Twenty years of migraines cured

Mrs. Z. was plagued with severe migraine headaches, which occurred as often as every day. She had a history of headaches for over 20 years. As she was a receptionist in a doctor's office, the headaches often interfered with her work. Due to the pain, her quality of life was reduced significantly. She had been all over the country seeking help, including the Mayo Clinic and several centers specializing in the treatment of headaches.

Food intolerance testing proved that she was highly allergic to wheat and rye. By removing these foods from her diet and providing the appropriate nutritional support, her headaches were brought under control. Today, Mrs. Z. is headache-free. If she errs on her diet and eats anything containing wheat or rye, such as a pancake or a piece of toast, her headaches return.

Four trips to famous medical clinics across the country, including the Mayo Clinic, provided Mrs. Z. with little or no help. Yet, it is amazing that results this striking can be achieved simply by removing a few allergenic foods from the diet.

Wheat Allergy Could Mean a Wild Kid

Those who have children deemed to be "hyperactive," take note. It is likely that the child has allergies, and wheat is one of the top offenders. Wheat affects the brain by two mechanisms. First, it may cause a drop in blood sugar. This is especially true of refined wheat products such as pasta, bread, buns, and cookies. Wheat products which are heavily refined contain little or no fiber. Without fiber the starch from the wheat is rapidly turned into sugar. This causes excess amounts of insulin to be released, leading to a drop in the blood sugar level. When the blood sugar drops, mental symptoms are likely to occur. Glucose is the brain's only fuel, and its function is greatly affected when blood glucose levels fall precipitously. Secondly, once entering the bloodstream, wheat proteins can be carried to the brain, where they attach to brain cells at sites called *receptors*. Various types of receptors exist on the cell membranes of brain cells, but most important are those which receive insulin. Incredibly, these are the receptors to which the wheat proteins attach. Insulin is needed to commandeer glucose into brain cells, and without it, the brain cannot be properly fueled. When the insulin is blocked by the wheat proteins, disturbance of mental function occurs. This may be manifested by poor concentration, learning impairment, irritability, mood swings, and/or behavioral disorders. Wheat is trouble if you are allergic to it.

Wheat Is Everywhere

It is nearly impossible to buy packaged, canned, or frozen food from the supermarket without finding within it some wheat or wheat derivative. It is reasonable to state that at least 60% of all processed foods contain either wheat, wheat flour, breading, malt, or other unspecified wheat derivatives. Flour is often added by food manufacturers as a thickening agent, although this information is not always listed on the label.

Don't panic if you suspect you are allergic to wheat. There are a wide variety of other foods left such as fruits, vegetables, meats, nuts, and milk products. The panic of avoiding wheat or disparaging about a limited diet without wheat is often due to a simple fact: wheat addiction. In other words, some individuals are so addicted to it that avoiding it is like going through withdrawal. Yet, it is always important to remember to concentrate on what you *can* have, not what you cannot have. This will make life much easier.

Nuts and Seeds

Intolerance to peanuts is the most common nut or seed allergy. Actually, peanuts are not nuts, belonging instead to the legume family. Sensitivity to peanuts often begins in early childhood. Individuals can also be sensitive to walnuts, pecans, cashews, pistachios, sunflower seeds, filberts, and sesame seeds. Nuts, especially walnuts and peanuts, contain fatty acids which, if rancid, can be toxic to white blood cells. This toxicity can then lead to an allergic response. However, individuals may also react to the protein in nuts. Symptoms of nut/seed allergy include headaches, backaches, sore throat, sinus problems, rash, agitation, depression, fatigue, bloating, heartburn, fluid retention, and spastic colon.

Spices

Spice sensitivity seems to be on the rise. This may be explained by the fact that the majority of commercial spices are irradiated. Radiation alters the internal chemistry of food, making sensitivity more likely. Certain spices may also contain contaminants such as fungicides and herbicides. In particular, mint causes allergic intolerance, as does black pepper. If you are sensitive to several spices, this may be a sign of a weakened immune system. Some spices contain chemicals, such as alkaloids (found in black pepper) or certain rancid oils, which react negatively with the immune system.

Spice allergy would perhaps be less common if the spices were not irradiated. Residues of radioactive chemicals are found within all commercial spices, and these substances are likely to provoke significant immunological reactions.

Natural Chemicals

Other chemicals naturally occurring in foods can evoke allergic reactions. It is interesting to note that there are a greater number of natural chemicals in existence than synthetic ones. A single food may contain hundreds—perhaps thousands—of naturally occurring chemicals. Only a few of these natural chemicals are powerful enough to cause allergies. However, many allergic reactions go unnoticed, and a form of tolerance to the causative substance develops. This is true with coffee and cocoa. Both of these beans contain hundreds of chemicals, caffeine being the most well known of these. In addition, cocoa contains a substance known as *theobromine*, which can be harmful to the digestive tract, brain, adrenal glands, and immune system. Because of the powerful chemicals it contains, allergic intolerance to cocoa bean is incredibly common, affecting as many as one in four individuals. Coffee itself can be toxic, especially if it is consumed in excess.

Case history:
Coffee causes irritable bowel syndrome

Mrs. G. was a 10- to 20-cup-a-day coffee drinker. She had a history of irritable bowel syndrome. This condition often resulted in mucous and blood in her stool along with severe abdominal pain. After she quit consuming coffee, the irritable bowel attacks subsided. Some years later she happened to get a job in my office. On occasion her colon problems flared up. She was not sure what caused these flareups, but she did admit to having an occasional cup of coffee. The Food Intolerance Test showed she was extremely sensitive to several natural chemicals, including salycilates and coffee. Upon eliminating her occasional cup of coffee, the flareups disappeared.

Synthetic Chemicals

Today, hundreds of thousands of synthetic chemicals are manufactured by various chemical companies. Over 6,000 different chemicals are legally added to our foods. It seems that food manufacturers and processors have an open fist policy. They dump as many chemicals into the foods as they like. There is now a trend due to consumer demand to provide additive-free foods. Yet for many, the damage has already been done. A vast number of individuals have developed allergic intolerance to the chemicals in the food. This is readily explained. The immune system recognizes the chemical as being foreign and, therefore, attacks it. A biochemical reaction then occurs between the toxic chemical and the immune system. The result is symptoms ranging from flu-like sensations to headaches. Eventually, exposure to the chemical will automatically result in an allergic response. Some of the more common chemicals that can be tested include saccharin, aspartame, MSG, sulfites, pesticides, and herbicides.

Fats and Oils

Food allergy or intolerance can occur to animal and/or vegetable fats. Butter allergy is common. This is due in part to the chemicals put in butter, especially *Butter Yellow,* a hydrocarbon made from coal tar. Allergies to olive, safflower, corn, sunflower, and cottonseed oil can also develop. Most margarine is made from corn, soy, and/or cottonseed oil. If you are allergic to either of these, this would be another good reason to avoid margarine. Allergies to these foods are highly common. As a rule, if you are allergic to a food, you also must avoid the oils that are made from that food. For example, an olive allergy means that olive oil must be avoided.

Case history:
Butter causes stuffy sinuses

A 33-year-old male was plagued with chronic nasal drainage. His nose became easily congested, and he often developed sneezing spells. At times his nose would run so profusely that he was forced to leave his place of work due to the embarrassment. He was also highly susceptible to colds and flu.

Testing showed that he had the maximum reaction to butter. Whenever he ate large amounts of it he noticed an increase in nasal discharge. Apparently, natural chemicals in the butter caused a depression of his immune system, since both his allergy symptoms and immune function improved dramatically when he avoided it. Removal of butter alone led to a 90% improvement in his symptoms.

The Role of the Adrenal Glands

People who have numerous allergies (to me, numerous means 30 or more of a possible 205) have weakened adrenal glands. The adrenal glands are the most important organ for fighting allergies. They produce hormones, such as cortisone and DHEA, which help prevent allergic reactions and/or decrease their intensity. The adrenals can be strengthened with the appropriate types of nutrients. Stress reduction and removal of the offending foods are also important. Eating excessive quantities of sugar and starch weakens the adrenal glands. This is why the reduced carbohydrate diet described in this book is so beneficial.

Proper function of the adrenal glands is dependent upon excellent nutrition. The glands are dependent upon a regular supply of certain nutrients, and the most important of these are as follows:

- vitamin A (helps in the synthesis of adrenal cells)
- vitamin C (prevents the breakdown of adrenal hormones and aids in hormone synthesis)
- pantothenic acid (invaluable in preventing damage to the adrenal glands; it is required for the synthesis of adrenal hormones)
- vitamin B_6
- thiamine
- sodium (needed to help the adrenals maintain fluid and electrolyte balance)
- magnesium
- manganese
- potassium
- selenium (prevents the adrenals from being damaged or infected)
- vitamin E
- bioflavonoids (helps prevent the adrenal cells from degenerating)

Many allergic patients actually have a deficiency in sodium. Often, such individuals crave salt. The reason is that the weakened adrenal glands can no longer produce enough of the hormone which causes the kidneys to retain salt. This hormone is known as *aldosterone*. Thus, without sufficient aldosterone, salt is readily lost into the urine. In such patients food should be cooked with salt and a heavy hand should be used with the salt shaker. In addition, salty snacks are advisable.

Royal jelly is perhaps the greatest nutritional means to strengthen weakened adrenal glands. This is because it is naturally rich in steroids and contains the most complete balance of natural steroids of any substance. Interestingly, royal jelly contains some 50 different natural steriods, the same quantity found in the normal adrenal gland. Royal jelly is more potent if combined with pantothenic acid. This is because pantothenic acid is a critical nutrient for the normal functioning of the adrenal glands. This vitamin is absolutely required for the glands' production of natural cortisone, aldosterone, DHEA, and other steroids.

It is important to realize that not all royal jelly is the same. The majority of products available are relatively low in active ingredients, which is measured by a steroid known as 10-hydroxydecanoic acid. *Royal Kick* is a high potency royal jelly, containing a 10-hydroxydecanoic acid content of nearly 6.5%. Commercially available products are usually lower than 3.5%. Furthermore, Royal Kick is fortified with pantothenic acid, which greatly boosts its energizing powers. If you suffer from adrenal weakness, take Royal Kick, two or three capsules twice daily.

Allergies and Intestinal Malabsorption

Food allergies cause a reaction which leads to inflammation in the intestinal wall. Excess quantities of mucous are formed by cells lining the intestine to blunt the damage. This inflammation, along with the excess mucous, promotes a malabsorption of vitamins, minerals, and other nutrients. Wheat allergy is often associated with zinc malabsorption. Multiple grain allergies, known medically as *gluten intolerance,* causes a malabsorption of virtually all the vitamins and minerals. Gluten intolerance provokes the destruction of the intestinal walls, leading to wholesale nutrient malabsorption. Allergy to milk or milk products can cause severe malabsorption of minerals and many vitamins. Bean or legume allergy may cause widespread destruction of the intestinal membranes similar to that seen in gluten intolerance.

I'll bet you are wondering what your allergy profile is. When you find out what your allergies are, this chapter will serve as your guide.

CHAPTER 11
Alcoholism:
The Number Three Killer?

Alcoholism is one the world's greatest epidemics. Despite all efforts to treat this disease, the incidence continues to climb dramatically. An interesting statistic is that over 30,000 new alcoholics develop each year in New York state alone. In the U.S. today there are some 25 million to 30 million alcoholics. That is nearly one out of every 10 people. What's more, there are millions of others who should be regarded as "borderline" alcoholics, and these individuals could readily become full-fledged alcoholics at any moment. Thus, it should not be a surprise that approximately 60 billion dollars are spent each year because of the physical, medical, mental, and social repercussions of this rampant disease.

Alcoholism is the number three killer, because it kills in numerous ways. It is unique as a disease in that death can be caused by a variety of mechanisms. Furthermore, the disease creates the scenario where both the alcoholic and the innocent are victimized. Alcoholism causes or contributes to the death of over 300,000 people annually. Statistics show that the major factor in fatal industrial accidents is imbibing on the job. A much greater concern is that nearly one out of every two deaths from car accidents is alcohol related. Also, a high percentage of mass transportation accidents, including airline and train disasters, are related to the drinking habits of the crew.

The most predominant way alcohol kills is through its direct effects upon the human body. Alcoholics suffer fatalities from both the number one and number two killers: heart disease and cancer. In addition, prolonged alcohol consumption induces its own brand of fatal disease: cirrhosis of the liver.

163

The current approach to treating the alcoholic, which has relied primarily upon psychological and behavioral therapies, is highly ineffective. It is astonishing that alcoholism is the only major disease for which physicians refer care to the lay public. The standard approach has been drug detoxification, counseling, and group therapy. Extensive educational programs both for the alcoholic and his/her family members are also administered. During these sessions the importance of diet and nutrition is never discussed. On the contrary, the attendees follow the most atrocious dietary habits, eating all manner of sugary and starchy foods, plus they smoke incessantly. Thus, it is no surprise that the results are incredibly poor. In the very best centers less than 12% are cured. Therefore, it is important to use every means possible to resolve this disastrous problem.

The nutritional and dietary basis of this condition has been completely neglected by the medical establishment as well as the treatment centers. This is despite the fact that poor nutrition has as much to do with the development of alcoholism as does any other factor. Actually, it is often the primary factor. In other words, alcoholism is primarily a physical disease rather than a psychological one, and it should be treated directly by the medical profession, not the lay public.

Nutritional factors contributing to the cause of alcoholism were studied extensively in the 1940s. However, since then the issue has been neglected, and researchers, as well as physicians, failed to pursue this concept until recently. Now, Lieber and others are bringing forth definitive proof that poor nutrition plays a major role in the cause of alcoholism. For instance, Lieber has determined that all alcoholics suffer from massive deficiencies of B vitamins, particularly niacin and thiamine.

The lives of many alcoholics who *wish to be helped* can be saved by the principles discussed in this chapter. The current facts describing the tremendous havoc which alcohol causes in respect to the body's nutritional status will be reviewed. You will be given numerous pearls of wisdom on how to most effectively treat this dreadful disease.

What is Alcohol?

Alcohol is nearly 100% carbohydrate. It originates primarily from starches. The starches are highly refined, meaning they are low in nutrients such as vitamins and minerals. Starches are fermented by the addition of yeasts, and alcohol is formed as a by-product. At best, alcohol is a fuel devoid of essential nutrients. As thoroughly described by Lieber, alcohol is an "empty" calorie food. In other words, it is devoid of valuable nutrients.

Most alcoholic beverages are derived from grains which themselves are originally nutritious. To produce it brewers and distillers remove the germ and outer coatings (bran) of these grains, using only the starchy portion. The nutrient-rich parts fail to ferment easily, they resist rotting, and, thus, they must be discarded. This constitutes a loss of nearly all the fat soluble vitamins, which are located in the fatty germ and most of the B vitamins, which are found both in the germ and the bran. Hard liquor, being distilled, is entirely free of nutrients. The process of distilling generates only the volatile alcohol; flavorings and colorings are added later. The minerals, vitamins, and trace elements from raw materials such as corn mash, rye, or barley, are left behind in the residues. These are discarded or used as a nutritious feed for cattle. Even worse are beverages such as brandy, rum, and liqueurs, which are made from distilled alcohol *plus added sugar.* Refined sugar itself is 99.9% nutrient free. Often, when individuals mix drinks, they actually add sugar to what is already nothing but pure nutrient-free carbohydrate.

Thus, it is accurate to say that alcoholic beverages are essentially protein, fat, vitamin, and mineral free. Contrary to popular belief, beer is little better. Most beer is made from the starchy part of barley. It is much lower in B vitamins than many are led to believe. Beer, with its diuretic effect, purges from the body more vitamins and minerals than it provides. What little nutrition it does possess comes from the yeast it contains, which is added during the fermentation process.

Wine also contains a minimal amount of nutrients. Red wine is more nutritious than white wine, because the skin remains on the grapes during fermentation. However, usually only the juices from the fruits are used. Thus, the majority of the original nutrients are left behind in the skins and pulp. Even so, some wines are high in iron, especially red wines. As discussed in Chapters Seven and Eight this extra iron may cause more harm than good, especially in men.

Addictive Actions

The highly refined nature of alcohol accounts for much of its addictive power. This also accounts for its drug-like action on human chemistry and behavior. It should be noted that the same is true of narcotic drugs, which are also of plant origin. They too are highly refined in order to make them more potent. It is a general rule that the more refined a narcotic is, the more powerful its addictive nature. Crack is an example, since it is even more refined than cocaine. The same is true of alcohol. In all sense of the word alcohol cannot be defined as a food. Rather, it is a drug, and it acts like a drug within the body. Thus, the various organs of the body, rather than being nourished by alcohol, are "affected" by it. Alcohol can be defined as a food-derived chemical with addictive and drug-like action.

How Alcoholism Develops

Most alcoholics develop their disease gradually. Some individuals, particularly teenagers, become alcoholics literally overnight. Binging on alcohol creates such a massive disruption in nutritional status that the teenagers seemingly become addicted immediately. In most cases a pattern develops wherein there is a profound craving for alcoholic beverages as well as for sugars and starches. These cravings indicate the existence of an imbalance in body chemistry. This imbalance makes the individual highly vulnerable to developing the addiction.

Are You Genetically Susceptible?

It is now generally believed that those who have a significant family history of alcoholism are more vulnerable to the development of the disease. The alcoholic gene, as it is often described, appears to involve a craving for alcohol and other refined carbohydrates such as sugar and grains. The more deficient in nutrients individuals with this gene become, the more likely it is that they will crave alcohol as a stimulant. They may seek alcohol for the temporary high that it gives. These susceptible individuals are usually also genetically inclined towards hypoglycemia or low blood sugar. Thus, they may crave alcoholic beverages to fill the need for refined carbohydrates, alternating with perhaps sweets or starches. However, eventually most alcoholics prefer the booze over sweets.

Social Drinking—The Beginnings of Alcoholism?

Many alcoholics fall prey to the typical social drinking norms. Advertising by the alcohol industry would have us believe that consuming its beverages is synonymous with having a "good time," and, in the case of fancy wines or hard liquors, being "sophisticated." Individuals, especially teenagers, feel pressured by peers to begin drinking. Today, even grade school children, that is children less than 12 years old, are succumbing to these pressures. The fact is alcoholism is rife within the public school systems. This may account for the rising incidence of violence within these schools.

Much alcoholism has its origin in colleges, where there is intense peer pressure to party and indulge through the use of addictive substances. Often, combined with a diet high in sugar and starch (the typical college diet has 50-70% of its calories as carbohydrates), the stage is set for long-term addiction.

Once an individual becomes an alcoholic, he/she begins to gradually replace food calories with alcoholic ones. As the disease progresses, the alcoholic shows a greater aversion to food, particularly wholesome food.

Alcohol eventually displaces food. In extreme cases it can account for up to 80% of an alcoholic's caloric intake.

How Alcohol Affects the Body

Alcohol is a simple molecule. Once it enters the stomach and intestines it is absorbed rapidly. The presence of food in the stomach slows its absorption. Within one to two hours nearly all of the ingested alcohol gets into the system. Once in the blood, most alcohol is taken up by the liver, which attempts to break it down. The remainder is excreted unchanged by the lungs (in the breath), the kidneys (in the urine), and through the pores of the skin.

Liver damage can occur even from as few as two or three drinks per week. This condition is known as fatty liver. You may be wondering how this could occur. The liver is the only organ containing large quantities of the enzyme (known medically as *alcohol dehydrogenase*) which can metabolize alcohol. Thus, it bears the brunt of the damage.

Niacin Deficiency and the Alcoholic Body

In the liver alcohol is decomposed for purposes of becoming a fuel, since the body can find no other useful function for it. These reactions lead to the formation of a potent chemical known as *acetaldehyde*. This chemical is a powerful poison, which must be removed from the body rapidly to avoid inevitable tissue damage. The liver attempts to detoxify acetaldehyde through a reaction which requires niacin (vitamin B_3). If there is a deficiency of niacin, potentially toxic levels of this chemical accumulate. The result is damage to the liver cells. Once damaged, these cells cannot metabolize alcohol or other sugars adequately, meaning the alcohol and sugars cannot be transformed into useful fuel. As a result, the liver cells are forced to synthesize these carbohydrates into fats, and, ultimately, the liver cells become infiltrated with fat. The fat forces all of the life-giving cellular components out, and the liver cell looks under a microscope like a miniature water balloon. This is called *balloon degeneration* of hepatocytes (i.e. liver cells). Eventually, the fat damages these cells to such a degree that they become scarred and damaged irreversibly. This is cirrhosis of the liver.

You may recall from Chapter Two that most Americans are deficient in niacin. The alcoholic is even more likely to have a major niacin deficiency. Some of the primary signs of niacin deficiency include weight loss, fatigue, irritability, diarrhea, skin rash, loss of memory, senility, and extreme cravings for carbohydrates and/or alcohol.

Direct Toxic Effects

Alcohol itself is directly toxic to cells and cell membranes. The cell membrane's fatty acid coating is disrupted by the alcohol molecules. This is because alcohol is a solvent, and solvents corrode human fatty acids. When the fatty acids within the cells are repeatedly damaged by solvents, such as alcohol, the risk for developing organic diseases, particularly cancer and heart disease, rises dramatically. Alcohol also causes direct damage to the stomach and intestinal wall as well as to the brain and spinal cord. It is important to note that a single alcoholic beverage may destroy as many as one million brain cells. Imagine the damage that is done as a result of hundreds or thousands of drinks. The pancreas is also readily damaged by alcohol, and it is no surprise that alcoholics are highly likely to develop hypoglycemia, diabetes, pancreatitis, or even pancreatic cancer.

Hypoglycemia—The Alcoholic's Curse

Hypoglycemia is a major problem in maintaining alcohol addiction. Put simply, this is a condition wherein the brain cannot get enough sugar to function normally. When blood sugar levels drop, the alcoholic becomes nervous and/or agitated and seeks to correct this by having a drink. Blood sugar imbalances can lead to violence, mood swings, and erratic behavior. Normally, blood sugar levels are lowest in the morning which, for the alcoholic, can be a horrible time. This is also a difficult time for close family members, who have to deal with the alcoholic's mood swings, depression, and potential violence. Alcoholics also experience blood sugar drops during periods of psychological or emotional stress and are then more vulnerable to having drinking binges and fits of violence. Imagine hurting or even killing a person because of a preventable or curable physical condition like a hypoglycemic attack. With alcoholics, low blood sugar is likely the primary cause of their violent tendencies. In such compromised individuals even mild exercise can lead to a significant drop in blood sugar levels. This is how delicate the blood sugar mechanism is in most alcoholics. **Therefore, the suggested treatment for alcoholics is to eliminate refined sugars or starches in any form**. In fact, they may not even be able to handle natural sources of sugar or starch, such as an orange, apple, or baked potato, without having blood sugar fits.

The Right Alcoholic Diet

We talked briefly about the wrong alcoholic diet, i.e. one high in alcohol, sugar, and starch. The right diet is rich in protein, fresh vegetables, nuts, seeds, and some fruits. The best diet is one in which grains are omitted entirely. The reason is that the majority of alcoholics are allergic to grains. This is why it is necessary for each alcoholic to have a Food Intolerance Test, since allergies to grains and other foods may play a role in the cause of the disease, as is demonstrated by the following case histories.

Case history:
Weekend beer binger kicks the habit

Mr. E., an aspiring building contractor, was heading for disaster. After a week of hard work, he celebrated the weekend by drinking a beer. The problem was that once he started drinking he couldn't stop. He would chug up to 20 beers at a sitting. By definition, this behavior qualifies him as an alcoholic.

Upon the insistence of his wife, he came to my clinic for testing. It was found that he was allergic to barley and brewer's yeast, the two major ingredients of beer. In addition, he was highly sensitive to cane sugar, molasses, and rye, all of which are used to make alcohol. By removing these allergic foods, Mr. E. has been able to control his drinking binges entirely. His home is a happier place, and he and his wife are now the proud parents of their first child.

Case history:
Chronic alcoholic in DTs successfully detoxified

When I first saw Mr. McD., he was in obvious distress. He was as pale as a ghost, and what was most obvious was that he was trembling uncontrollably. His hands and arms were shaking so badly that he was even making me nervous. Anyone who lives with a chronic alcoholic knows that this is a sign of *delirium tremens* (DTs), which means that the alcoholic is in serious trouble and that his/her life is in danger.

The normal treatment for DTs is, of course, drugs. These drugs are used to suppress the nervous agitation, tremors, and any potentially violent behavior. Yet, the drugs do nothing to treat the primary cause of the DTs: *nutritional deficiency* .

DTs are nothing more than a manifestation of end-stage damage to the nervous system resulting from severe vitamin/mineral deficiencies, alcohol induced, of course. The deficient nutrients are primarily thiamine, vitamin B_5, folic acid, niacin, vitamin B_{12}, vitamin C, magnesium, and selenium, although thiamine deficiency is the main player. This was the basis for the treatment administered to Mr. McD. He too had allergies, with positive reactions to brewer's yeast and malt.

Mr. McD.'s case was so severe that the administration of intravenous vitamin therapy was necessary. He was also given large doses of vitamins by mouth and was placed on a strict anti-alcoholic diet. With the use of drugs, Mr. McD.'s tremors were successfully eliminated, and within two weeks he was completely off alcohol. He hasn't had a drink since and this was without AA meetings or support groups. Just nutrition and positive, firm advice from his doctor were used—that was Mr. McD.'s formula for a cure.

A wide range of food allergies occur in alcoholics and, to a degree, these allergies are responsible for their addictive behavior. For this reason it is difficult to design a proper diet without knowing what the allergies are. However, the following are some general guidelines that can be helpful:

1. Avoid all grains and grain derivatives. This includes whole grains.

2. Eliminate sugars, molasses, malt, maple syrup, and other sweeteners from the diet.

3. Control the hypoglycemia by eating a high-protein breakfast and at least two between-meal snacks per day. Follow the diet and recipes contained in this book, adding snacks between meals of nuts, seeds, sliced vegetables, and meats.

4. Throw all your booze, beer, and wine away.

Rice Bran and Rice Polish

Rice bran and rice polish are the only grain-like foods allowed on this diet. In fact, rice is a seed rather than a grain. Rice bran, the husk of the bran, is extricated in the process of producing white rice. Rice polish is the substance remaining when the brown rice is refined into white rice. It was formerly used as the main treatment for beriberi as well as alcoholic tremors. Few people realize that alcoholism is in essence a form of beriberi, and rice polishings were the remedy first used to cure this disease. Rice bran and polishings can still be used to cure and can greatly help the alcoholic recover from his/her disease.

Why is rice bran so effective? Because it is one of the top natural sources of thiamine (vitamin B_1), niacin (vitamin B_3), and magnesium which are the three major nutritional deficiencies seen in the alcoholic. The recommended amount is two heaping tablespoons of rice bran three times per day added to juice or over food. In stubborn cases try taking two heaping tablespoons every four hours. Rice bran, as well as the germ and polish, is also rich in chromium, a mineral critical for maintaining proper blood sugar levels.

It is superior to use all of the rice coating components for combating this condition. All of these components are found in Nutri-Sense protein/rice bran extract drink mix. Nutri-Sense is the only mix containing rice bran, polish, and germ, plus it is fortified with lecithin and crushed flax. The latter are sources for the essential fatty acids so sorely needed by alcoholics. Because it is free of all of the typical alcoholic-sensitive grains, such as wheat, rye, corn, and malt, this is universally tolerated by alcoholics. Remember, it is the natural vitamins that heal.

Add this wonderful tasting source of natural B vitamins to milk, juice, or water. Or, add to yogurt, cottage cheese, soup, or casseroles. Make a special cereal simply by pouring whole milk and/or cream over a few tablespoons of Nutri-Sense. The point is get as much of the Nutri-Sense into the diet as possible. It may well be lifesaving to do so.

Deficiencies Galore

Alcoholics develop a wide range of nutritional deficiencies. In addition to vitamins and minerals, they become deficient in essential fatty acids and proteins. No surprise then that the structural changes in an alcoholic's liver mimic those seen in a starvation victim. The following is a partial list of the nutrients which are deficient in most alcoholics:

1. vitamin A
2. vitamin C (the number one cause of scurvy in alcoholism)
3. vitamin E
4. vitamin D
5. vitamin K
6. vitamin B_1
7. vitamin B_2
8. vitamin B_3
9. vitamin B_5
10. vitamin B_6
11. biotin
12. vitamin B_{12}
13. folic acid
14. essential fatty acids
15. amino acids and proteins
16. enzymes
17. zinc
18. cobalt
19. selenium
20. calcium
21. phosphorus
22. magnesium
23. manganese
24. potassium
25. chromium

It is easy to see that alcoholics are deficient in virtually every nutrient known. However, certain of these nutrients are particularly crucial, as described on the following pages:

Nutrients for Decreasing Alcoholic Cravings

Harrison's Textbook of Medicine states that most alcoholics are deficient in protein. This is no surprise, since they are simply not getting enough of it in their diets. In addition, alcohol interferes with the absorption of amino acids, the building blocks which make up proteins.

Dr. Roger Williams aptly described how glutamine, an amino acid found in high-protein foods such as eggs, milk, and meat, has a protective effect against the cravings for alcohol. Glutamine was first studied in rats which were given alcohol to drink. These rats eventually craved alcohol so much that they preferred it over water. The administration of glutamine eliminated these cravings, and the rats returned to drinking water. With humans, similar decreases in cravings have been seen, although doses as high as 3 to 4 grams of glutamine per day may be necessary. Another nutrient proven to decrease cravings is the fatty acid found in evening primrose oil. This natural oil is called *gamma-linoleic acid* (GLA). It has been effective in minimizing alcoholic withdrawal symptoms and helps heal alcohol-induced damage to brain tissue and nerves, restoring memory, proper thinking, and reaction time.

Certain herbs, particularly rosemary, royal jelly, and sage, also decrease alcohol craving. Royal jelly is powerful, because it strengthens weakened adrenal glands, and the latter are always disabled in alcoholics. Royal Kick premium royal jelly, which is fortified with that crucial anti-alcoholic vitamin pantothenic acid, is particularly effective. The Royal Kick is fortified with pantothenic acid, which makes it exceptionally potent. Take four to six capsules in the morning, and use it as needed during the day. While Royal Kick boosts energy, incredibly, it also calms the nerves, a function desperately needed by alcoholics. Royal Oil is a special type of crude fresh royal jelly. It is the ideal anti-addiction tonic. Royal Oil is stabilized liquid royal jelly which tastes great, plus it is easy to take. Simply take a squirt or two under the tongue as needed. It immediately halts both sugar and alcohol cravings. Sage is also incredibly powerful for combating alcohol cravings. It does so by boosting adrenal function. Take five drops of the edible Oil of Sage (North American Herb & Spice) three times daily. Ideally, add the sage oil to hot water and drink as a tea.

B Vitamins to the Rescue

B vitamins are the most crucial nutrients for detoxifying, curing, and healing the alcoholic. Niacin alone has been shown to be curative by some physicians and researchers. Most alcoholics have a severe niacin deficiency.

Normally, some niacin can be manufactured from the amino acid tryptophan. The bowel contains bacteria which synthesize niacin from this amino acid. However, prolonged alcohol consumption leads to a tryptophan deficiency and also causes the destruction of the helpful bowel bacteria. Thus, alcohol destroys niacin in numerous ways, and it interferes with its absorption. As a result, alcoholics are desperately deficient in this nutrient. This explains why alcoholics respond so well to it. Dr. Robert Smith described a 50-60% success rate using niacin alone in curing alcoholic priests. Over half of some 500 priests enjoyed freedom from alcoholism five years after the initial treatment. No doubt, niacin helps detoxify alcoholics and makes it easier for them to overcome the addiction.

Smith's work indicates that for niacin to exert prolonged benefits it must be taken daily. However, Smith used only synthetic niacin, the type found in vitamin pills. Had he utilized natural niacin, such as the type found in Nutri-Sense, it is likely that a more progressive long-term result would have occurred.

On autopsy, the brain and other organs of an alcoholic show signs of pellagra, the original disease caused by niacin deficiency. Such a critical situation demands that the alcoholic take at least a minimal daily dose of niacin for life such as 100 to 200 mg. Higher amounts might prove more helpful but not too high. Extreme doses of niacin, such as 3 grams or more on a daily basis, have been shown to cause hepatitis, so avoid taking massive amounts of this vitamin. Preferably, take large amounts of Nutri-Sense; it is safe in any amount. In addition, foods rich in niacin are highly recommended, particularly rice bran, although calve's liver, rabbit, chicken, fish, peanuts, and sunflower seeds are also excellent sources.

Niacin's beneficial effects upon the alcoholic are wide in scope. Enriching the diet with niacin-rich foods as well as taking niacin/rice bran supplements can help prevent the alcoholic from dying young.

Thiamine—The Morale Vitamin

Alcoholics are routinely deficient in thiamine. Alcohol thoroughly destroys this vitamin. In addition, the typical diet followed by the alcoholic is exceptionally low in thiamine. Alcoholics should add thiamine-rich foods to their diets on a regular basis. Nutri-Sense is a fine source of natural thiamine, because it contains all of the top three sources of natural thiamine: rice bran, rice germ, and rice polish. Other good sources include sunflower seeds, pine nuts, wheat germ, soybeans, peanuts, liver, eggs, and sesame seeds. These and other foods naturally rich in thiamine are not normal constituents of the alcoholic's diet.

Alcoholics develop a wide range of symptoms secondary to thiamine deficiency. These symptoms include depression, mood swings, hypoglycemia, anxiety, paranoia, insomnia, muscle weakness, indigestion, nerve pains, nausea, poor appetite, indigestion, and nervousness. Later, as the deficiency becomes more profound, alcoholics may develop a degenerative disease of the brain and/or spinal cord. Thiamine is needed for the proper function of both of these organs. In fact, the function of all nerves in the body is dependent upon this vitamin.

Supplements are required to normalize thiamine levels. An excellent protocol is to take three tablespoons of Nutri-Sense three times daily along with a B complex tablet. The Nutri-Sense is critical, because it provides a high density of crude thiamine in an easy to digest form. Be sure to also aggressively add thiamine-rich foods in the diet such as roasted peanuts, peanut butter, pine nuts, eggs, and liver. In addition, a pharmaceutical grade type of thiamine is available, which is far superior to the standard type. Known as fat-soluble thiamine, this special type of synthetic thiamine offers the benefit of being more readily absorbed than the type typically found in B vitamin supplements, that is thiamine hydrochloride. The latter is water-soluble and, thus, may be difficult to retain within the tissues. Fat-soluble thiamine is available from NutritionTest.com

B_{12} and Folic Acid

Vitamin B_{12} and folic acid are intimately connected nutritionally. If one of these vitamins is deficient, it disrupts the function of the other. This illustrates how destructive alcohol is, because it aggressively depletes the reservoirs of both of these vitamins from the liver, where they are normally stored. As little as a single drink of alcohol can measurably diminish these critical nutrients.

When levels of these vitamins are severely depleted, the alcoholic develops a form of anemia. With this type of anemia there are enough red cells, but the size and shape of these cells, as well as their function, is abnormal. In essence, these cells become bloated, and their nuclear material degenerates. This deadly disease is known medically as *macrocytic* or *pernicious anemia.* Symptoms of this dangerous blood abnormality are tiredness, poor digestion, abdominal bloating, graying of the hair, poor appetite, numbness of the extremities, sore tongue, diarrhea, and weight loss.

Alcohol wreaks havoc on the metabolism of B_{12} and folic acid in a variety of ways. While in the intestines, it directly interferes with the absorption of folic acid. The absorption of B_{12} and folic acid is dependent upon a healthy stomach lining. This is yet another example of alcohol's nutritional and organ toxicity. Not only does it destroy these vitamins, but it also causes severe damage to the lining of the stomach. The stomach lining produces a substance, known as intrinsic factor, that is absolutely necessary for B_{12} and folic acid absorption. Eventually, alcohol so thoroughly disrupts stomach function that $B_{12,}$ and folic acid absorption is essentially annihilated.

To restore the proper levels of folic acid alcoholics should consume large quantities of fresh green leafy vegetables. Meat, particularly liver, is also an excellent source. There are only a few good dietary sources of B_{12}. Alcoholics must consume as many B_{12}-rich foods in the diet as possible, and the top sources are fresh red meat, liver, eggs, sardines, salmon, tuna, and cheese. Furthermore, since the absorption in alcoholics is compromised, it is often necessary to take supplemental B_{12}. What's more, they need a form of the vitamin which is readily absorbed such as sublingual or intranasal B_{12}. Other food sources of B_{12} are clams, haddock, catfish, crab, and caviar. In addition, injections of B_{12} and folic acid would be invaluable and in some instances lifesaving. If you are an alcoholic, your doctor may be willing to administer them. Alcoholics should get at least two shots a week for the first month, tapering off to a shot at least once or twice per month as a maintenance.

Minerals are Important

Alcohol interferes with the absorption of several minerals. It also causes the loss of minerals in the urine. Alcoholics lose a great deal of magnesium in their urine. Magnesium deficiency predisposes alcoholics to sudden death from heart attacks or strokes. Magnesium supplements are important, but it is also important to add foods rich in magnesium to the diet. These foods include rice bran, green leafy vegetables, apricots, figs, chick peas, wheat germ, peanuts, nuts of all types, and spices. Magnesium is responsible for the hot flavor of certain spices. Magnesium-rich spices include coriander leaf, cayenne pepper, dill weed, celery seed, sage, fennel, and mustard. Many of these spices, particularly coriander and dill weed, are rich in potassium as well, another mineral sorely needed by alcoholics. Calcium is also rich in many spices. Basil, rosemary, sage, and chervil are super-rich sources. Wild oregano is a superb source of calcium. Oregamax contains crude calcium, as well as magnesium and phosporus, in a highly absorbable form. Alcoholics are prone to develop fractures. The minerals in Oregamax provide potent support for the skeleton.

For those who cannot tolerate spicy food there are nutritional supplements made from herbs/spices which are high in natural potassium. Perhaps the best are Herb-Sorb, Oregamax, and Gene's wild greens powerdrops (see Appendix B). Use lots of spices in your cooking. Recipes with spices are included in the recipe section of this book. The added magnesium and other minerals will boost overall health. You might be surprised at the results.

Zinc May Be the Missing Link

Virtually all alcoholics have profound zinc deficiencies. Zinc controls numerous functions, which, when disrupted, predisposes individuals to alcoholism. It is my contention that zinc deficiency causes certain individuals to become alcoholics. Without adequate zinc, the ability to taste or smell food is compromised. Therefore, the normal appetite for eating wholesome foods is disturbed. As a result, the individual rejects rich wholesome foods in favor of rather bland, empty calorie foods such as starches, sugary treats, and alcohol. Zinc is also needed for the digestion of protein. In this regard it is required for the activity and synthesis of numerous digestive enzymes. Zinc is a component of insulin, and it is required for its synthesis. This may explain why alcoholics, so desperately deficient in this mineral, suffer from blood sugar disorders. It is also needed for the proper metabolism of essential fatty acids as well as protein assimilation. Zinc is a required component for normal prostate cell health. A lack of zinc predisposes to the development of prostate inflammation as well as prostate cancer, another epidemic among alcoholics.

Zinc deficiency leads to the craving of foods rich in carbohydrates and low in protein such as white flour products and sweets. The deficiency may also lead to ravenous cravings for alcohol. The zinc-deficient individual often avoids healthy foods which are rich in nutrients, aroma, and taste. It has been shown that supplementing the diet with zinc gradually restores these functions to normal and decreases the abnormal cravings for alcohol and sugar.

Alcoholics lose up to eight times more zinc in their urine than do normal individuals. The ability of the body to absorb and transport zinc is diminished because of the toxic effects of alcohol upon the liver. In addition, zinc is required by the liver for the metabolism of alcohol, but alcohol cannot be quickly detoxified in the event of a deficiency. Without zinc, alcohol readily poisons liver tissue.

Because they are severely deficient in zinc, alcoholics cannot properly utilize numerous other nutrients which are zinc dependent such as fatty acids, vitamin B_6, amino acids, and vitamin A. The scope of symptoms in alcoholics related to zinc deficiency include anorexia, loss of taste/smell, hair loss, mental disturbances, depression, anxiety, agitation, sugar cravings, dry skin, fatigue, impotence, susceptibility to colds or flu, bacterial infections, and poor wound healing. Hangnails, white spots on the nails, premature graying of the hair, and stretch marks on the skin also warn of zinc deficiency. For a thorough approaching to discerning your degree of zinc or other mineral deficiency see the Web site, NutritionTest.com.

Summary

Alcohol is a poison. It is toxic to tissues and organs throughout the body. It damages the liver, brain, heart, stomach, and intestines. If used in excess, it predisposes to heart disease, sudden death, senility, and cancer. It has been directly related to the cause of cancer of the esophagus, throat, stomach, pancreas, and colon. In women it is a primary cause of breast cancer. Alcohol creates its own disease: cirrhosis of the liver. It is a physical disease and its consequences are physical. If you avoid alcohol, it may seemingly lower the opinion some of your peers or associates have of you. However, by doing so you may well save your life. Furthermore, few people are belittled more than the drunkard. He/she is derided continuously and is the butt of every conceivable joke. By halting the drinking habit you'll earn the love and respect of the people who mean the most—your family, friends, and business associates, who care about your health and happiness.

CHAPTER 12
Fats Are Not the Killer

Fatty foods are necessary for optimal health. That's right, it's safe to eat fats. The point is that many foods *naturally high* in fats are healthy to eat. Whether from vegetable and animals sources, fats are essential for the health of the cells and organs of the human body.

It is realized that this is exactly the opposite of what you have been taught or told. The media and medical profession have created widespread fat paranoia. People are afraid to even look at foods naturally rich in fats, such as eggs, cream, butter, meats, almonds, and avocados, let alone eat them. This is ludicrous. Eggs, meats, butter, and other foods naturally rich in fats are among the most wholesome foods available. They are nutrient dense, that is they are rich in vitamins, minerals, protein, and fuel fats. On this diet it is possible to eat as much naturally fat-rich foods as is desired. In fact, you need to include as many natural fats in the diet as possible. As described in Chapter Five, there is a tremendous need for dietary fats, both as a source of fuel/energy as well as the essential fatty acids.

Of course, certain fats must be avoided. These are the bad fats, that is the synthetic fats and/or refined fats. This is largely because eating the wrong kinds of fats is destructive to the cells in our bodies, because the bad fats prevent the good fats from being utilized. The bad fats are also difficult to digest. These noxious fats include margarine, partially hydrogenated oils, cottonseed oil, refined soy oil, refined corn oil, and refined sunflower oil. Canola oil is also heavily refined and is inferior as an edible oil compared to butter and extra virgin olive oil.

As described in the first chapter, the majority of North Americans

179

are severely deficient in essential fatty acids. Therefore, it is wise to eat as many foods naturally rich in these fatty acids as possible on a daily basis. Top food sources of essential fatty acids include flaxseed, wild game, almonds, filberts, walnuts, pine nuts, peanuts, sunflower seeds, rice bran, rice germ, and pure cold-pressed vegetable oils.

The safe fats are a healthy, critical component of the diet. It is safe only to eat natural fats. These may be called the *good fats*. The dangerous fats may be described as the *bad fats*.

Bad fats should be avoided at all costs. These fats have little or no nutritional value. Here is a list of fatty foods and fat sources you must avoid:

- Margarine
- Baked goods
- Lard
- Hot dogs
- Sausage
- Bratwurst
- Pork rinds
- Bologna
- Mayonnaise
- Salad dressing
- Processed cheeses (Cheez Whiz, Velveeta, American)
- Deep-fried foods
- Vegetable oils (which are not cold-pressed)
- Crisco
- Shortening
- Peanut butter with added hydrogenated fats
- Potato chips or other fried snacks
- Creamy dressings

The bad fats, such as those found in the above foods, are harmful because they interfere with the proper function of the human body. They disrupt digestion by irritating the liver and gallbladder. In fact, they are indigestible. Because they cannot be properly digested or eliminated, they can clog arteries, sticking to the inside of the arteries and leading to hardening of the arteries, high blood pressure, and heart disease. Bad fats weaken the immune system and disrupt the function of the white blood cells. They interfere with brain function, an organ dependent upon natural fatty acids. The consumption of certain of these fats, notably hydrogenated oils and salad dressing oils, is associated with an increased risk for cancer, which was thoroughly proven by Walter Willet, M.D., and colleagues at Harvard University.

Recently, the food processing industry has added another vegetable oil to the marketplace: canola oil. This is made from a plant seed known as rapeseed. While touting the oil for its high content of mono and polyunsaturated fats, they have neglected one fact: canola oil contains the highly toxic *erucic acid*. Erucic acid is *unfit for human consumption*. For this reason, canola oil is not the ideal cooking or food oil. What's more, canola oil tends to turn rancid when cooked or added in processed foods. In contrast, good fats are those found naturally occurring within certain wholesome foods. A list includes:

Almonds	Macadamia nuts
Avocado	Olives
Beef	Organ meats
Brazil nuts	Peanuts (roasted)
Butter	Peanut butter
Cheese (hard and feta cheeses)	Pecans
Cottage cheese	Pine nuts
Chicken (with skin)	Pistachios
Duck	Pumpkin seeds
Eggs	Rice germ
Filberts	Sesame seeds
Goat's milk (whole)	Sunflower seeds
Goose	Walnuts
Hazelnuts	Wheat germ
Lamb	Yogurt (from whole milk)

Because these are natural healthy fats, you can eat as much of these foods as you desire *without concern*. This is providing that you are not allergic to any of them. These foods are healthier than typical low-fat foods like pasta, bread, rice, oats, and other starchy foods because, pound for pound, they contain a greater concentration of nutrients. Plus, they are far more nutritious than the worthless snack foods that many of us eat without the least bit of concern. These nutrient-poor snacks include cookies, pastries, crackers, chips, candy, French fries, pizza, fruit drinks, and soft drinks. In addition, the fats found in the good fat foods actually protect you against heart disease, arthritis, cancer, and many other degenerative diseases, because these fat-rich foods provide a great supply of nutrients as well as fuel for the internal organs.

It's Fats that Give You Energy NOT Carbohydrates

If you desire more energy, then eat lots of the good fats. Fats are the most efficient energy source. The best example of this I have seen is the national champion college wrestling team—the Iowa Hawkeyes. I observed their dietary habits firsthand, since at that time (1976) I was a college wrestler at the University of Northern Iowa. Due to the standards in sports nutrition at that time, our team had been instructed to eat *only carbohydrates* before the match. While my team was eating pancakes covered with sugary syrup, to my amazement the Iowa Hawkeyes were eating steak and eggs. During that period the Hawkeyes were the strongest, most powerful college wrestling team ever known. In retrospect

I am certain that much of their competitive edge was due to their ignorance of the sports nutrition "party line" at the time – that pre-game meals should be high in sugar and starch and low in fat.

You too can achieve many of these same benefits—more energy and, if you are an athlete, tremendous strength and endurance—by eating foods naturally rich in fats. In fact, if more athletes took advantage of these concepts and applied them in their routines, their performance would soar dramatically.

There are many reasons fats are an excellent source of energy. They are well absorbed and easily utilized as fuel. Fats contain double the caloric energy of proteins or carbohydrates.

Mitochondria: Cellular Power Plants

Within the cells of the human body exist tiny factory-like organs known as *mitochondria*. Mitochondria are responsible for over 90% of the cellular energy production. These microscopic organs efficiently use fats as a source of energy. In fact, they prefer fat over carbohydrates as an energy source.

You can actually have more energy from eating foods rich in fats than from carbohydrate- or sugar-rich foods. Try this yourself. Tomorrow, eat a breakfast high in carbohydrates such as cereal with skim milk and orange juice. The next day eat a high fat and protein breakfast such as three eggs cooked in olive oil or butter with a hamburger patty. Compare how you feel. If you experience an energy lag between 10:00 a.m. and 2:00 p.m. on the first day and felt fine on the second, you'll understand the point. Fats sustain energy longer by providing a greater concentration of cellular energy per pound and by preventing blood sugar swings. In contrast, fluctuations in blood sugar levels are commonly caused by carbohydrate-rich foods, especially if these foods are eaten early in the morning or late evening.

The good fats and fat-rich foods previously listed are important food sources. They are of particular value for people with the following diseases:

- Cholesterol elevation
- Hardening of the arteries
- Hypoglycemia
- Triglyceride elevation
- Diabetes
- Heart disease
- Obesity

These are precisely the diseases for which fats have been prohibited. Contrary to popular belief, these diseases respond better to fat-rich foods than to carbohydrates. Fat is a natural part of a healthy diet. Without it, body dysfunction as well as disease is likely to occur. A good example of this is the recent scientific survey comparing the health aspects of high-fat milk products versus skim milk products. A team of eight researchers in Massachusetts found that low-fat milk products such as skim milk, low-fat yogurt, and low-fat cottage cheese increase the risk of cancer. Regarding cancer it seems that the milk sugar, galactose, is the culprit rather than the fat. The point is the irritating effects of galactose only occurred when the fat was removed from the milk. Obviously, the whole unaltered food, as existing naturally, is superior to the man-made or altered food.

The complex carbohydrate diet, highly touted by nutritionists across the country, is a tremendously poor choice for people who suffer from fatigue as well as heart disease, cancer, stroke, and diabetes. A high *natural* fat diet, enriched with large amounts of vegetables and low-sugar fruits is the preferred choice. The following case history illustrates how this works.

Corporate executive loses 30 pounds and drops over 90 points on his cholesterol

Mr. C. is a top executive at a major insurance company. His primary concern was that he had a persistent problem with elevated cholesterol. In addition, he had gained 30 pounds and had difficulty losing it. The extra weight looked disfiguring, since Mr. C. is a tall man with a medium bone structure, and all that fat went right to his waist. His memory was also failing, and he was plagued particularly with problems in short-term recall. There was some concern that this was having a negative impact on his work.

Previously, Mr. C. tried the standard low-fat, low-cholesterol diet, eliminating all foods containing fat such as eggs, cheese, meats, avocados, nuts, etc. While his weight did drop by 15 pounds, his cholesterol stayed the same. Previously, his diet consisted primarily of beans and pasta with fruits and vegetables eaten occasionally.

Mr. C. was placed on the high healthy-fat diet as outlined in Chapter 13. He omitted all refined sugars and starches as well as alcoholic beverages from his diet. The results were spectacular. Within three months his cholesterol dropped nearly 100 points, and he lost 30 pounds. This was without any exercise. His memory also improved, and he notes that it is better than it has been in years.

How could such a dramatic improvement in weight loss, cholesterol, and circulation (better memory) occur? In Mr. C.'s case it was because his body is able to metabolize healthy fats better than carbohydrates, whether they were healthy ones or not.

There is another factor—remember Chapter Five—how processed foods are laced with refined vegetable oils and hydrogenated fats? These fats disrupt the metabolic machinery. They interfere with thyroid function, and this is the master gland of metabolism. They distort the structure and chemistry of cells within the liver, leading in many cases to elevations in cholesterol despite their being advertised as causing its reduction. The diet outlined in this book eliminates all foods containing these fats and replaces them with large amounts of essential fats, fats which help normalize the metabolism.

It has even been shown that the essential fats help drive the bad fats right out of the cells. In Mr. C.'s case this is precisely what happened and explains the dramatic improvement in metabolism he experienced. Now Mr. C. can eat natural sugars and starches without automatically putting on weight. Even so, he was advised to stay on the fat-rich diet for the long term. He has more energy, better memory, and improved weight control.

In Chapter 13 you will be given two sample weeks of this diet. If you follow this program, 50% to 70% of your food calories will probably come from fats. However, there is no need for concern. In fact, if your diet consists mostly of processed foods, you are getting that much fat in the diet anyway. The following chart illustrates how this can happen:

Processed Foods	**% of Calories from Fat**
• Italian dressing	.96
• Cream cheese	.92
• Thousand island dressing	.90
• French dressing	.87
• Imitation sour cream	.86
• Sausage	.82
• Hot dog	.81
• Bologna	.81
• Bratwurst	.81
• Liverwurst	.78
• American cheese	.77
• Cole slaw	.73
• Chocolate-covered almonds	.70
• Potato chips, Pringles type	.69
• Cheese spread	.68
• Coffee creamer, non-dairy	.67
• Chicken nuggets	.65
• Chocolate-covered candy bar with peanuts	.64

Processed Foods   % of Calories from Fat

- Frozen egg substitute (made with hydrogenated oils) 64
- Potato chips, regular type 62
- Brownies 60
- Potato salad 59
- Chicken thigh, deep-fried 58
- Chocolate kisses 58
- Corn chips 57
- Wheat crackers 56
- Cheese puffs 56
- Beef tacos 53
- Chocolate eclair 53
- Cheese and sausage pizza 52
- Doughnut, raised type 51
- French fries, deep fried 51
- Vanilla ice cream 50
- Danish pastry 50
- Fish sandwich (with cheese, tartar sauce, and fries) 50
- Double burger (with sauce and fries) 50
- Tortilla chips 49
- Coconut custard pie 48
- Macaroni and cheese 48
- Pumpkin pie 48
- Doughnut, plain, cake type 44
- Peanut butter cookie 42
- Waffle, plain 36

Natural Foods (and Spices)   % of Calories from Fat

- Butter 100
- Olives 95
- Macadamia nuts 93
- Pecans 88
- Avocados 88
- Walnuts 88
- Coconut meat 87
- T-bone steak, broiled 82
- Pistachios 77

- Sunflower seeds 76
- Almonds 76
- Pumpkin seeds 76
- Pine nuts 75
- Poppy seeds 75
- Lamb chop 74
- Feta cheese 73
- Peanuts 71
- Hamburger patty, cooked 64
- Fresh egg 63
- Ground nutmeg 62
- Ground lamb, cooked 61
- Herring (without added oil) 59
- Celery seed 58
- Mustard seed 55
- Coriander seed 54
- Roasted chicken with skin 53
- Salmon 52
- Sardines 48
- Cottage cheese 39

Note that many natural foods which have been denigrated nutritionally, such as eggs, meats, cheese, whole milk, avocados, etc., contain no more fat than the processed foods. For example, some egg substitutes are higher in fat than fresh eggs. Natural foods are always the superior choice, regardless of their fat content. Most people are familiar with naturally healthy foods rich in sugar and/or starch. These include corn, peas, beans, whole grains, fruits, and fruit juices.

Nuts are among the most healthy of all natural fats. They contain a rich array of fatty acids which are useful for building healthy cells. Pumpkin seeds are extremely healthy and are a rich source of essential fatty acids. A special type of pumpkinseed oil is available. Called Pumpkinol, this is a special type of pumpkinseed oil made from a unique type of pumpkin seed which is exceptionally rich in essential fatty acids. Pumpkinseed oil is superior to flaxseed oil as a nutritional supplement. It is a rich source of alpha linoleic acid, but it also contains its companion oil, alpha-linolenic acid. What's more, it is super-rich in natural vitamin E, including the highly sought after gamma tocopherol. Furthermore, in contrast to flaxseed oil, Pumpkinol is a superb source of chlorophyll. This is evidenced by looking at it, because it is a rich forest-green color. For more information see the appendices.

Many people are afraid of consuming natural fats. However, from the aforementioned information it is evident that these natural fats are essential for overall health. Do not purposely avoid the intake of fatty foods. If you do, your health will suffer severely.

Now you can become familiar with how tasty, how appetizing, and how nutritious a high natural-fat diet really is. Good fats add both nutrition and taste. Plus, they help make you feel full. *Bon appetit!*

CHAPTER 13
Two Weeks of Eating Right

Eating right means eating foods you tolerate well. The problem is each individual varies in what he/she tolerates best. This sample menu does not take into account any specific food allergies the individual may have. In order for the diet to be most effective, each person's food allergies should be determined. Even so, this diet serves as an example of how eating a diet free of processed foods makes an enormous difference in how you feel. The elimination of junk/processed foods from the diet is a major improvement in nutrition. These harmful foods are so readily available, so habit-forming, and so convenient that anyone who consistently avoids them must be commended. This program will give you the tools to accomplish this rather stupendous feat.

You will notice that these menus also eliminate foods naturally rich in carbohydrates such as apples, rice, beans, potatoes, and whole wheat bread. Even though these foods are wholesome and natural, it is preferable to eliminate them for the first 90 days. This will give your pancreas, liver, intestines, and adrenal glands a chance to rest from all the years of sugar overload. After 90 days, gradually add carbohydrate-rich foods into the diet. Start with the starches, since they are less stressful to the pancreas and liver than high-sugar foods such as oranges and apples.

A diet low in sugars and starches can make an enormous impact upon how you feel. It is likely that you will notice a significant increase in energy and stamina and that you will be less tired in the morning or evening. Another benefit is that you will be less sleepy during the day. There may also be a noticeable improvement in memory and concentration, and mental fog will likely be eradicated. With these and

189

many other benefits forthcoming, it is advisable to practice these principles rigorously for at least 90 days. After this time you can introduce high-carbohydrate foods such as whole grains, potatoes, peas, beans, lentils, corn, grapes, pears, apples, oranges, and honey. However, introduce these foods gradually with your guide being whether or not eating them causes the return of any of the typical symptoms associated with food allergy or carbohydrate intolerance such as fatigue, mental dullness, mood swings, depression, irritability, weight gain, muscle or joint soreness, indigestion, colitis, bloating, skin rash, stuffy sinuses, runny nose, etc.

There is a special consequence of following this diet. You will probably lose weight. The longer you adhere to it, the more weight you will lose. If you are already thin or if you lose more weight than you need to, you may not necessarily lose extra weight. However, if you do, add carbohydrate-rich foods such as potatoes, rice, fruit, and honey back into the diet.

It is crucial to regard snacks as a serious part of the diet. They are probably the most important portion of the menu. These snacks prevent the blood sugar level from dropping. When the blood sugar level falls, cravings for sugary or starchy foods become irresistible. As a result, the individual is likely to succumb to potentially dangerous eating binges. In order to make this program work be sure to eat the snacks.

An asterisk (*) indicates that recipes can be found in the recipe section (Part II, Section 1).

One Week Menu
Day One

Breakfast
Scrambled Eggs Mediterranean Style*
one-half cantaloupe or honeydew melon
glass of V-8 or tomato juice

Mid-morning snack:
Nutri-Sense protein/B vitamin shake

Lunch
steamed vegetables with dip
salad sprinkled with tuna or salmon—add as much as you like

(olive oil and vinegar dressing)
one-half grapefruit
glass of unsweetened papaya or pomegranate juice

Mid-afternoon snack:
almonds or pecans
Drink: Strawberry-Guava Punch*

Dinner
Roast leg of lamb*
squash, baked
green beans, steamed or cooked in a small amount of water
herbal tea
Dessert: Melon Smoothie*

Day Two

Breakfast
patty of ground turkey or chicken, cooked
two raw carrots
raw sunflower seeds, handful
grapefruit juice (fresh-squeezed is preferable)

Mid-morning snack:
hard-boiled egg or handful of olives; mineral water

Lunch
Italian Mushroom-Vegetable Soup*
salad with extra virgin olive oil and vinegar
bowl of cottage cheese (or, cup of either kefir or homemade yogurt – add
    diced melon or strawberries for extra taste)
herbal tea

Mid-afternoon snack:
almonds or pistachios plus sliced vegetables, tomato juice, or
mineral water

Dinner

grilled salmon with herbs and lemon-butter (or olive oil)

Cole Slaw Salad (without added sugar)*

broccoli and/ or cauliflower, steamed

kiwi fruit

Day Three

Breakfast

feta cheese omelet with two or three eggs (with or without spinach), basted in extra virgin olive oil

one whole grapefruit, peeled

small bowl of Greek olives

glass of V-8 or tomato juice

Mid-morning snack:

handful of pumpkin seeds, plus sliced vegetables

glass of mineral or purified water

Lunch

one-half baked chicken (preferably organic) plus spices

Carrots Piquant*

salad topped with zucchini and sliced onions, vinaigrette dressing

mineral or purified water

Mid-afternoon snack:

slices of red and green peppers

handful of almonds (raw, or preferably, roasted with salt)

purified or mineral water

Dinner

lamb chops (second choice: veal chops)

salad topped with onions, Greek olives, and feta cheese (olive oil, garlic and balsamic vinegar dressing)

spinach, steamed or boiled in small amount of water—drink juice.

small sweet potato (a special treat unless you are a diabetic, dieter, or are intolerant to carbohydrates)

glass of grapefruit juice

Day Four

Breakfast

Diced zucchini in olive oil*

wedge of watermelon

Nutri-Sense protein/B vitamin shake

Mid-morning snack:

slices of feta or goats cheese topped with peanut butter

Drink: Carrot and Cream Cooler*

Lunch

homemade Beef Stew (without potatoes; use turnips instead)*

salad, topped with slices of cheese (extra virgin olive oil, vinegar, and
   herb dressing)

herbal tea or decaffeinated coffee

Mid-afternoon snack:

macadamia nuts or pumpkin seeds; herbal tea or tomato juice

Dinner

Grape Leaf Rolls without rice (a very special treat)*

Mediterranean Salad*

Hummus*

sliced raw vegetables (carrots, romaine lettuce, and celery—dip into the
   hummus)

tomato juice

Day Five

Breakfast

beefsteak, any type

one-half cantaloupe

cucumber slices, peeled

purified water

Mid-Morning Snack

Nutri-Sense shake, sliced vegetables (carrots, celery, zucchini, turnips, etc.)

Lunch

tuna salad in avocado boat

fruit garnish (melon, strawberries, grapefruit)

glass of fresh-squeezed or frozen vegetable juice (frozen juices are available at most health food stores)

Mid-afternoon snack:

cup strawberry-flavored kefir or homemade yogurt*

Dinner

Green Bean Stew*

Brussels Sprouts Carrot Celery Salad*

Diced Fruit in a Bowl (kiwi, papaya, strawberries, and melon)*

herbal tea or decaffeinated coffee (with real whipping cream if desired)

Day Six

Breakfast

sliced turkey breast

Grapefruit Medley*

glass of carrot or grapefruit juice

Mid-morning snack:

Gazpacho Drink*, handful of almonds or pecans

Lunch

fresh broiled fish or can of sardines

Lemon Cole Slaw*

steamed green vegetables (broccoli, green beans, Brussels sprouts, etc.)

kiwi fruit

Mid-afternoon snack:
boiled egg or one cup of plain yogurt,
Strawberry-Almond Coolers*

Dinner
stir-fry chicken (or shrimp) sautéed in olive oil
    (served on a bed of slivered almonds and pine nuts, lightly toasted)
carrot juice, fresh, canned or frozen
Diced Fruit in Bowl*

Day Seven

Breakfast
Diced Zucchini in Olive Oil* plus two scrambled eggs
one-half cantaloupe or wedge watermelon
slices of tomatoes, cucumbers, and bell peppers (add salt, if desired)
herbal tea

Mid-morning snack:
red pepper slices
handful of pistachios
mineral water

Lunch
Pumpkin Soup*
Sauteed Brook Trout with Onions, Walnuts, and Spices*
fresh steamed vegetables (broccoli, cauliflower, cabbage, string beans,
    etc.)

Mid-afternoon snack:
slices of feta or Swiss cheese
Greek olives
V-8 juice

Dinner

Kufta (Mediterranean Meatballs) with Sauce*

Mediterranean Yogurt and Cucumber Salad

Stuffed Cabbage Rolls (optional)*

tomato juice with lemon or lime

Week Two
Day One

Breakfast

cheese slices topped with peanut, pecan, or almond butter (use goat, cheddar, or gouda)

celery and carrot sticks

herbal tea

Mid-morning snack:

roast beef slices

Drink: Cranberry Juice Creamy Surprise*

Lunch

Poached Sweetbreads*

tossed salad (topped with Creamy Garlic-Avocado Dressing)*

purified water with twist of lemon or lime

Mid-afternoon snack:

Protein Drink*

sliced vegetables

Dinner

Squash Soup*

Whitefish in Lemon-Dill Sauce*

tomato slices topped with fresh or dried mint

Green Beans in Olive Oil (optional)*

carrot juice, canned, frozen, or fresh

Day Two

Breakfast
Nutri-Sense shake
Herbed Turkey Sausage*
grapefruit juice, preferably fresh-squeezed

Mid-morning snack:
sliced chicken breast
Drink: Strawberry-Almond Cooler*

Lunch
Salmon with Spring Vegetables and Hot Mustard*
Dilled Broccoli/Cauliflower Combo*
purified or mineral water with wedge of lime

Mid-afternoon snack:
Nut and Olive Salad*
tomato juice

Dinner
Artichoke Salad*
Simple Baked Onions*
Stuffed Lamb Loin*
Hummus*
Low-Carb Fruit Platter*

Day Three

Breakfast
Green Beans or Zucchini in Olive Oil* (add 1/4-pound ground lamb or
     beef, if desired) or two-three poached eggs
wedge watermelon
V-8 or tomato juice

Mid-morning snack:
chicken drumstick or breast
pink grapefruit juice

Lunch
chef's salad topped with tuna, mackerel, or salmon
Pumpkin Soup*

Mid-afternoon snack:
nut mix (pecans, almonds, pumpkin, and sunflower seeds)
glass of purified or mineral water

Dinner
Onion Steak*
Italian-Mushroom Vegetable Soup*
Grilled Squash Medley*
slices of papaya and melon

Day Four

Breakfast
ground beef patty
Zucchini in Olive Oil*
glass of grapefruit juice

Mid-morning snack:
handful of olives
Protein Drink*

Lunch
Spaghetti Squash Lasagna*
Sauteed Collard or Beet Greens*
purified water

Mid-afternoon snack:
slices of lamb or beef roast
celery and carrot sticks
purified water

Dinner
Caper-Almond Salad*
Roast Duck with Melon Sauce*
Red Cabbage Curry*
Sesame-Garlic Tomatoes*
Dessert: Watermelon Smoothie*

Day Five

Breakfast
Yogurt-Cucumber Salad*
nut butter on carrot and celery sticks
mineral or purified water

Mid-morning snack:
Blender Gazpacho*, cheese slices
herbal tea

Lunch
Asparagus Soup*
Watercress Salad*
Crab Cakes*

Mid-afternoon snack:
pecans or almonds
Drink: Melon Smoothie*

Dinner
Cabbage Soup*
Radish Salad*
Indian Chicken with Coriander Sauce*
mineral or purified water

Day Six

Breakfast
bowl of cottage cheese with diced melon
Protein Drink*

Mid-morning snack:
handful of pumpkin or squash seeds
grapefruit juice

Lunch
tossed salad with olive oil and vinegar
Indian Coconut Curry*
bowl of strawberries or kiwi fruit
Cranberry Juice Creamy Surprise*

Mid-afternoon snack:
slices of roast beef or lamb
carrot and celery sticks
purified or mineral water

Dinner
grilled salmon or tuna, with lemon-butter or olive oil
Lemon Cole Slaw*
Squash Stir-Fry*
Fruit 'n Nut Salad*
herbal tea

Day Seven

Breakfast
Scrambled Eggs Mediterranean Style*
whole grapefruit, peeled
glass of tomato or V-8 juice

Mid-morning snack:
Nutri-Sense drink

Lunch
Lamb-Stuffed Artichokes*
Cabbage Soup*
Bermuda Onion/ Beefsteak Tomato Delite*

Mid-afternoon snack:
cucumber and tomato slices
slices of chicken or turkey breast
glass of grapefruit juice

Dinner
Turkey/Pumpkin Stew*
Sautéed Collard Greens*
sliced kiwi and strawberries
purified water

Oh, What a Wonderful Menu!

This completes your first two weeks of tasty, healthy cuisine. The menu outlines the basic principles of the diet. Use these principles, the recipes in Section II, and your own recipes to create additional weekly menus.

Notice that you can eat fairly large quantities of food. In fact, if any of the menus are not filling enough, you can add additional salads or vegetable dishes as listed in the recipe section. Even if you are dieting, you need not starve. This is true as long as you eat *wholesome* foods and as long as you don't cheat by adding *junk* foods. If you eliminate the junk/processed foods, you can enjoy the benefit of *eating until you are full* without risking your health or gaining excess weight.

Now Keep it Going

As always, a word of caution: after a few weeks on the diet, many people reach a plateau where they feel so good and are so happy with their accomplishments that they decide to reward themselves. The reward, of course, is eating junk foods or possibly loading up on their allergenic foods. The level of health within the body will determine how often the individual can "cheat" without sliding backwards. However, for most people, cheating on the diet will soon lead to a reversal of whatever progress is made. The body is forgiving and can withstand a certain amount of abuse. However, most of the individuals reading this book have already suffered a decline in health and desire to prevent any further decline. Thus, it is crucial to remain disciplined and keep the cheating to an absolute minimum.

Is it Good to Eat Meat Every Day?

It isn't necessary to eat meat every day to be healthy. In fact, it is a good idea to occasionally go without meat. Even so, foods such as beef, lamb, chicken, and fish are included in these menus for good reason. They are important sources of nutrients and are *wholesome, unprocessed foods.* They are a far more valuable food source than the foods which commonly displace them such as doughnuts, muffins, breads, pasta, cookies, candies, crackers, chips, and soft drinks. Also, in contrast to the foods just mentioned, fresh meats do not cause damage to the body. Any drawbacks to meat are due to the addition of chemicals such as estrogens and antibiotics. A good compromise would be to buy "organic" meats. These are from cattle raised by farmers who do not use hormones or chemicals. It is interesting to note that Europeans only allow the importation of U.S. beef which is hormone-free, although our government is attempting to force them to import it. We should adhere to the same standard for our own population.

Is Fasting Important?

The majority of Americans are unaccustomed to fasting, yet, this is one of the missing links to excellent health. Certainly, no one will starve to death by missing a meal. However, the real benefits are achieved by fasting for a prolonged period, like a week or a month. Fasting is invaluable for the prevention of disease and for health improvement. There are several types of fasts. I do not recommend complete fasts, consuming only water. Such fasts can cause potentially dangerous disruptions in electrolytes, especially in the elderly. A healthier alternative is juice fasting. Watermelon fasting is another healthy option. Be sure to use sea salt occasionally on the watermelon fast, as this will balance the high amount of natural potassium in the melon and will also help boost adrenal function. However, the Islamic fast is the best type. This is accomplished by consuming no food or drink of any type for a prolonged period every day such as a 12- to 14-hour span. In this fast you must arise early and eat a modest breakfast. Then, totally fast from all foods and beverages until nightime. Have a light meal with, perhaps, fresh vegetable juices. Thus, a complete resting of the gut is accomplished, which is not achieved by fasts which allow drinking.

Rest your system from solid foods at least twice per year by fasting for at least a week or two. If you wish to fast for a month, do so, but be sure to do it in a controlled fashion. As a result, you will enjoy more vigorous, vital health.

CHAPTER 14
Conclusion

Eating right means using your common sense to make choices that are healthy. It means following the laws of nature. It means avoiding fad or restrictive diets. This book illustrates how it is possible to eat wholesome foods of all types—meat, poultry, fish, fats, vegetables, grains, and fruits—without concern. Eating right is just as easy as eating wrong. Once you become accustomed to eating right it will become difficult to revert to old eating habits. This usually happens about 90 days after strictly following the dietary guidelines outlined in this book.

"Eating wrong" means consuming substances that can harm the body. This includes all types of heavily processed foods. It includes white flour products, sugary desserts, sugar-laden drinks, processed meats, as well as alcohol and cigarettes. While these foods and substances may seemingly taste good, provide a temporary feeling of elation, and/or have visual appeal, they are entirely devoid of nutritional value. In fact, with time you will soon find that they become tasteless, and you may even come to abhor them.

Ill health could be a concern of the past, providing you follow the simple principles outlined in this book. Of course, no one is immune from natural disasters or accidental injury. This book only addresses the issue of premature deaths which are preventable—deaths from cancer, heart attacks, strokes, diabetes, neurological diseases, or any other potentially fatal degenerative disease. Such illnesses can kill rapidly. However, they may cause another form of "death"—a slow, writhing, painful existence, which eventually cripples or kills the individual.

205

Why get cancer when you can prevent it? Why have a heart attack when you can avoid it? Why develop arthritis when you can abort it? Why develop a paralyzing neurological disease when it could be prevented? It just does not make sense to allow yourself to develop these or other diseases when there is so much information available on health improvement and prevention. The point is sickness is preventable. Don't become one of the victims.

The statistics are scary. The rate at which new diseases are developing is unprecedented, whether in modern or ancient history. Alzheimer's disease is a relatively recent phenomenon, as is AIDS. Heart disease is only a century old. Many cancers commonly seen today were unheard of 40 years ago. Life-threatening "modern" diseases such as lupus, scleroderma, rheumatoid arthritis, and Crohn's disease, were essentially unknown as little as 100 years ago.

Bizarre neurological disorders such as multiple sclerosis, ALS (Lou Gehrig's disease), and muscular dystrophy, are all 20th century phenomena. Diseases of the colon are modern day creations due largely to a diet low in fiber and high in sugar. Asthma and emphysema were relatively rare until the turn of the century. Obviously, something has to change. Otherwise, it will only get worse.

The individual must ask him/herself, what can be done to avoid being one of the statistics? The primary issue is to significantly change the way you personally live. No doubt, the world is quickly becoming a toxic nightmare. There is only so much each individual can do about that. However, you can take action to clean up your personal environment. You have to make the necessary changes in lifestyle. Something has to break.

Change is not always easy. However, following some simple rules makes change much easier. Here are some rules for changing your immediate environment:

1. Avoid eating anything that could harm you. Your body has a right to remain healthy. You have a responsibility to, above all, avoid harming it. Incidentally, this is the Hippocratic oath that all physicians must swear to abide by. During the 7th century A. D. this oath was also propounded by Prophet Muhammad, who said that, in essence, the human body "has certain rights that must honored", that is each individual has an obligation to take care of his/her body. What's more, Biblical philosophy confirms this, i.e. "your body is your temple."

2. Prohibit yourself from using margarine, hydrogenated, or partially hydrogenated fats. This also includes lard and shortening.

3. Never use commercial vegetable oils. Use instead extra virgin olive oil or cold-pressed oils.

4. Reduce your intake of sugar and sweets by at least 90%. Those with a major disease should eliminate sugar entirely. If you must have sweets, use honey or other unprocessed natural sweeteners such as carob molasses, grape molasses, or crude cane sugar. Regarding the latter be sure it is raw and unfiltered. Don't fool yourself into believing that processed sugars in the health food store, such as fructose, barley malt, fruit syrup, corn malt, or corn syrup, are any better than white sugar.

5. Buy only wholesome foods for your home. Quit buying junk food. Stock your refrigerator with fresh meats, milk products, eggs, vegetables, and fruits.

6. Avoid buying food which is in a cardboard box. Exceptions include dried vegetables or fruits and whole grains. Most of these foods are highly processed and are adulterated with chemicals and additives.

7. Make every attempt to include foods grown without pesticides, herbicides, antibiotics, hormones, or other chemicals as part of your diet. These "organic" foods should make up at least 50% of your daily food intake. Another reason for needing the organic foods is that, pound for pound, they provide significantly more vitamins and minerals than commercial foods.

8. Supplement your diet with the minimal antioxidant program described on page 277-278.

9. Clean up your water with a water purifier, a most important step.

10. Take large amounts of antioxidants to counteract air pollution, toxic chemicals, and radiation in the environment. Also, take on a regular basis supplemental herbs with oxidative powers, that is the powers to help the body kill harmful germs.

I hope we can all work together to do something about the damage that is being done to the environment. However, I believe you must take care of yourself first. At least do that. Then, when we are all strong and healthy enough, we can go to battle for Mother Earth:

God made the earth beautiful; it is a bountiful resting place for humanity. He provided the human race with everything we need: water to drink, food to eat, air to breath, herbs and medicines to heal.

Human beings, in their ignorance, as well as arrogance, have upset her fine chemistry, causing damage that is impossible to repair.

You know how immense the oceans are. As hard as it is to believe, these bodies of water are now thoroughly polluted. The pollution of coastal waters is a monstrous dilemma. Those who have visited the East or West Coast may have noticed there are few if any seashells on the shores. As little as 30 years ago these shells abounded on the beaches. Due to the pollution of the ocean and the shoreline by toxic wastes, radioactive chemicals, PCBs, agricultural runoff, sewage, global warming, and many other manmade insults, the number of gentle creatures which inhabited these shells and which have been found on the beaches for centuries have dwindled dramatically. The 1990s have become the decade of the dolphin. Thousands of these precious creatures are being washed ashore, dead. A mysterious AIDS-like virus is to blame, so the newspapers reported. The real cause is immune depression from toxic chemical poisoning, leaving the dolphins vulnerable to infections by dangerous organisms—organisms which otherwise could not have gained a foothold. This for the dolphins is the consequence of their "bathing" every second of their lives in a sea of poisons. This proves that despite the immense dilutional factor of the water in the ocean, the toxic substances are effectively destroying portions of it. How can we clean up billions of gallons of salt water? It is virtually impossible. The minimum that needs to be done is to stop any further dumping of chemical and human waste. We must hope that the earth herself will restore the oceans to normal.

You can see the enormity of it all. This is why I suggest that the focus be on the individual. In this book you have been provided with several simple rules. The time bombs have been discussed, and you are aware of the ones which can be avoided. Here are some other important keys to living right.

1. Keep the digestive and elimination systems in optimal health. Poor bowel function leads to disease. Don't abuse your body by eating toxic or harmful foods. Ideally, the individual should have at least one bowel movement daily. The regular consumption of high fiber foods aids this process. Don't use harsh laxatives to force a bowel movement. If elimination is sluggish, take an enema. Ideally, determine why the constipation exists and resolve it. Try the remedies listed in Part II of this book. Also, take sufficient amounts of fiber daily if you tend towards sluggish bowels. Herbal laxatives which are gentle in action are often helpful. Carob molasses is superior to the herbal laxatives, plus it is not habit-forming. Ground flaxseed is an excellent fiber supplement, since it provides fiber and essential fatty acids, both of which improve colon function. However, if you eat right and take natural sources of fiber, the bowel function will normalize. Elimination of refined sugar intake greatly aids bowel function. Gene's powerdrops, either the wild greens or wild berry types, greatly aids intestinal/colon function and is my favorite intestinal herbal remedy. To cleanse the intestines and naturally bulk the stools take 5 to 10 drops twice daily. With a healthy diet and the proper supplements it is possible to achieve the bowel habits of

primitives: two to four soft bulky stools daily.

2. Regularly include in the diet a plethora of natural herbs, either fresh or as supplements. Opt primarily for the edible herbs like cilantro, arugula, parsley, garlic, onion, oregano, sage, cumin, cloves, cinnamon, and rosemary. These are safer and more nourishing than the "medicinal" herbs such as ginseng and goldenseal.

3. Fast at least once per year. Go on a modified fast, abstaining from food and drink for at least 12 hours during the day. Do this for several days. Or try a juice fast, drinking only fresh-squeezed juices for 5 to 7 days. I do not recommend complete fasts using only water. I know this is done in some clinics and spas. Although a few may have benefited from these fasts, most of us would become too weak to withstand them.

4. Realize that life is a choice. You can choose to eat right, or you can continue to eat the way you do now. You can smoke cigarettes, drink alcohol to an excess, eat poorly, eat too much sugar, or you can choose to stop all of these health-robbing habits. This book has provided the tools necessary to replace the bad with the good.

5. Above all, be consistent. If you are going to fast, don't just do it once. Put a date on the calendar, and do it every year. Take your nutritional supplements on a daily basis, and follow the diet religiously. Take as many preventive measures as you can so you can stay healthy, be well, and live a long and productive life.

PART II

Recipes
and
Remedies

PART II

Recipes for Eating Right

Entrees: Meats, Fish, Eggs and Poultry

Beef Stew

1 cup water
1 lb beef or veal, cut for stew (1/2 inch pieces)
1 celery stalk, diced
1/2 medium onion, chopped
2 carrots, sliced
1 /2 cup fresh green beans, chopped in 1-inch sections
3 tablespoons rice bran (optional)
1 teaspoon salt
1 teaspoon pepper
1 or 2 bay leaves

Combine ingredients in Dutch oven or quart casserole. Cover and bake in oven at 300 degrees for 2 1/2 hours. Remove bay leaf.
Makes 4 servings

Turkey/Pumpkin Stew

1 lb turkey, cooked

2 tablespoons olive oil or cold-pressed vegetable oil

1 green pepper, diced

1 red pepper, diced

1 cup pumpkin puree

4 cups chicken or turkey stock

1/2 onion, diced

3 1/2 cups fresh pumpkin, peeled and cubed

3 sage leaves, minced

parsley leaves, minced (for garnish)

pinch cayenne pepper

1 teaspoon honey (optional)

Cut turkey into cubes. In a Dutch oven sauté turkey in oil until browned. Remove and place in a bowl. Sauté peppers and onions in same oil for 5 minutes. Mix pumpkin puree with stock, honey, and cayenne; then mix into pot with peppers and onions. Bring to a boil and add cubed pumpkin. Lower heat and add sage and turkey. Simmer for 30 to 45 minutes until all vegetables are tender. Serve garnished with parsley.
Makes 8 to 10 servings

Crackerless Meat loaf

1 lb ground beef

3 tablespoons *Nutri-Sense*

1/4 cup onion, finely chopped

1/4 cup celery, finely chopped

1/4 cup sweet red pepper, finely chopped (optional)

1/2 teaspoon salt

1/8 teaspoon sage

one 6-oz. can tomato paste

Combine ingredients and mix well. The Nutri-Sense provides additional nutrients, particularly B vitamins and trace minerals, plus it is a low starch and wheat free replacement for crackers. Spoon final mix into a 9 x 5 inch loaf pan. Press lightly. Bake at 325 degrees for one hour.
Makes 4 servings

Sweet and Tender Lamb Stir Fry

Have you ever heard of combining meat with fruit? This recipe does so in a unique way. Papaya contains special enzymes, which aid in the digestion of meat. The papaya is also rich in vitamin C, which is lacking in most meat dishes. Garlic and onions assist the digestion of fat, plus they help prevent fat accumulation in the blood. This extra-light, digestible meat dish represents an innovative method of preparing meat.

5 cloves garlic, finely chopped

1/2 large red onion, thinly sliced

1/2 lb lamb meat, cut into 1-inch chunks

2 tablespoons extra virgin olive oil

1 teaspoon coriander seed, ground

1 cup papaya, chopped

In a medium non-stick skillet, combine garlic, onion, lamb, and oil. Lightly stir over medium high heat until lamb is browned. Add coriander and papaya and continue cooking just until papaya is hot.
Makes 2 to 4 servings

Salmon Cakes

Salmon is a tremendously healthy food. It is a top source of protein and essential fatty acids. It is an unusual food, because it is rich in the majority of essential nutrients. Unlike most meats, it is an excellent source of vitamins D and E. The bran or Nutri-Sense provides important B vitamins and the yogurt adds extra protein. This recipe is a tasty way to get your nutrients.

8 ounces fresh or canned salmon (if canned, drain juice)

1/4 cup green pepper, chopped

1/4 cup oat or rice bran or 3 Tbsp Nutri-Sense

1/4 cup plain yogurt (optional: add small amount of vanilla flavoring to the plain yogurt)

1/4 cup onion, chopped

1/4 teaspoon dried mustard

1/4 cup chopped celery

1 egg, beaten

salt to taste

dash of pepper

dash of ground cumin (optional)

Combine all ingredients and spoon into four greased custard cups. Bake at 325 degrees for 30 minutes. Serve with sauce.

Sauce:

1/2 cup vanilla-flavored or plain yogurt

1/2 cup cucumber, finely chopped (peel and remove seeds)

2 tablespoons chopped onion

1/2 cup sour cream

1/2 teaspoon dried dill weed or 2 teaspoons fresh dill weed

Combine ingredients in saucepan. Heat and pour over salmon cakes. *Makes 4 servings.*

Kufta (Mediterranean meatballs)

5 lbs ground round or hamburger (80% lean) or 2-1/2 lbs. ground round with 2-1/2 lbs ground lamb

1 tablespoon salt

1 teaspoon black pepper

1 tablespoon dried parsley or 2 tablespoons if fresh-chopped

1 tablespoon dried mint leaves or 2 tablespoons if fresh-chopped

3/4 cup finely chopped or shredded onions

2 eggs

In a large bowl add meat, salt, pepper, parsley, mint, and eggs. Mix all ingredients thoroughly with hands until the ingredients hold together. Make into balls with melon scooper or hand press to about one half the size of a walnut. Place in long cake pan (15 x 10) greased with a few drops of olive oil. Put the meatballs close together. Broil until brown, 3 to 4 minutes on each side. Cool and set aside.

Sauce:

2 fresh tomatoes, peeled and cubed (or 1 small can whole tomatoes, drained)

1 cup tomato sauce

1 large can V-8 or tomato juice

1 lb ground round or 80% lean hamburger

2 medium onions, coarsely chopped

1 tablespoon salt

1 teaspoon black pepper

1/2 teaspoon garlic powder or 4 cloves fresh garlic, finely grated

1/4 cup olive oil

4 cups water

In a Dutch oven sauté onions in olive oil for 2 to 3 minutes. Add hamburger and brown until the meat is no longer pink. Sprinkle meat mixture with salt, black pepper, and garlic. Cook on medium heat for about 7 minutes. Add fresh or canned tomatoes, tomato sauce, V-8, or tomato juice, and water. Bring to a boil. Turn to medium heat and cook for one half hour, stirring every 5 to 10 minutes. Add meatballs and cook an additional 5 minutes. Serve over toasted pine nuts and brown rice. *Makes 20 servings*

Grape Leaf Rolls

3 lbs. coarse ground beef (80% lean)

2 tablespoons salt

1 teaspoon black pepper

1 teaspoon garlic powder

1 cup fresh chopped parsley (or 1/2 cup dried parsley flakes)

1/4 cup fresh chopped mint (or 1 tablespoon dried mint)

2 tablespoons olive oil

1 teaspoon garam masala (a spice sold in specialty stores—
    use allspice if this is not available)

1/2 cup green onions, chopped

1 teaspoon dried basil (or 1 tablespoon fresh chopped basil)

1/2 cup pine nuts (browned in a few drops of olive oil)

1 lb jar grape leaves (sold in specialty stores and some supermarkets)

FILLING: Add together uncooked meat, salt, pepper, garlic, parsley, mint, olive oil, garam masala, green onions, basil, and pine nuts; mix all ingredients together until well blended.

HOW TO ROLL LEAVES: Drain grape leaves in a strainer. Take each leaf, stem facing you and lay it on a board. Spread 1 tablespoon of filling and roll tightly like a cigar with your fingers. Makes about 90 grape leaves. Takes approximately 1 hour to roll.

COOKING: If using a pressure cooker, cook all 90 rolls at once; otherwise, use two medium-sized pans. Put small pieces of beef rib or chuck roast bones on the bottom. Place first layer of rolled grape leaves in a row. Crisscross the remainder of the rows as you fill the pan. Once the pan is full, peel 6 whole cloves of garlic and put on top of the rolls. Sprinkle 1/4 teaspoon of salt and pour on 1 cup of lemon juice and 1/2 cup water. Cut one whole lemon in half, squeeze the juice, and put the lemon halves on top.

TO COOK IN PRESSURE COOKER: Put the tightly sealed lid on the pressure cooker and make sure the vent is open before putting the pressure knob on the lid. Turn on high heat. Let boil for 5 to 10 minutes after the pressure knob starts to squeak. Reduce heat to medium and cook for 15 minutes. Turn off stove. Let pressure cooker cool.

CAUTION IN SERVING: Do not open lid of pressure cooker when cooking or while it is still emitting steam. You can speed up the cooling process by running cold water over the cooker until steam disappears. Then it is safe to remove the lid. Serve warm as is or dip in hummus or homemade yogurt. Extras may be frozen.

Spaghetti Squash Lasagna

All lasagna lovers will relish this wheat and noodle-free recipe, especially those who are allergic to wheat. Spaghetti squash is different from other types of squash. When cooked, the flesh can be fluffed into strands which are very similar to noodles.

With this recipe you receive the culinary benefit of noodles but without all the starch. Plus, spaghetti squash, pound for pound, is much higher in valuable nutrients, such as beta carotene, potassium, calcium, magnesium, and phosphorus, than the majority of vegetables.

1 large spaghetti squash

1/2 lb ground beef (85% lean)

1/2 teaspoon dried whole basil

1 clove garlic, crushed (or 1/8 teaspoon garlic powder)

1 eight oz can whole tomatoes, drained

1 six oz can tomato paste

1 ten oz carton regular (not low fat) cottage cheese

1/4 teaspoon pepper

1/2 teaspoon salt

1/2 lb sliced mozzarella cheese

1/4 cup fresh Parmesan cheese, grated

1 egg, beaten

Preheat oven to 350 degrees. Wash squash; pierce several times with fork and place on cookie sheet. Place in oven and bake for 1 hour or until soft. Once cool, cut squash in half and remove seeds. Using a fork, lift out the spaghetti-like strands. Measure out 4 cups of strands.

In a large heavy skillet cook ground beef until browned. Be sure to crumble well. Drain off grease. Add spices, tomato paste, and tomatoes; simmer without covering for 30 minutes or more.

Mix together cottage cheese, Parmesan cheese, and egg in a bowl. Just as you would with regular lasagna, layer the three ingredients—the spaghetti squash, the cottage cheese mixture, and the ground beef mixture. Use a 12 x 8 x 2-inch baking or casserole dish. Bake at 375 degrees in a preheated oven for 25 to 30 minutes. Let stand for a few minutes and serve.

Makes 4 servings

Lamb-Stuffed Artichokes

8 large globe artichokes

juice of 1 lemon

1 medium-sized onion, finely chopped

1 lb ground lamb

1/4 cup pine nuts

1 tablespoon olive oil

2 teaspoons salt

1 tablespoon parsley, finely chopped

2 cups water

3 tablespoons butter

2 tablespoons lemon juice or 4 capsules Red Sour Grape (Resvitanol™)

pepper

Wash artichokes thoroughly. Remove tough outer leaves and trim carefully around base just enough to look neat. Open leaves carefully with fingers to expose choke, and remove this with a teaspoon. Drop prepared artichokes into a bowl of cold water with half the lemon juice added.

Sauté onion in olive oil until clear, then add pine nuts and stir over medium-low heat until lightly browned. Combine meat with onion and pine nut mixture, adding 1 teaspoon of salt and parsley. Add pepper to taste. Continue cooking until lamb is no longer pink.

Drain artichokes and fill centers with meat mixture, forcing in as much as they will take and piling the meat at top. Arrange artichokes in a large pan, add water, and sprinkle remaining lemon juice/Red Sour Grape (Resvitanol™) over them. Sprinkle with an additional teaspoon of salt.

Cover and bring to a simmer. Gently simmer for 50 to 60 minutes until artichokes are tender. Drain off liquid into measuring cup. Keep artichokes hot.

SAUCE:

Melt butter. Add to one cup of drained water mixture along with either lemon juice or Red Sour Grape (Resvitanol™). Pour over artichokes and serve.

Makes 8 servings

Beef or Lamb Liver

Liver is a top source of a wide range of nutrients which are difficult to receive in the diet. Its rich nutrient armamentarium includes pantothenic acid, pyridoxine, vitamin B_{12}, folic acid, biotin, niacin, choline, carnitine, vitamin A, potassium, and magnesium, in other words, virtually every nutrient known. Only liver from organically raised animals is fit for human consumption. If this is unavailable, calf's or lamb's liver might be a suitable option.

1 lb beef or lamb liver

1 large onion, sliced in rings

8 fresh mushrooms, sliced (or one medium can)

1/2 cup olive oil

salt

pepper

garlic powder

1/2 teaspoon curry powder (optional)

6 capsules Red Sour Grape (Resvitanol™) (optional)

Slice liver, then cut slices in halves. Sprinkle onion and mushroom slices with salt, pepper and garlic powder.

In a large frying pan add 1/4 cup olive oil, and heat on medium-high heat. Add liver and brown both sides. While cooking, sprinkle with curry powder and Red Sour Grape (Resvitanol™), if desired. The latter gives it a tart taste and moderates some of liver's strong flavor. CAUTION: avoid over-cooking the liver as most of its nutritional value will be lost. Remove liver and place on serving plate. Wipe oil out of pan and add the other 1/4 cup oil. Brown onions and mushrooms. Place mushrooms and onions on top of liver and serve immediately.

Makes 4 servings

Green Bean and Lamb Stew

2 lbs lamb roast (although lamb is preferable, you may use chuck roast)
trim visible fat and cut into cubes

4 cloves fresh garlic, diced

1 large onion, diced

8 fresh tomatoes (or 1 large can of whole tomatoes), chopped

3 lbs fresh or frozen green beans

1 small can tomato sauce, unsweetened

2 teaspoons salt

1 teaspoon pepper

1/4 cup olive oil

Wash and cut beans into pieces, being sure to remove stems. Put olive oil into 6-quart pot and heat for one minute. On medium heat add meat cubes, salt, pepper, and brown for ten minutes or until there is no visible redness. Add onions and garlic and stir constantly for 2 minutes. Add tomatoes, and if canned, reserve juice. Continue stirring for 1 to 2 minutes. Add tomato sauce and reserved tomato juice. Stir and add green beans. Note: If you are using frozen beans, cook sauce on medium heat 1/2 hour before adding beans. Water may be added, if needed. Garnish with parsley.
Makes 8 servings

Whitefish in Lemon-Dill Sauce

Whitefish of any type (whitefish, flounder, walleye, orange roughy, etc.) will fit well into this recipe. Whitefish itself is an excellent choice, since it is rich in certain fish oils known as omega-3 fatty acids. These help improve circulation and prevent degenerative disease.

2 tablespoons butter

1 tablespoon fresh lemon juice and/or three capsules Red Sour Grape

5 slices lemon with rind

1 tablespoon freshly chopped dill (or 3/4 tablespoon dried dill)

1 small onion, sliced thin

1 lb fresh or frozen whitefish fillets

Heat butter, dill, lemon juice, Red Sour Grape, salt, and onion in large skillet over medium-low heat; sauté for about three minutes. Add whitefish and lemon slices; cover and cook for 7 to 9 minutes and baste

occasionally. Pour sauce over fish and serve.
Makes 2 to 4 servings

Salmon With Spring Vegetables and Hot Mustard

Are you happy to hear that mustard is good for you, and that it belongs to a family of vegetables known to prevent cancer? Brown mustard is a nutritious addition to food selections. It is high in certain vitamins as well as essential fatty acids and protein. Coarse brown mustard is the preferred type, since it undergoes the least amount of processing. Both coarse mustard and salmon provide essential fatty acids.

1 lb Alaskan salmon

2-3 tablespoons butter

1 cup julienned carrots

1 cup finely julienned white part of leek

1 cup julienned (peeled) celery

1/2 teaspoon black pepper

1/2 cup julienned zucchini

1 cup fish stock

salt

1/3 cup all-natural brown mustard

2 capsules HerbSorb (optional)

In a large saucepan or skillet melt butter. Scatter half the carrots, leeks, celery, and zucchini in pan and turn to medium heat. Sprinkle pinch of salt and emptied contents of capsules. Place salmon fillets into the pan beside the vegetables, and add pepper and the remaining vegetables. Slowly pour in fish stock. Cover and simmer for 5 to 6 minutes only. Remove from heat. In a small saucepan add 1 tablespoon butter and melt. Add mustard and cook until hot. Serve over fish, or as a dip for fish and/or vegetables.
Makes 4 servings

Poached Haddock Portuguese Style

1 lb. haddock fillets

1 medium onion, finely chopped

1/4 cup fresh parsley, finely chopped

2 tablespoons tarragon vinegar

2 cloves garlic, crushed

1 teaspoon wild oregano (from Greek oregano bunches)

1/4 teaspoon crushed black pepper

3 tomatoes, diced

1 teaspoon olive oil

Crumble wild oregano from the bunch and set aside. Place fish in water in a heavy pan or electric skillet and cover with the remaining ingredients, including spices. Bring mixture to a boil, then cover and simmer for 10 to 12 minutes. Remove the fish carefully so it doesn't break apart and keep warm by covering with foil while the sauce is heated and boiled down. Once reduced by half, pour sauce while it is hot over the fish, and serve.

Makes 4 servings

Sauteed Brook Trout With Onions, Walnuts, and Spices

Trout and walnuts provide valuable amounts of essential fatty acids. The trout provides the fish oils, and the walnuts provide linoleic and linolenic acids. The fatty acids from these foods are highly digestible and valuable for human nutrition.

4 whole brook trout, boned

2 limes (use 1/4 cup vinegar or 8 capsules Red Sour Grape if you are citrus sensitive)

3 medium onions, peeled and cut into 8 wedges each

1 cup walnuts, coarsely chopped

1/4 cup olive oil

1/2 teaspoon ground turmeric

1/4 teaspoon ground cinnamon

1/4 teaspoon ground cumin

salt and pepper

1/4 cup cold-pressed vegetable oil (peanut, walnut, or olive oil)

Squeeze the juice of one lime and set aside. Thinly slice the other lime and set slices aside. In a medium-sized saucepan, heat olive oil over low heat. Add onions and sauté for 10 to 15 minutes until limp, but do not brown. Remove the pan from heat and stir in walnuts, turmeric, cinnamon, cumin, and 1/2 teaspoon salt. Set aside and keep warm.

Wash trout under cold water and pat dry. Lightly sprinkle the cavity and skin with salt and pepper. In a large skillet, heat vegetable oil over medium-high heat, but be careful not to burn the oil. Add trout, 2 at a time, cooking until golden brown and cooked through.

To serve, spoon onion mixture into the cavity of each trout, pour remaining sauce over the trout and garnish with lime juice and slices.
Makes 4 servings

Stuffed Lamb Loin

3 tablespoons olive oil

1/4 cup onion, finely chopped

2 garlic cloves, crushed

1 cup spinach, shredded

1/4 cup fresh parsley, finely chopped

1/4 cup fresh basil, shredded

2 tablespoons sun-dried tomatoes, finely chopped

2 tablespoons pine nuts (or sunflower seeds), chopped

2 teaspoons lemon pepper

1 teaspoon salt

1/2 cup crumbled feta cheese

1 3/4 to 2 lbs fresh lamb sirloin roast, boned

In a medium skillet, heat 2 tablespoons olive oil; sauté onion and garlic for 2 to 3 minutes. Mix in spinach, parsley, basil, sun dried tomatoes, pine nuts, and one teaspoon of lemon pepper (Red Sour Grape is preferable, if available). Cook additional 2 to 3 minutes or until spinach and parsley are wilted. Mix in feta cheese; set aside. Preheat oven to 325 degrees. Remove all visible fat from meat. Make a slice one half way through the meat lengthwise down the center. Cover with plastic wrap and with meat mallet, pound to 1-inch thick. Place filling down center of meat; roll and tie with string at 2-inch intervals.

Brush with a tablespoon olive oil and sprinkle with a teaspoon lemon pepper and salt. Place on rack and roast to desired degree of doneness. This can be tested with a thermometer. For medium-rare, roast for 1 1/2 hours (150 degrees), or for medium, roast for an additional 10 minutes (160 degrees).
Makes 6 to 8 servings

Indian Chicken With Coriander Sauce

2 onions, peeled and quartered

10 tablespoons olive oil or cold-pressed peanut or sesame oil

3 whole skinless, boneless breasts of chicken (preferably organic)

1/4 cup slivered almonds

3 tablespoons ground coriander

1 teaspoon ground cardamom

1 piece fresh ginger, about 2 inches long, peeled

2 cups plain yogurt

2/3 cup fresh coriander leaves (or 2 tablespoons dried)

1 teaspoon black pepper, preferably freshly ground

1/4 teaspoon salt

1 cup water

sliced almonds (to garnish)

Using a food processor, finely chop the onions and set aside. Use it again to finely chop the coriander leaves and ginger; set aside. Heat 2 tablespoons oil in a large deep skillet over medium heat. Add chicken breasts and cook until lightly brown (about one minute each side). Remove and set aside.

Add the remaining oil and heat; add onions and cook until limp but not brown. Stir in 1/4 cup almonds and cook for 2 additional minutes. Next, add coriander/ginger mixture; mix well. While still on medium heat, add the rest of the spices, yogurt, reserved chicken breasts, and 1 cup of water; bring to a boil over high heat. Cover and reduce to a simmer for 25 to 30 minutes or until the chicken is thoroughly cooked. Remove from heat and let stand for 30 minutes to enhance flavor.

Reheat chicken mixture over low heat while at the same time sautéing the remaining almonds in a teaspoon of oil in a small skillet until lightly browned. Serve by pouring sauce over chicken and topping with almonds.

Makes 3 servings

Broiled Chicken Pieces With Spices

1 whole chicken, cut into pieces (leave skin on)

3 tablespoons olive oil

2 cloves garlic, sliced (or 1/4 teaspoon garlic powder)

1/2 teaspoon salt

1/8 teaspoon pepper

paprika

4 capsules of HerbSorb (optional)

Empty capsules of HerbSorb and set aside. Place chicken pieces on cookie sheet. Add olive oil, garlic, salt, HerbSorb, and pepper to a small bowl and mix. Spread mixture over front and back of chicken pieces. Sprinkle paprika on back side. Lay chicken with the skin down and place into broiler. Broil on each side until brown (about 5 minutes); sprinkle paprika on front side after turning over. Place into preheated oven (350 degrees) and cook for an additional 25 to 30 minutes. Baste juices or additional oil over chicken if necessary.

Makes 4 servings

Indian Coconut Curry

Coconut milk is very filling due to its high fat content. It complements vegetable cookery and aids in digestion by improving the absorption of vegetable pigments and carotenes, which are fat soluble. Try this all-vegetable curry for a change of pace from meat-containing entrees.

2 cups fresh coconut, cut in 1/2 inch cubes (or, 1 cup canned coconut milk)

1 cup water

1 cup chopped onion

1/2 cup chopped green pepper

1/4 cup peanut oil (cold-pressed)

1 teaspoon curry powder

1/4 teaspoon salt

1/2 teaspoon cardamom seed, crushed

2 cups cauliflower

1 cup broccoli

1/4 cup fresh-squeezed lemon juice

2 cups sweet potatoes, cubed (optional)

Place coconut and water into blender, and blend at high speed until smooth. Strain through two thicknesses of cheesecloth, squeezing out liquid. (You have just made fresh coconut milk.) In a large, heavy skillet heat oil and sauté onions and green pepper until clear. Add all spices.

Next, add sweet potato, cauliflower, broccoli, and water as needed. When vegetables are tender, add coconut milk and lemon juice. Cover, let stand for 5 minutes and serve.

Additional suggestions: for extra vegetable protein, pour curry over toasted pine nuts or slivered almonds. A fitting drink would be any of the creamy coolers which are listed in the drink section.

The next four recipes are compliments of Chefs Felice Martinelli, Steven Dunn, and Robert Jones of *Amourette,* located in Palatine, Illinois.

Crab Cakes

8 oz fresh crab meat, shredded

1 whole egg

1 teaspoon brown mustard

2 tablespoons of mayonnaise (sugar-free brands made with cold-pressed oils are available in health food stores)

dash of salt

dash of white pepper

dash of Tabasco sauce

1 heaping teaspoon rice bran or Nutri-Sense

1 teaspoon clarified butter

In a large bowl combine crab meat, egg, and mustard; mix thoroughly. Add mayonnaise and mix until mixture is paste-like. Add salt and pepper, rice bran/Nutri-Sense, and Tabasco sauce.

To cook, mold crab mixture in the size of a silver dollar. Sauté in skillet with clarified butter until golden brown on both sides. Serve with a cayenne-flavored mayonnaise or mustard.

Makes 2 servings

Roast Duck With Melon Sauce

One 3-1/2 to 4 lb duckling

1/3 cup vegetable oil (cold-pressed)

1 teaspoon dried thyme

2 bay leaves

1/4 teaspoon salt

black pepper

Cut off excess fat from around duck body. Crush bay leaves and sprinkle inside duck cavity. Add thyme, salt, and sprinkle pepper inside cavity. In a large pan heat the oil and sear the duck first on the bottom, then turn over and sear the side until light brown. (This will prevent the duck from sticking to the pan while roasting.) Drain excess oil.

Heat oven to 425 degrees, and place duck in oven for 11/2 hours.

Melon Sauce

1 honeydew melon, remove seeds and retain juice
1 tablespoon shallots, chopped
2 tablespoons honey (optional)
2 tablespoons butter

Puree melon and set aside. Heat butter in saucepan and add shallots; sauté until limp. Add pureed melon and honey; simmer for 10 to 15 minutes. Strain in a fine sieve and try to get all the juice out by pressing down with a ladle. Return juice to pan; bring to a boil. Reduce heat and cook until mixture thickens.

Cut roasted duck from carcass. Spoon sauce over duck and garnish with melon balls.
Makes 4 to 6 servings

Poached Sweetbreads

1 lb. of sweetbreads (soaked in cold water overnight)

1-1/2 qt water

1/2 onion

1 small carrot, chopped

1 rib celery, chopped

1 leek end (use white only)

bay leaf

2 sprigs of fresh thyme (optional)

juice of one lemon

cracked black pepper

Add all ingredients together in pot (except sweetbreads). Bring to boil. After boiling for a few minutes, add sweetbreads. When water comes back to a slow simmer, remove from heat and let cool. Leave ingredients in stock and refrigerate.

SAUCE:

1/2 to 3/4 cup balsamic vinegar

3-1/2 cups olive oil or cold-pressed vegetable oil (sesame, peanut, or olive oil)

1/4 cup shallots, minced

1 egg yolk (use 1 tablespoon of pureed avocado if you have an egg yolk allergy)

2 tablespoons of brown (all-natural) mustard

1/4 cup fresh parsley, chopped

1 teaspoon salt

1/4 teaspoon white pepper

2 tablespoons water (if needed)

Add all ingredients in mixing bowl except oil and vinegar. Now add small amount of vinegar and mix well. Pour in oil a little at a time, while whisking the mixture rapidly to form an emulsion. When it starts to thicken, add a little more vinegar to thin. Now add the oil and water alternately until all is in bowl. If mixture is too thick or strong, add water to thin or lighten flavor.

TO SERVE: Heat sweetbreads in stock until hot and remove. Strain vegetables and place over sweetbreads. Pour on sauce as desired, and serve.
Makes 4 servings

Onion Steak

1/4 cup freshly squeezed onion juice

1/2 large onion, sliced

1/4 teaspoon garlic powder (or 2 cloves garlic, crushed)

1/2 teaspoon salt

2 steaks of your choice

Marinate steaks in mixture of onion juice, salt, and garlic powder for at least 2 hours. When ready, cook in oven, or fry in skillet on medium heat. Caution: do not overcook the meat as this will reduce its digestibility and destroy most of its nutritional value. Fry onion slices in skillet on medium-low heat for 3 to 4 minutes, or until clear. Top steaks with onions and serve. Add sautéed mushrooms, if desired.
Makes 2 servings

Grilled Marinated Steak With Red Pepper Sauce

3 tablespoons olive oil

1 medium red onion, diced

3 cloves garlic, chopped

1 small fresh hot chili pepper, seeded and finely chopped

4-6 large, sweet red bell peppers

3 to 4 lbs New York strip or sirloin steak

1/8 teaspoon salt

1/8 teaspoon black pepper

Marinade:

1-1/2 cup olive oil

1/2 cup balsamic vinegar

3 sprigs fresh thyme

Red Pepper Sauce: Over an open flame sear red bell peppers, turning with tongs to scorch skin on all sides (or broil, turning frequently). Place roasted peppers in paper bag, folding the top closed. Preheat oven to 200 degrees and cook peppers in oven for 50 minutes. Remove peppers and cool with running water. At the same time, remove any burned outer skin. Core the peppers, discarding core and seeds. Chop coarsely. In a food processor or blender puree peppers until smooth.

In a non-stick skillet heat olive oil and sauté onion, garlic, and chili pepper until chili pepper is softened (4 to 5 minutes): set aside. In a small bowl combine bell pepper puree with onion-garlic mixture. Season with salt and pepper. Let sauce stand 2 hours at room temperature to blend flavors.

In a large pan combine marinade ingredients. Add steaks and turn to coat. Let stand at room temperature for at least 2 hours (or for 8 to 12 hours in refrigerator). Cook steaks over grill until medium or medium rare. Serve topped with heated pepper sauce.
Makes 10 to 12 servings

Roast Leg of Lamb

1 leg of lamb (or lamb shoulder)

1/4 cup olive oil

4 cloves garlic, crushed

1/2 lemon

1/2 orange

1/4 teaspoon salt

1/4 teaspoon pepper

1 teaspoon crumbled wild oregano (from Greek oregano bunches)

2 onions, peeled and quartered

2 stalks celery, cut into 3 inch pieces

1 cup water

Place leg of lamb in a roaster. Alongside, add quartered onion and celery. In a bowl add juice of lemon and orange along with crushed garlic, olive oil, salt, oregano, and pepper. Mix for a few seconds. Pour mixture over meat, making sure to cover meat evenly. Add water to the bottom of roaster.

In a preheated oven (350 degrees), heat uncovered for about 2 hours. Check roast frequently during this period, basting it in its juices. At the 2 hour interval, baste roast with 2 tablespoons of olive oil. Cover and cook for an additional 3 hours (a total of 5 hours) and serve.
Makes 6 servings

Meatballs on Squash Almandine

1 large winter (spaghetti) squash

1/2 cup slivered almonds

1/2 cup onion, chopped

6 cloves of garlic, crushed

1 lb hamburger meat (85% lean) or 1/2 lb ground beef and 1/2 lb ground lamb.

1/2 cup fresh parsley, finely chopped

1/4 cup green or red peppers, chopped

1/4 cup celery, chopped

1/4 cup capers (optional)

1/2 cup Nutri-Sense or 1/2 cup cooked wild rice

1/2 teaspoon salt (or preferably 1 teaspoon sea salt)

1 tablespoon olive oil

2-16 oz cans tomato sauce (unsweetened)

Combine onions, garlic, parsley, peppers, celery, capers, salt, Nutri-Sense (or wild rice), and hamburger together in large mixing bowl. Gently mix with hands until well combined. Make into large meatballs. Brown meatballs in heavy skillet in olive oil. Drain oil and fat from meatballs and discard. Add tomato sauce, and simmer until meatballs are light pink in the center.

Bake squash until outside is soft. Scoop out interior and set aside. In a small skillet, heat a small amount of olive oil and add slivered almonds. Cook until browned and combine with squash. Serve meatballs and sauce over spaghetti squash and almonds. You may also serve over wild rice if spaghetti squash is not available.

Makes 6 to 8 servings

Scrambled Eggs Mediterranean Style

For the egg lover this is a wonderful treat. If at all possible, try to use farm-fresh eggs.

3 eggs, extra-large

1/4 cup olive oil

1/4 cup green onions, diced (use entire onion)

1 clove garlic, crushed

Crack eggs into bowl. Using a non-stick skillet, heat olive oil on medium-low heat, and add onions and garlic. Sauté until lightly browned. Add eggs and scramble. Avoid cooking eggs excessively, as this will reduce their nutritional value. Serve hot.

Makes 2 servings

Soups

Asparagus Soup

1 lb asparagus stalks

3 cloves garlic, minced

4 green onions, diced

1 tablespoon extra virgin olive oil

2 cups water or chicken stock

1 tablespoon fresh parsley, chopped

2 teaspoons lemon juice, fresh

1 teaspoon ground coriander or 3 capsules HerbSorb

dash of white pepper

1/4 teaspoon salt

Slice off hard ends of asparagus stalks, and chop the rest into 1 inch chunks. Reserve the tips. In a saucepan sauté onions and garlic in olive oil

over medium-low heat until limp. Add water or stock, asparagus, parsley, lemon juice, and spices. Cook until asparagus is tender. Put in electric blender and blend until smooth. Return to pan and add reserved asparagus tips; add spices, cook until hot, and serve.
Makes 4 to 6 servings

Peanut Butter–Tomato Soup

1/2 cup chopped onion

1 cup diced celery

2 cups stewed tomatoes

2 tablespoons butter (use olive or peanut oil if you are butter-sensitive)

2 tablespoons pure peanut butter

4 cups water

1 teaspoon salt, or to taste

Press tomatoes through a colander or process in blender. Sauté onion and celery in butter in a heavy skillet until tender. Thoroughly mix tomatoes with peanut butter and add along with other ingredients. Simmer until well blended and serve.
Makes 6 to 8 servings

Pumpkin Soup

1 cup chopped green onions (include stems)

2 cups mashed, cooked pumpkin (or one 16-oz. can)

2 tablespoons chives

3 cups chicken stock

1 cup grated carrots

1/4 teaspoon nutmeg

1/2 teaspoon ginger

dash of pepper

1/3 cup whipping cream

1/2 cup water

2 tablespoons fresh parsley, chopped

Sauté onions in a nonstick pan until limp. Add remaining ingredients except whipping cream and parsley. Cover and simmer for 20 minutes. Stir in whipping cream and serve. Garnish each bowl with fresh parsley.
Makes 6 to 8 servings

Italian Mushroom–Vegetable Soup

1/2 tablespoon basil

2 tablespoons olive oil

1 large onion, chopped

2 large cloves garlic, minced

3 ribs celery, sliced

2 cups mushrooms, sliced

1 tomato, finely chopped

1 large carrot, finely chopped

1 can tomato sauce, unsweetened

1 can tomato juice from canned tomatoes

4 cups chicken stock

4 cups various sliced vegetables (such as zucchini, yellow squash, and green beans)

Sauté onion, garlic, celery, and carrot in olive oil until almost soft. Add mushrooms and cook until barely tender. Add liquids, vegetables, and basil. Bring to a boil and simmer until vegetables are tender.
Makes 12 servings

Cabbage Soup

3 cups cabbage, coarsely chopped

3 cups tomato juice

1 cup water

1 carrot, peeled and sliced

2 tablespoons fresh parsley, chopped

1/2 cup onion, chopped

1/4 cup red or green pepper, chopped

1/2 cup celery, chopped (include leaves)

1/8 teaspoon salt

dash of pepper

dash of basil or thyme to taste

Bring juice and water to boil. Add vegetables and seasonings. Boil again and simmer for 15 to 20 minutes.
Makes 6 servings

Squash Soup

3 lbs winter or butternut squash

3 tablespoons butter

1/3 cup chopped onion

1 clove garlic, crushed

1 teaspoon coriander, ground

1/4 teaspoon ground cardamom

1/2 teaspoon salt

chopped parsley

3 cups water or stock

Simmer squash in water or stock 10 minutes or until tender. Set aside. Sauté onion and garlic in butter until soft. Stir in seasonings and add to squash mixture. Put all ingredients (except parsley) into blender and process until smooth. Make into two batches if necessary. Place in saucepan and heat. Garnish with chopped parsley and serve.
Makes 4 servings

Watercress–Tomato Soup

2 tablespoons butter or olive oil

1 leek, sliced

1/4 cup chopped onion

1 teaspoon minced garlic (fresh), or 1/2 teaspoon garlic powder

2 cups canned, peeled, whole tomatoes (cut into pieces)

1-1/2 cups chicken stock

1 bunch watercress, stems removed

2 tablespoons fresh parsley (chopped)

dash pepper

salt to taste

In a medium-sized saucepan sauté leek, onion, and garlic in butter or olive oil. Cover and cook over low heat for 10 minutes. Add tomatoes and chicken stock and bring to a boil. Reduce heat and simmer for 15 to 20 minutes. Add watercress, parsley, and spices. Simmer for an additional 5 to 10 minutes and serve.
Makes 4 servings

Noodleless Minestrone

3 large onions, finely chopped

4 tablespoons olive oil

1 quart vegetable stock

1 quart water

1 large can tomatoes, chopped

3/4 teaspoon garlic salt

3/4 teaspoon celery salt

1/2 teaspoon basil

1/2 teaspoon oregano

1/4 teaspoon thyme

1 cup zucchini, sliced in julienne strips

Sauté onions and vegetables in oil. Add stock and water; bring to a boil. Add tomatoes and spices. Simmer for 10 minutes. Sprinkle with Parmesan cheese, if desired.

Makes 10 servings

Healthy Heart Soup (A Cold Soup)

This soup is good for the heart, because it is rich in three heart-nourishing nutrients — carnitine, coenzyme Q-10, and selenium. Avocados are the richest known plant source of carnitine, and garlic is an excellent natural source of coenzyme Q-10. Garlic is also high in the heart-saving mineral selenium, especially if it is grown in selenium-rich soil.

2 ripe avocados

2 large cloves garlic, crushed

1 tablespoon olive oil

1-1/2 tablespoons red wine vinegar

2 ripe tomatoes, peeled

3/4 cup Very Veggie (spicy type, made by Knudsen Juice Co: V-8 juice may be substituted)

1/2 teaspoon sea salt

1/2 medium white onion cut in large pieces

2 tablespoons green onion tops, chopped

Peel avocados and cut into pieces. Add avocado to blender and blend until smooth. Coarsely chop tomatoes and onions and place in blender. Add garlic, salt, olive oil, Very Veggie juice, and vinegar and

blend entire mixture until smooth. Serve as is or chilled. Garnish with green onion tops.
Makes 4 servings

Chicken "Cure a Cold" Soup

This soup contains all sorts of ingredients useful in relieving the symptoms of colds—and some which can help the immune system cure it. The soup is high in vitamins A and C, plus it contains lots of garlic and onions—Nature's antibiotics. The garlic and onions, proven to have tremendous antiseptic actions, are the key ingredients. However, the aromatic oils from the leaves/seeds of oregano, coriander, and bay provide additional antiseptic action. Chicken broth and fat provide essential fatty acids, which also have antibiotic-like action. The Cure a Cold Soup is far superior to any over-the-counter medicine or remedy for providing relief. Watch your sinuses and breathing passages open up after eating this hearty, nourishing soup.

18 cloves garlic, crushed or finely diced

1 or 2 extra-large yellow onion, diced

2 teaspoons Hungarian paprika

2 teaspoons coriander

2 teaspoons salt

small handful freshly crushed oregano leaves (from wild oregano bunches, non-irradiated)

3-4 bay leaves

1/2 cup parsley, minced

4 medium-sized carrots, peeled and diced into large chunks

2/3 cup celery, diced

1 large red sweet pepper, cored and diced

1 cup cooked Brussels sprouts, whole (remove any discolored outer leaves)

1 cup fresh or frozen green beans, stems removed

1/2 medium-sized turnip, peeled and diced

1/2 chicken, whole with skin on

Wash chicken thoroughly. In a large pot place chicken in water and boil for 20 to 30 minutes. Skim top layer off water. Add garlic, oregano, coriander, bay leaves, salt, and onion; continue cooking over reduced heat. Add vegetables and cook for an additional 10 to 20 minutes or until flavors blend.
Makes 4 to 6 servings

Hot or Cold Tomatillo Soup

Tomatillos are also known as strawberry tomatoes. They are a tasty and more wild version of regular tomatoes. Tomatillos are native to Mexico and are commonly used in Mexican cooking. They are low in calories and high in fiber.

6 tomatillos, sliced.

1/4 cup green pepper, diced

1 large red sweet pepper, chopped in large pieces

4 cloves garlic, finely sliced

1 cup Very Veggie

1/4 cup green onions, diced (whites and greens)

dash cardamom (optional)

1/2 teaspoon salt

2 teaspoons olive oil

In a medium skillet, sauté over low heat garlic, onions, and all vegetables in olive oil until tender, being careful not to overcook. Add Very Veggie, salt, and cardamom and cook until hot. Serve immediately or refrigerate and serve cold.
Makes 2 servings

Salads

Radish Salad

This salad is especially good for those with digestive problems. Radishes contain substances which stimulate digestive juices and help heal the lining of the stomach and intestines. In addition, they are useful for the cardiac patient or for anyone with a concern or family history of cancer, since they are a rich natural source of the mineral selenium. Try to get radishes grown in states with selenium-rich soil, such as the Dakotas, Iowa, Missouri, Kansas, Nebraska, Arizona, Colorado, Oklahoma, Texas, and some parts of California.

1/2 cup red radishes, diced

1/2 cup daikon radish, diced

red radish sprouts (optional), handful

1/2 cup cucumbers, chopped

1/2 cup red onion, chopped

1 cup cherry tomatoes, sliced in quarters

1/4 cup balsamic vinegar

3 tablespoons olive oil

2 tablespoons fresh parsley, finely chopped

Combine all ingredients in a salad bowl and gently toss. Serve as is or topped with crumbled feta cheese.

Watercress Salad

Watercress has long been known to have valuable medicinal and nutritional values. As indicated by its name, watercress grows naturally in water. It has a very high water content (93%) and almost no calories. A one cup serving of watercress provides almost as much calcium as a cup of milk. In addition, it is low in phosphorus, which makes it an ideal calcium source. Watercress is also very rich in vitamins A and C. What's more, the plant is rich in a variety of sulfated compounds, which are potent cancer fighters. It should be on the top of your list of anti-cancer foods.

10 sprigs of watercress

1/2 head lettuce, shredded

1 tablespoon chopped sweet red pepper

1/2 cup diced cucumber

8 radishes, thinly sliced

1/2 cup grated goat's milk cheese or white cheddar cheese

onion or garlic salt to taste

Toss all ingredients together in a bowl just before serving. Use a dressing of your choice.
Makes 4 to 6 servings

Nut and Olive Salad

If you are nuts over nuts, you will love this salad. Nuts are an excellent addition to salads, because they are crunchy and are more filling than vegetables alone. Olives are also very filling due to their high fat content.

12 large black or green olives, pitted

2 tablespoons walnuts, chopped in large chunks

2 tablespoons pecans

1 tablespoon raw or roasted sunflower or pumpkin seeds

1 head lettuce, chopped or torn

1/4 cup chopped celery

1/4 cup finely shredded red cabbage

1/4 cup shredded carrots

parsley sprigs (as garnish)

salt to taste

Toss lettuce and vegetables in large bowl. Add salt to taste. Mix nuts in a separate bowl. Put salad mixture in salad bowls and top with nuts. Chill or serve as is with or without a dressing of your choice.
Makes 6 to 8 servings

Bermuda Onion/Beefsteak Tomato Delight

This salad is tremendously nourishing and invigorating, particularly on a hot summer day. Both onions and tomatoes are cooling, as is parsley. Try it as part of your dinner menu or as a snack by itself.

4 extra thick (1/3 inch) slices of Bermuda onion

2 large tomatoes, cut in extra thick slices

2 tablespoons fresh parsley, chopped (or 1 tablespoon parsley flakes)

1/3 cup goat's feta (crumbled), or shredded Swiss cheese

1 clove garlic, crushed

1/4 teaspoon black pepper

dash salt

olive oil and vinegar

On two plates, alternate a layer of tomatoes and onions at an angle. Mix parsley, garlic, salt, and pepper with olive oil and vinegar (balsamic and tarragon are excellent choices), and pour over plates. Top with cheese and a few pine nuts, if desired.
Makes 2 servings

Variety Lettuce Salad
With Pine Nuts and Goat's Cheese

When making a salad, it is always best to use several types of vegetables. By using several varieties of lettuce, the nutritional value of the salad is increased. Fresh salad greens are a top source of vitamin C as well as certain B vitamins, notably riboflavin, folic acid, and pyridoxine. Pine nuts are one of the finest vegetable sources of high quality protein, and they are easily digested.

1/2 cup pine nuts

1/2 lb green beans

1 head radicchio lettuce

1 head of Boston lettuce

1/2 head Bibb lettuce

1/2 head romaine lettuce

1/2 lb. goat or feta cheese

1 quart water

1/2 teaspoon salt

Wash vegetables and lettuce thoroughly in cold water, drying off any water. Trim edges of green beans. Preheat oven to 400 degrees. Place pine nuts on cookie sheet and put in oven for 6 minutes to toast, shaking pan several times.

Bring water to a boil and add salt. Add the green beans and cook until the beans are tender but still crisp (about 4 to 6 minutes). Drain, refresh under cold water, and set aside.

Tear lettuce into bite-size pieces, and add all ingredients in large bowl. To serve, place in salad bowls and top with crumbled cheese and pine nuts.

Use olive oil and vinegar, vinaigrette, or any other dressing found in the recipe section.

Makes 6 to 8 servings

Carrots Piquant

This recipe contains sesame and poppy seeds, both of which are rich sources of essential fatty acids. The carrots provide a significant amount of vitamin A (as beta carotene), and the turmeric serves as a top source of bioflavonoids. The garlic provides trace minerals, such as sulfur, selenium, calcium, and germanium. Chili powder is very high in magnesium, and there is hardly a better source of potassium than coriander—and it tastes good.

1 lb of carrots

2 teaspoons of fresh ginger, finely diced

4 cloves garlic, finely diced

1/4 cup green onions, diced

4 teaspoons poppy seeds

2 teaspoons sesame seeds

1/2 teaspoon chili powder

1/2 teaspoon turmeric

1 teaspoon cumin

2 teaspoons ground coriander seeds

1 tablespoon sesame or olive oil

Wash carrots well and peel. Cut carrots in half through the width and slice into thin strips lengthwise. In a large nonstick skillet sauté carrots and onions in oil until just tender. Remove carrot/onion mixture and set aside. Add ginger, garlic, poppy, and sesame seeds in skillet and stir over medium heat for 2 to 3 minutes. Add water if necessary. Stir in the rest of the ingredients including carrot/onion mixture, cook for an additional 3 to 4 minutes, and serve.

Makes 6 to 8 servings

Brussels Sprout Salad
With Avocado-Vinaigrette Dressing

Brussels sprouts are an excellent, although little used, food. They are both tasty and nutritious, being one of the richest vegetable sources of vitamin C. They are also an excellent source of potassium. Brussels sprouts are almost 90% water and contain only a few calories (only 50 calories per cup).

2 cups Brussels sprouts

1 carrot, shredded

1 grapefruit, peeled and sectioned (or use 1 cup diced cantaloupe or honeydew)

1/4 cup walnuts, chopped

Dressing:

2 tablespoons vinegar

1 tablespoon avocado

1/2 teaspoon brown mustard

1/4 cup cold-pressed soy or sunflower oil

Salad: remove membranes from grapefruit and set aside. Wash sprouts and remove discolored outer leaves. Steam Brussels sprouts until tender and cool. Once cooled, slice the steamed sprouts using a sharp knife. Combine with carrot, grapefruit (or melon), and walnuts.

Dressing: add vinegar, mustard, and avocado in blender or food processor, and blend till smooth. Gradually add oil while blending until mixture is thick.

Add enough dressing to moisten salad and toss. Reserve leftover dressing for other salads.
Makes 4 servings

Brussels Sprout-Carrot-Celery Salad

This makes a good crunchy salad from winter vegetables. Carrots are added to increase the vitamin A value of the salad, since Brussels sprouts are only a moderately good source. Walnuts provide valuable amounts of essential fatty acids.

2 cups Brussels sprouts

1 cup chopped celery

1 cup carrots, diced

2 tablespoons walnuts (optional)

Wash sprouts and remove discolored outer leaves. Steam until tender and chill. With a sharp knife, thinly slice sprouts. Combine ingredients and toss with enough vinaigrette dressing to moisten. Add walnuts, if desired. Serve immediately.
Makes 6 servings

Yogurt-Cucumber Salad

1 large, thin cucumber (or 2 medium-sized)

1/4 teaspoon garlic powder (or 1 garlic clove, crushed)

1/2 teaspoon salt

1/2 teaspoon dry, crushed mint (or, 1 tablespoon fresh mint leaves, diced)

2 cups homemade or 2 small cartons yogurt (plain)

Cut cucumber into quarters and slice. Add cucumber slices, garlic, pepper, salt, and mint; mix well. Mix in yogurt and serve.

Spinach Salad

2 lbs spinach, chopped

2 cucumbers, sliced in half circles

1/2 cup fresh lemon juice (use vinegar if you have a citrus allergy)

3 garlic cloves, crushed

3 green or red peppers, sliced into strips

2 avocados, cubed

1/2 teaspoon onion powder.

Mix all ingredients in a large bowl. Refrigerate for three hours and serve.
Makes 6 servings

Caper-Almond Salad

butter lettuce (enough for 2 servings)

3 green onions, sliced

2 tablespoons almonds, slivered

capers

vinaigrette or olive oil and vinegar dressing

beet slices

Toss torn butter lettuce with green onions. Top with capers and slivered almonds. Garnish with beet slices.
Makes 4 servings

Mediterranean Salad

1 large head of lettuce

4 leaves romaine lettuce

2 tomatoes, cubed

1/2 red sweet pepper, cut in strips

1/2 green pepper, cut in strips

2 cucumbers, peeled and sliced

1 stalk celery, sliced

3 stems green onions, sliced (optional)

Dressing:

1/8 teaspoon black pepper

1 clove garlic, finely minced (or 1/8 teaspoon garlic powder)

1 tablespoon fresh or dried mint

1 teaspoon salt

juice of 1/2 lemon

2 tablespoons fresh parsley, finely chopped (or 1 tablespoon parsley flakes)

Dressing: In a bottle, combine olive oil, salt, lemon juice, mint, black pepper, garlic, and parsley. Tighten lid and shake well. Refrigerate overnight to blend flavors.

Salad: Cut lettuce in half. Slice each half into strips and chop core into cubes. Wash in a strainer twice and let drain. Add the remainder of ingredients and refrigerate for at least 2 hours. When ready to serve, add dressing and eat immediately for the finest taste.
Makes 4 to 6 servings

Cabbage Salad With Onions

1 head cabbage, shredded

1/4 cup onion, shredded

1/2 teaspoon salt

1/4 teaspoon black pepper

1/2 lemon, squeezed

1/4 cup chopped parsley

pinch garlic salt (optional)

In a large salad bowl add onion, salt, pepper, parsley, and lemon juice. Mix well. Seasoning can be modified as desired.
Makes 8 servings

Steamed Cabbage Salad Vinaigrette

4 cups finely shredded cabbage

2 tablespoons cold-pressed olive or sunflower oil

1 tablespoon cider vinegar

1/4 teaspoon brown mustard

garlic salt to taste

Steam cabbage for 3 to 4 minutes, just until crisp-tender. Combine oil, vinegar, and mustard and pour over hot cabbage. Serve immediately or chilled.
Makes 6 to 8 servings

Lemon Coleslaw

3/4 head green cabbage, grated

1/2 head purple cabbage, grated

2 large carrots, grated

3 stalks celery, chopped

1 cup green or red pepper, chopped

Mix the above together.

In a blender or food processor, mix:

juice of two lemons

1/2 tomato

1 clove garlic

1/4 cup extra virgin olive oil

1 tablespoon dill weed

1 tablespoon caraway seed (optional)

1/2 teaspoon cumin (optional)

Blend until smooth and toss with cabbage salad.
Makes 6 servings

Artichoke-Avocado Salad

1 ripe avocado

1 small jar marinated artichokes

1/2 cup salsa or picante sauce

1/3 cup onion, chopped

1/2 cup radishes, sliced

2 tomatoes, diced

2 tablespoons extra virgin olive oil

1/4 teaspoon pepper

salt to taste

lettuce

Drain artichokes and discard oil. Combine artichokes, picante sauce, onion, olive oil, and radishes in a large mixing bowl. Add pepper and salt. Cover and chill for 2 to 3 hours. Add tomatoes. Cut avocado into strips and add. Serve on a bed of lettuce.
Makes 2 servings

Vegetable Dishes

Green Beans in Olive Oil

1 large onion, diced

6 cloves fresh garlic, grated (or 1 teaspoon of garlic powder)

1 large tomato, cubed

2 lbs fresh or frozen green beans

1/2 cup olive oil

1/4 cup fresh parsley (or 2 teaspoons parsley flakes)

1/2 teaspoon black pepper

1 tablespoon salt

1/2 teaspoon lemon pepper or, preferably, Red Sour Grape (from capsules)

1/4 cup lemon juice.

If using fresh green beans, remove stems and cut into 2-inch pieces; set aside. Heat oil in a large frying pan for one minute; add onions. Cook for 2 to 3 minutes or until tender. Add tomatoes, green beans, black pepper, parsley, lemon juice, salt, and lemon pepper (or Red Sour Grape). Stir for one minute and cover. Cook for 25 to 30 minutes on medium heat. Serve immediately.
Makes 8 to 10 servings

Red Cabbage Curry

1 tablespoon olive oil

2 teaspoons mustard seeds

1 teaspoon curry powder or turmeric

1 small red onion, quartered and sliced thin

1 small head red cabbage, thin sliced

2 tablespoons lemon or lime juice, fresh squeezed (use 6 capsules of Red Sour Grape (Resvitanol) if citrus sensitive)

1/2 teaspoon salt

In a large skillet heat oil. Add spices and mustard seeds; simmer for a short time. Add onion and simmer for several minutes, stirring often. Add cabbage and salt. Mix and cook until cabbage begins to wilt. Add lemon or lime juice and serve hot.
Makes 4 servings

Walnut/Pine Nut Stuffed Onions

4 medium Spanish or red onions

1/2 cup pine nuts

1/4 cup celery, chopped

2 tablespoons fresh parsley, minced

2 tablespoons walnuts, chopped

2 tablespoons green or red bell pepper, diced (optional)

1 teaspoon tarragon

1/2 teaspoon coriander

Bake onions in their skins in a preheated oven at 350 degrees for 25 to 30 minutes. Cut off tops and scoop out most of the insides, leaving 2 or three layers of onion plus the skin. Set aside scooped onion. Take a thin slice off the bottom (root end), being careful not to cut into the cavity so that the onion will stand upright.

Chop the set aside onion centers, and in a medium bowl add to the remaining ingredients. Stuff onion shells and place in oven for 25 to 30 minutes or until onions are tender.

Makes 4 servings

Simple Baked Onions

Onions are an excellent food choice. If you love them, do not hesitate to eat some every day. Onions stimulate digestion, improve circulation, and are a wonderful energizer. They also help protect against the number one and two diseases—heart disease and cancer. Use them as an addition to entrees as often as possible.

2 large yellow or red onions

In a preheated oven at 350 degrees bake onions in their skins for 30 to 40 minutes or until tender. Serve as is, and let each person cut into their own juicy onion.

Makes 2 servings.

Sautéed Beet Greens

Beet greens, also known as beet tops, are a fine source of beta carotene, and also contain significant amounts of potassium, calcium, magnesium, iron, and vitamin C. They are also an excellent source of fiber. This recipe will work well for other greens such as spinach, turnip tops, or mustard greens.

1 large bunch beet greens

2 tablespoons lemon juice, fresh squeezed

1 medium onion, coarsely chopped

2 cloves garlic, crushed

1/4 cup olive oil

1/4 teaspoon salt

1/8 teaspoon black pepper

In a wok or an extra-large, deep skillet add olive oil and onions, but do not heat. Dice stems of beet greens and beet leaves into bite-sized pieces. In a bowl add lemon juice, salt, pepper, and garlic. Mix well. Heat oil on medium heat, and cook onions until limp but not brown. Add onions and garlic; sauté for 1 to 2 minutes. Add lemon juice, salt, and pepper; stir. Add leaves and stems; toss constantly using two spatulas. Cook until leaves turn bright green (about 2 to 3 minutes).
Makes 4 to 6 servings

Sautéed Collard Greens

Collards are a highly nutritious vegetable which originate from the cabbage family. In fact, collard greens may be regarded as a form of wild cabbage. This fact is important in understanding why collards are so nutritious. Unlike most vegetables available in the marketplace, collards have been changed very little by domestication. Collard greens are one of the richest vegetable sources of calcium. They are higher in protein than most vegetables and contain about the same amount of protein per serving as do grains—but without the starch. One cup of stems and leaves provide nearly 100 mg. of vitamin C, 2.4 mg. of niacin, 10,000 I.U. of vitamin A, 468 mg. of potassium, and 300 mg. of calcium. So eat your heart's desire of collard greens—you will be well rewarded for it.

1 large bunch collard greens plus stems

1 large onion, coarsely chopped

4 cloves garlic, crushed

1 teaspoon salt

1/8 teaspoon pepper

3 tablespoons lemon juice, fresh squeezed (or 3 tablespoons vinegar, if you are allergic to lemon)

1/4 cup extra virgin olive oil

Wash collards well in water. Cut stems from leaves, and slice leaves in half. Chop collard leaves and stems into bite-sized pieces and set aside. In an extra-large, nonstick skillet or a wok, heat oil on medium heat; add onions, garlic, and sauté for 1 to 2 minutes. Add lemon juice, salt, and pepper and stir. Add leaves and stems, and toss constantly using two spatulas. Cook until leaves turn bright green (about 2 to 3 minutes).
Makes 4 to 6 servings)

Squash Stir-Fry

This recipe offers the advantage of having several types of squash, as well as a number of other vegetables, thus increasing the quantity and variety of nutrients available. Yellow squash is a rich source of vitamin A. Zucchini is a good source of calcium and phosphorus. Red sweet peppers are very high in vitamins A and C. Onions provide high amounts of sulfur, which is needed for healthy skin, hair, and nails. They also contain a substance known as *adenosine*, which helps in the production of cellular energy. Squash is 90-95% water, and this is the reason why it becomes so soft when cooked.

2 tablespoons butter

1 large zucchini, sliced thin

1 medium red onion, diced

1 sweet red or yellow pepper, diced

4 medium-size yellow squash, sliced thin

3 tomatoes, peeled and quartered

1/8 teaspoon garlic salt

dash of pepper

1 cup Parmesan, or 2/3 cup grated goat's cheddar cheese (optional)

Melt butter in wok or large heavy skillet but be careful not to burn. Add onion and pepper; stir for a few seconds. Add zucchini and yellow squash and cook until crisp-tender. Add tomatoes, salt, and pepper and stir well. If desired, sprinkle cheese over vegetables and toss gently until cheese melts.
Makes 8 servings

Zucchini in Olive Oil

3 medium-sized zucchini, cubed

2 medium tomatoes, cubed

1 medium onion, diced

2 cloves garlic, crushed

1/4 cup extra virgin olive oil

1/4 teaspoon black pepper

1/2 teaspoon salt

1 tablespoon fresh parsley, chopped (or 1 tablespoon parsley flakes)

1/8 teaspoon dried or fresh basil

In a large frying pan heat olive oil for 1 minute. Add onions and fry for two minutes, stirring constantly. Add salt, pepper, garlic, and tomatoes. Stir for one minute, adding zucchini, parsley, and basil. Stir occasionally for 15 minutes over medium-low heat. Serve hot.
Makes 4 servings

Blender Gazpacho (Gazpacho Drink)

1/2 cup onion, chopped

3 tomatoes, quartered

2 cloves garlic, diced

1 medium green pepper, chopped

1 small cucumber, peeled and sliced

1 teaspoon salt

4 tablespoons lemon or lime juice

2 tablespoons extra virgin olive oil

1/2 cup water

2 tablespoons picante sauce

Add all ingredients into blender or food processor. Blend until vegetables are finely chopped. Serve in chilled bowls or cups. You can make this into a gazpacho drink by thinning it with tomato or V-8 juice.
Makes 4 one-cup servings

Molded Gazpacho

2 envelopes unflavored gelatin

1 cup water

1 lb. tomatoes

1/2 cup green pepper, chopped

1/2 cup onion, finely chopped

2 tablespoons parsley, chopped

2 tablespoons fresh lemon juice

2 tablespoons apple cider vinegar

1/8 teaspoon cayenne pepper

2 cloves garlic, crushed

salt to taste

Add gelatin to 1/3 cup water and soak. Bring other 2/3 cup to a boil. Add gelatin and stir well until dissolved. Let cool. Add remaining ingredients and refrigerate.
Makes 6 servings

Sesame-Garlic Tomatoes

2 teaspoons sesame oil

1 teaspoon sesame seeds

1 clove garlic, minced

2 cups cherry tomatoes

1/3 medium onion, finely chopped

1/4 teaspoon coriander

Heat oil in skillet and add garlic and onions, stirring to keep them from scorching. Reduce heat and add tomatoes plus coriander; cook for 5 to 10 minutes, stirring occasionally. Serve hot and top with sesame seeds.
Makes 4 servings

Zucchini Canoes

3 zucchini, whole

1/2 cup zucchini, chopped

1 cup celery, chopped

1 cup yellow squash, chopped

6 tomatoes, chopped

2 onions, chopped

3 garlic cloves, minced

1/2 block tofu, crumbled (optional)

1 medium red pepper, diced

Sauté in small amount of olive oil one onion and tofu—set aside. Sauté second onion, red pepper, and celery for 4 minutes. Add zucchini and yellow squash, and cook for an additional 4 minutes. Season with salt and pepper if desired.

Cut zucchini in halves and scrape out center. Fill zucchini with vegetable mixture, sprinkle onion-tofu mix on top, and bake for 1/2 hour at 350 degrees. Eat hot or use as a nutritious snack.
Makes 6 servings

Dilled Broccoli/Cauliflower Combo

1/2 pound broccoli, fresh

1 medium-sized head of cauliflower

1/2 teaspoon lemon juice (preferably fresh)

1/2 teaspoon dill weed

1 tablespoon butter

Cook vegetables in small amount of water or steamer until tender but still crisp. Add lemon juice, dill, and melted butter and toss.
Makes 4 servings

Grilled Squash Medley

Squash is an excellent food choice, as it is high in nutrients and quite low in starch and calories. Some types of squash, such as winter squash, are an excellent source of vitamin A (beta carotene). The squash varieties in this recipe provide good quantities of calcium, magnesium, potassium, vitamin C, and beta carotene. For this recipe, select squash no more than 1-1/2 inch in diameter.

2 zucchini squash, whole

2 Japanese eggplant

2 small yellow squash

extra virgin olive oil

garlic salt

pepper

Slice all squash and eggplant lengthwise. Brush with a little olive oil. Sprinkle garlic salt and pepper to taste. Grill over hot coals for 6 to 8 minutes on each side or until just tender.
Makes 6 servings

Roots and Such Stir Fry

Root vegetables are among the healthiest foods known to mankind. As the name implies, these vegetables draw nutrients directly from the soil. Thus, it is not surprising that root vegetables are extra-rich in certain trace minerals such as selenium, magnesium, potassium, sulfur, germanium, silicon, etc. This medley of roots and vegetables provides an abundance of potassium, selenium, phosphorus, calcium, beta carotene, and vitamin C.

3 small turnips

4 medium carrots

1 small green pepper

1 small red pepper

1 small red onion

2 medium parsley roots (save tops)

8 mushrooms, fresh

1 small sweet potato (optional)

1/4 head red cabbage, finely shredded

1/4 cup extra virgin olive oil

2 tablespoons Pomegranate Sauce

Chop coarsely all the above ingredients (except cabbage). Heat oil in skillet or wok until hot taking care not to allow oil to smoke. Add turnips, carrots, and peppers to oil, stirring constantly for 5 minutes. Add remaining ingredients and cook until slightly tender (about 2 minutes). Then add cabbage and Pomegranate Syrup (sauce). Stir for one minute and serve immediately. For an entree add 1 cup cubed chicken or turkey.

Note: The pomegranate syrup contains natural sugar calories, and the sweet potato contains a significant amount of starch calories. Although both are rich food sources of nutrients, for most people following this diet it is safer to omit these from the recipe. They may be added at a later time, when tolerance for natural sugars and starches improves.
Makes 6 servings

Pickled Turnips

Most people have never eaten turnips. If you try to purchase them at a grocery store, usually the checker won't know what they are. This recipe offers a convenient and delicious way to get a weekly dose of turnips. There are only a few ways to make turnips into a tasty part of a cooked meal, so it is best to eat them raw. This recipe provides a form of raw turnips which are both delicious and more digestible than they would be otherwise. The pickling process using vinegar, garlic, and spices breaks down the fibers of the turnip, making it easier for the digestive mechanism to liberate the nutrients. Why eat turnips on a regular basis? Because they are one of the richest vegetable sources of selenium, provided they are grown in selenium-rich soil. They also contain significant amounts of vitamin C, calcium, and potassium.

Turnip greens are one of the most nutritious vegetables known. They may well be the richest vegetable source of vitamin A (beta carotene), containing over 15,000 I.U. per cup. In addition, they contain very high amounts of calcium, magnesium, potassium, phosphorus, iron, zinc, vitamin E, vitamin C, and folic acid.

When you finish all your pickled turnips and turnip greens, be sure to drink the juice. As you can imagine, it is loaded with nutrients.

6 to 10 medium-sized turnips

1/4 cup vinegar

2 to 3 teaspoons salt

3 cloves garlic, thinly sliced

1 quart-sized mason jar (with new lid)

1 medium beet

turnip leaves (a few)

1 tsp wild, dried oregano, optional (from oregano bunches)

Wash turnips, beet, and turnip leaves thoroughly. Peel turnips and cut into wedges. Add to jar. Peel beet and boil in small amount of water until it softens—save the juice. Cut beet into wedges. Add turnips, beet wedges, and garlic to jar. Follow with salt, vinegar, oregano, and beet juice. Fill with water (must be boiled) if necessary. Stuff with turnip leaves and seal tightly. Once cured, use as a snack or as a vegetable dish with meat entrees.

Pickled Red and Green Peppers

1 large red sweet pepper

1 large green pepper

1 small hot red pepper (optional)

3 cloves garlic, finely sliced

1/4 teaspoon pickling spice

1/4 cup vinegar

1 tablespoon salt

1 quart-sized mason jar with new lid

Wash peppers well. Core peppers, remove seeds, and cut into slices. Place pepper and garlic slices in jar. Add spices, vinegar, and hot pepper (if desired). Fill with water (must be boiled), and seal tightly. Once cured, use as a snack or with entrees.

Fruit Dishes

Grapefruit Medley

The idea of combining grapefruit with vegetables originated in Guatemala. When properly combined, fruits and vegetables can be very tasty, as this recipe demonstrates.

3 large grapefruits
1 small sweet red bell pepper, cored and diced
2 teaspoons fresh onion, minced
2 tablespoons fresh parsley, minced
1/2 teaspoon red pepper (hot), crushed
1/2 teaspoon salt

With a serrated knife peel the grapefruits taking care to remove all the white outer lining. Cut the membranes, and take out the inner grapefruit segments, discarding the membranes. Cut the segments in halves or thirds and place in 2-quart bowl. Add remaining ingredients and mix gently. Refrigerate for at least 1 hour before serving.
Makes 6 to 8 servings

Low-Carb Fruit Platter

Certain fruits are relatively low in carbohydrates and, thus, are not fattening. Even the weight conscious individual can relish this fruitful delight. The fruits found on this plate contain 10% or less sugar.

1 cantaloupe, cut in halves
1/2 honeydew melon
1 papaya, peeled
1 pint strawberries, tops removed
parsley and sweet red pepper slices (as a garnish)

Always wash fruit carefully before preparing. Peel melons and cut into long slices 1-inch wide. Cut papaya into 1-inch cubes. Cut strawberries into halves. Arrange fruits on a large platters and garnish with parsley and red pepper slices.
Makes 4-6 servings

Diced Fruit in a Bowl

8-10 strawberries
1/2 cantaloupe
1 kiwi fruit
1 large wedge watermelon or honeydew melon

Wash all fruit well. Cut tops off of strawberries and slice in half. Remove peel from cantaloupe and dice into cubes 1/2-inch long. Peel kiwi and slice. Dice watermelon or honeydew melon into cubes 1/2 inch long. Gently mix fruit until uniformly blended. Chill and serve.
Makes 2 to 4 servings

Fruit 'n Nut Salad

1/2 honeydew melon

1/2 cantaloupe

1 large wedge watermelon

1/2 grapefruit, peeled

1 kiwi fruit

15-20 strawberries

1 whole papaya

1 whole guava (optional)

3 tablespoons pecans, chopped

3 tablespoons walnuts, chopped

1 tablespoon coconut, shredded (unsweetened)

2 one-half pint containers of real whipping cream (optional)

Make melons into melon balls. Take grapefruit sections and remove membranes. Peel kiwi fruit, and slice. Cut these slices in half and cut strawberries in half. Peel papaya and guava and cut into segments. Add all fruit to a large bowl and mix gently. Top with pecans, walnuts, and coconut. If desired, use whipping cream as a topping. Pour whipping cream into bowl and whip with a hand or regular mixer.

Drinks and Smoothies

Energy Shake

This high-protein shake provides a boost of energy for several reasons. Nutri-Sense is a rich natural source of vitamin E, phospholipids, and fatty acids, all of which help increase cellular energy and stamina. Lecithin itself, which is also found in Nutri-Sense, is a tremendous energizer. The protein or milk powder helps sustain energy levels by preventing blood sugar levels from falling. Finally, the sugars in the honey, juice, and/or fruit provide an easily digested, rapidly absorbed source of fuel for the body.

8 to 12 oz. water or juice

1 tablespoon Nutri-Sense

1 tablespoon lecithin granules

3 heaping tablespoons protein powder or powdered milk

2 tablespoons raw honey (optional)

Added fruit (unsweetened strawberries, blueberries, one-half banana)

Mix in blender and drink as a breakfast or between meal energizer.

Protein Drink

10 oz. water or juice

2-3 heaping tablespoons protein powder (unsweetened or sweetened with fructose only)

1 tablespoon of rice bran or Nutri-Sense

Mix in blender or shaker and use as a between-meal snack.
Makes 1 large serving

Strawberry-Almond Cooler

1 pint fresh, ripe, strawberries (or 3/4 pint fresh frozen)

12 oz almond milk, chilled

Add strawberries and almond milk to blender. Blend until smooth and serve.
Makes 2 servings

Strawberry-Guava Punch

This drink will give you a punch in more ways than one. It is delicious and nutritious. For the weight conscious, it is low in sugar. For anyone with fatigue, it is the perfect booster—you can add some protein powder for an extra lift. Guavas are a rich source of vitamin C, and between these two fruits plus the lemon, you get over 200 mg of vitamin C per 10 oz serving.

12 to 15 fresh, chilled strawberries

1 guava

2 tablespoons fresh-squeezed lemon or lime juice (optional)

20 oz sparkling mineral water

Wash strawberries and remove tops. Add all ingredients to blender or juicer. Alter amount of water as desired. Serve immediately. Any remainder should be consumed within 48 hours since vitamin losses increase with time.
Makes 4 servings

Cranberry Juice Creamy Surprise

Pure, unsweetened cranberry juice is good for the body. Cranberries are an excellent source of bioflavonoids and a fair source of vitamin C as well as potassium. Of particular importance is the fact that cranberries contain a special bioflavonoid known as *anthocyanin,* the substance responsible for their brilliant red color. Researchers have found that anthocyanin inhibits the formation of tumors. This colorful substance exerts another remarkable action—it aids in restoring vision and helps improve the ability of the eyes to adapt from light to dark.

Cranberries are naturally low in sugar and so is pure cranberry juice. This presents a slight problem—it is so sour that few could drink it by itself. This recipe solves this problem with the addition of ripe honeydew melon, one of the most naturally sweet of all fruits. The key to the success of this recipe is to use the inner lining (the mushy part) of the melon, and to pour in any melon juice in the core.

1 large chilled, ripe honeydew melon

1/2 cup pure unsweetened cranberry juice

Cut melon in half and remove seeds, being careful to retain any juice. Scrape inner, mushy part of melon and measure two cups; place in blender and add any melon juice plus cranberry juice. Blend until smooth and serve.
Makes 2 servings

Carrot and Cream Cooler

This drink is both filling and nutritious. It is excellent as a refreshing drink on a hot day or as an addition to a meal. One serving of carrot juice provides the minimum daily requirement of vitamin A. The almond milk provides protein and minerals such as potassium and magnesium. This drink is far superior to any beverage available in the grocery store, not to speak of nutrient-free drinks like pop, Kool-Aid, fruit drinks, and alcohol.

5 oz. carrot juice, chilled (preferably fresh-squeezed or canned)

5 oz. almond milk, chilled

Mix in blender or by hand and serve.
Makes 2 servings
Note: This is an excellent drink for the person with blood sugar problems. Carrot juice should be used as a drink at a frequency no greater than every other day. Be sure to use it within 48 hours, since beta carotene oxidizes once exposed to air.

Apricots and Cream Delight

Apricots are another very rich source of beta carotene, and they are relatively low in sugar. What makes them fattening is all that sugar added to the apricot products which are found at the supermarket. Check your health food store to see if unsweetened apricot products are available.

4 oz unsweetened, chilled apricot juice or puree—dilute with water if too thick

6 oz almond or other nut milk, chilled

Add all ingredients in blender, mix for a few seconds, and serve.
Makes 2 servings

Tropical Fruit N' Cream

Some tropical fruits are low enough in sugar to be used on this program such as fresh papaya. Papaya is a digestive stimulant, since it contains enzymes which assist digestive processes. Papayas also contain a significant amount of potassium, vitamin A, and vitamin C. Coconut milk is not just for taste. It too contains valuable nutrients such as potassium, phosphorus, calcium, and medium chain triglycerides. The latter is a type of fat that is readily absorbed by the body and highly nutritious. Almonds provide the much needed mineral magnesium, being one of the richest natural sources of this important nutrient.

1/4 cup chilled coconut milk, fresh or canned
1 cup almond or other nut milk (chilled)
1 whole papaya, peeled and diced
water (as needed)

Cut papaya into slices and set aside. Put nut milks in blender and blend at low speed. Add papaya, a few pieces at a time, and blend until creamy. Add water or ice to change thickness. For an additional exciting flavor, add a few ripe strawberries.
Makes 2 servings

Melon Smoothie (Cantaloupe)

2 cups chilled cantaloupe, cut into cubes
3 ice cubes

Add ingredients to blender and blend until smooth. Serve garnished with mint leaves and a wedge of lemon or lime.
Makes 2 servings

Melon Smoothie (Honeydew)

1 whole honeydew melon
3 ice cubes

Wash outside of melon and slice in half. Scoop out seeds but save any juice. Remove outer peel and cube. Add melon, juice, and ice to blender and blend until smooth. Serve garnished with mint leaves and wedge of lemon or lime.
Makes 4 servings

Watermelon Smoothie

3 cups chilled watermelon, seeds removed
4 ice cubes

Place melon and ice cubes in blender; blend until smooth and serve.
Makes 2 servings

Dressings, Dips, and Sauces

Vinaigrette Dressing

1/4 cup vinegar

2 large egg yolks

1/2 tablespoon salt

1 teaspoon pepper, freshly ground

2 cups extra virgin olive oil or cold-pressed vegetable oil

Add 1/2 the oil and the rest of the ingredients to a food processor. Blend for 5 seconds. Transfer to a mixing bowl and gradually whisk in the rest of the oil. Add other spices if desired.

Carrot and Avocado Dressing

1 cup carrot juice

1 avocado, peeled

1 large red sweet pepper, cored and diced

2 tablespoons balsamic or apple cider vinegar

1/4 teaspoon salt

Place all ingredients in a blender or food processor and blend until smooth. Use as a dressing for salads or as a sauce or dip.

Guacamole

1 large ripe avocado

1-1/2 tablespoons fresh lemon or lime juice

1/4 cup onion, minced

1 tablespoon diced green chili peppers

1/2 teaspoon garlic, minced

1/2 teaspoon cayenne pepper

1/2 teaspoon sea salt

Combine all ingredients in food processor or blender and process until smooth.

Hummus (Garbanzo Bean Dip)

2 cans garbanzo beans (save 1/2 cup juice)

1/4 cup water

3 tablespoons tahini (sesame seed paste)

1 clove garlic

1/2 cup reconstituted lemon juice or 1/3 cup fresh lemon juice

2 tablespoons olive oil

parsley and paprika (for garnish)

Heat garbanzo beans and water in a saucepan for 2 to 3 minutes or until hot. Combine beans, tahini, lemon, garlic, and salt in a food processor and mix until smooth (about 4 minutes) . If too dry, add 1/4 cup of juice from beans. Serve in shallow bowl with olive oil poured on top. Sprinkle with paprika and chopped parsley.

Garlic-Dill Dressing

3 tablespoons lemon juice

2 tablespoons extra virgin olive oil

1 teaspoon garlic salt

1 teaspoon dill seed

2 tablespoons fresh, minced parsley

Whip all ingredients in blender. Add water if necessary. Use as a salad dressing.

Sugarless Mayonnaise

1/2 cup flax seed oil

1/2 cup extra virgin olive or cold-pressed sunflower oil

1 egg, whole

2 tablespoons vinegar (may use lemon juice instead)

dash white or cayenne pepper

Mix oils together in a cup. In blender break egg and add vinegar (or lemon juice), dash of pepper, and 1/4 cup of oil. Cover blender and blend at low speed. Just as it begins to thicken, add the remaining 3/4 cup of oil in a heavy stream while continuing to blend at low speed.
Makes 1-1/2 cups

Soybean Hummus

This recipe is lower in carbohydrates than garbanzo bean dip and should be the "hummus of choice" during the first 90 days of the diet. However, both are excellent and healthy dishes. The soybeans and tahini paste provide essential fatty acids which are so desperately needed and difficult to get through the diet. Eat this dish as often as you can.

1 cup cooked soybeans

1/3 cup sesame tahini

1/2 cup lemon juice, freshly squeezed

3 tablespoons water

4 to 6 cloves garlic

1 tablespoon extra virgin olive oil

1 teaspoon parsley and paprika (for garnish)

In a blender combine tahini, soybeans, lemon juice, water, and garlic, and process on low speed until smooth. Chill and serve as a dip or sauce. Top with paprika and chopped parsley.

Sugar-Free Tomato Sauce

1 onion, chopped

1/2 cup celery, chopped

2/3 cup green pepper, chopped

2/3 cup carrots, chopped

1/4 cup fresh parsley, chopped

3 cloves garlic, diced

1 large can (1 lb-12 oz.) whole, peeled tomatoes, pureed

2 large cans tomato sauce (unsweetened)

2 bay leaves

2 teaspoons oregano (from wild oregano bunches)

1 teaspoon dried basil leaves

1/4 teaspoon pepper

1/2 teaspoon salt

In a large saucepan sauté onions, vegetables, garlic and parsley in a small amount of olive oil for 4 minutes or until limp. Add remaining ingredients. Mix well. Bring to a boil then reduce heat. Keep uncovered and simmer for 30 minutes or until flavors blend. Freeze in small portions and use as needed.

Hearty Salsa Sauce

Salsa can be used as a sauce or dip. Spices may be tailored depending on how hot you like it. This salsa makes an excellent dip for sliced fresh vegetables or as a sauce over cooked vegetables.

One 4 oz can green chili peppers, seeded and chopped

4 tomatoes, chopped

4 green onions, chopped

1 clove garlic, chopped

1 teaspoon oregano (from wild oregano bunches)

1 tablespoon extra virgin olive oil

1 teaspoon mustard seeds

juice of half a lemon

salt

pepper

Combine all ingredients in a bowl and mix. Serve chilled or as is.

Vegetable Dip

2 cups vegetables (green beans, zucchini, carrots, broccoli, yellow squash, or cauliflower)

1 teaspoon minced onion

1 tablespoon minced green pepper

1 tablespoon vegetable seasoning

1/4 teaspoon dried dill weed (or 1/2 teaspoon fresh dill weed)

1/8 teaspoon sea salt

Cook vegetables in a steamer for about 5 minutes. Let cool. Blend on high speed and add onion, peppers, dill weed, salt, and seasoning. Serve with fresh vegetables for dipping.

Eggplant Dip

1 large eggplant

1/2 cup yogurt (if milk-sensitive, use 1/2 cup diced avocado)

1 clove garlic, crushed

1 tablespoon extra virgin olive oil

1 tablespoon fresh parsley, finely chopped

1 teaspoon wild oregano (from oregano bunches)

dash cayenne pepper

salt to taste

Cook whole eggplant under broiler or in oven until soft (400-450 degrees). Let cool and remove pulp, discarding skin. Place pulp in cheese cloth or kitchen linen and squeeze liquid out until eggplant is dry. Add together eggplant and remaining ingredients in a blender and blend until thoroughly combined. Chill and serve as a dip for vegetables and meats or as a side dish by itself.

Creamy Garlic-Avocado Dressing

3 cloves garlic, minced

1-1/4 cups cottage cheese

1 medium avocado, peeled

2 tablespoons fresh parsley, chopped

2 teaspoons vinegar

1/2 teaspoon onion salt

dash cumin (optional)

Remove the outer green peel of the avocado and dice. Add all ingredients to food processor or blender and blend until smooth.

Extra-Strength Horseradish Dressing

Horseradish is excellent for health, largely because of its rich content of powerful enzymes (the reason for its biting taste). Most notably, horseradish is rich in *peroxidase,* which is beneficial since it helps preserve tissues. In effect, peroxidase is a ***natural preservative*** for human cells. Recently, it has been shown that peroxidase and other enzymes can be absorbed through the intestines into the bloodstream to be used by the cells and organs. To enjoy optimal health, eat horseradish as often as possible.

3 tablespoons lemon juice, fresh

1 tablespoon mustard

2 tablespoons horseradish

1/4 teaspoon black pepper

1 tablespoon parsley, freshly chopped

1 tablespoon minced garlic, or 1 clove fresh garlic

2 tablespoons fresh onion, minced or 1 teaspoon onion powder

Place all ingredients in a food processor or blender. Blend until smooth. Use as a dressing on salads, or as a dip for meats or vegetables. Spread on steaks and chops, this dressing will greatly add to their digestion.

Fresh Tarragon Dressing

4 teaspoons egg yolks (use fresh farm eggs, if possible)

4 tablespoons tarragon vinegar

4 tablespoons fresh, minced tarragon

1 cup cold-pressed olive, sunflower, sesame, or walnut oil

dash pepper

dash salt

2 tablespoons fresh parsley, finely chopped

Combine all ingredients and one-half the oil in a food processor or blender and process until well mixed. While blending, slowly add the rest of the oil. Use as a dressing on salads or as a dip for vegetables.

Butters and Yogurt

Clarified Butter

Place one pound of pure, unsalted butter in heavy pan or skillet. Simmer until butter is completely melted. Let stand until white, foamy froth forms on top of mixture. Carefully skim off foam and discard. This is the part of butter that burns. A clear golden liquid will remain. Use this for cooking and sautéing.

Better Butter

This recipe makes butter much more rich nutritionally, since Austrian pumpkinseed oil is super-high in vitamins, minerals, and, particularly, essential fatty acids, which are lacking in butter. It also makes butter more smooth and easier to spread. It is a good option for those who are allergic to milk products, since the addition of pumpkinseed oil improves the digestibility of the butter. For those super-sensitive to milk products use coconut fat instead of butter.

1/2 cup butter

1/3 cup Austrian pumpkinseed oil (Pumpkinol)

a few drops of oil of edible fennel (optional; for a licorice-like taste; fennel also improves digestion)

Mix in blender at low speed until creamy. Use as a spread or in cooking.

Homemade Yogurt

1 gallon whole milk

1/2 pint of whipping cream or 1 pint Half-and-Half

3/4 cup yogurt starter

Use a 16-quart stainless steel pan. Rinse with cold water. Add milk and cream, then cover. Let boil on medium-high heat for 15 to 20 minutes. Stir every 5 minutes. Caution: Keep a constant eye on the milk during the last 10 minutes to avoid over-boiling. Keep pan lid ajar and let cool to lukewarm (approximately 2-1/2 hours). Add yogurt starter and mix well into milk. Cover and let stand 5 hours or overnight. Uncover and refrigerate 1 day. Your yogurt is now ready with active cultures. Eat plain and over meat dishes, salads, vegetables, or with fruits.
Makes 20 to 24 servings

Goat's Milk Yogurt

This recipe is especially valuable for those allergic to cow's milk. In this case use powdered goat's milk, as its taste is not too overpowering.

7 cups water

3 cups goat's milk (preferably powdered)

starter culture or 2 to 3 acidophilus capsules

Bring water to a boil in stainless steel pot. Let cool to about 100 degrees (just hot enough to touch without getting burned). Add acidophilus culture and cover, letting stand for 8 to 9 hours. Refrigerate and serve as needed. Be sure to save some starter for the next batch. When making yogurt, try to use water which is not chlorinated, since chlorine kills the acidophilus bacteria.

Special Remedies for Specific Ailments

Colds or Flu

1. *Avoid* eating solid foods, meats, or starches for the duration.

2. *Eat* mainly fresh fruits and vegetables.

3. *Have* several bowls of homemade chicken soup. Try the Cure a Cold Chicken Soup recipe.

4. *Take* raw honey (uncooked and unfiltered), 1/3 cup three to four times daily (If using wild medicinal honeys, use less, like 1/4 cup twice daily.)

   Note: This remedy works superbly. Pure honey contains numerous anti-infective agents which boost immune power. The natural sugar helps fuel white blood cells into action against viruses or bacteria. Top quality medicinal honeys are now available. These are imported from the Mediterranean. Although available only in a limited supply, these are first class raw honeys. Available types include wild oregano and thistle honeys from medicinal plants and neroli orange blossom honey from the sour orange tree. These honeys, which are completely pure and undiluted and are of the highest quality, are available via mail order: 1-800-243-5242. From personal use I can tell you that the quality and utility of these Mediterranean honeys is stupendous and they are incomparably superior to the types of honeys produced in America as well as Europe. Yet, this is to be expected, because when foods or herbs are procured directly from the wild, they are infinitely superior to the commercial varieties.

5. *Gargle* with salt water or preferably vinegar, 3 to 4 times daily.

6. *Sniff* water into your nostrils 3 to 4 times daily. Let the water drip back into the sinuses, then gently blow it out.

7. *Limit* your calorie intake (the old 7-Up and saltines remedy is out).

8. *Avoid* excessive nose blowing as this can drive the infection deeper into the sinuses, lungs, eardrum, or even into the brain.

9. *Take* oil of oregano, 5 drops three or more times daily. Or, take it under the tongue, a drop every hour if necessary. The latter is the most effective means to decimate a cold.

10. *Be sure* to take plenty of vitamin C. If using synthetic vitamin C, take 2 to 4 grams daily. Natural or crude, unprocessed vitamin C is now available. Called Flavin-C, the vitamin C and the

bioflavonoids, are purely from natural sources. These totally natural sources included sour immature oranges, tangerines, grapefruit, rose hips, and acerola cherries. Thus, it is more potent than the synthetic and it is also better tolerated. Take 2 or more capsules of Flavin-C every hour.

Cold Sores

1. *Apply* aloe vera (straight from the plant or as a gel) to affected area.

2. *Take* stabilized fresh royal jelly (Royal Oil), several drops under the tongue as often as needed. Royal jelly, rich in pantothenic acid, boosts natural cortisone output, which fights the cold sores.

3. *Take* large doses of vitamin C and bioflavonoids. Bioflavonoids are powerful in destroying the cold sore virus. Take 2 to 4 grams of each daily until the lesions clear.

4. *Avoid* foods high in arginine (an amino acid). This includes all nuts and seeds, cocoa, and beans.

5. *Consume* foods rich in lysine, including cheese, milk, and meats.

6. *Take* extra lysine, 4 to 6 capsules per day.

7. *Apply* oil of oregano (from wild, high-mountain oregano), a drop or two directly on the cold sore as often as needed.

Constipation

1. *Avoid* harsh laxatives.

2. *Eat* mainly fruits and vegetables and avoid all gluten containing grains.

3. *Start* your morning with 2 large glasses of warm water. Add to each either 1/2 cup fresh-squeezed lemon juice or vinegar. Or, empty the contents of four capsules of Red Sour Grape (Resvitanol) into the warm water and drink.

4. *Drink* eight 10 oz glasses of water daily. Constipation often indicates the existence of a mild state of dehydration. Be sure to drink only nonchlorinated water, since chlorine may cause constipation.

5. *Take* 1/2 cup honey morning and night for at least three days (Caution: diabetics must omit this one.)

6. *Add* 1 to 3 heaping teaspoons of acidophilus culture three times a

day mixed in water or juice.

7. *Try* Oregamax capsules, three capsules twice daily. Oregamax capsules provide natural herbal fibers plus the antiseptic power to cleanse the bowel of harmful germs.

8. *Take* Gene's Powerdrops, 10 drops twice daily. These rare drops are made from wild greens, and the wild greens help cleanse the colon of impurities, plus they help normalize bowel function.

Diarrhea

1. *Rest* the digestive tract by fasting and by avoiding all meat, nuts, and grains.

2. *Drink* lots of fluids, especially water and, to a lesser degree, juices. The finest antidiarrhea juices are peach, pear, and apricot.

3. *Avoid* citrus fruits or citrus juices as well as apple and grape juice.

4. *Eat* primarily fruit. Pureed vegetables are also allowed. Pure homemade yogurt and kefir, which are rich in lactobacillus culture, may be helpful. Drink the broth only of homemade chicken soup.

5. *Take* honey, 1/3 cup 3 to 4 times daily. If diarrhea intensifies, increase the dose to 1/2 cup four times daily. If taking wild Mediterranean honey, use less: 1/4 cup two or three times daily.

6. *Try* oil of oregano, a drop under the tongue 3 to 4 times daily and two drops internally three times daily. Mix the oregano oil with the honey. With these two potent remedies the diarrhea should be eradicated within a day or two.

7. *Take* HerbSorb, a wonderful Eastern spice formula for regenerating the colon. When nothing else works, HerbSorb often comes to the rescue; take 2 or more capsules as often as needed until the diarrhea halts. Note: I have used this formula successfully after contracting food poisoning while traveling. Food poisoning is an epidemic. If you become sick when traveling, it is likely due to germs from contaminated foods.

Insomnia

1. *Try* eating a snack right before bedtime. First, eat a high protein snack (cheese, eggs, sliced meat, nuts). The snack should be salty, because salt relaxes the adrenal glands and helps induce sleep. If this doesn't work, try three tablespoons of raw honey in a warm glass of whole milk.

2. *Take* calcium, 1000 to 2000 mg. one half-hour before bedtime. If you awaken, take another dose. Take also pantothenic acid, about 500 mg at bedtime.

3. *Take* Herbal Zeezzz, a potent, all-natural sleep aid and nerve tonic, 5 drops under the tongue as needed until sleep is induced. This is the most potent, effective sleep aid I have ever used.

4. *Try* sage tea. Simply boil water and add a bunch of sage. Drink plain or with raw honey. Or, for a more powerful effect add 5 to 10 drops of edible oil of sage (be sure to consume only the edible variety) to the hot water and drink. You should fall asleep shortly afterward.

5. *Rub* oil of wild lavender (emulsified in extra virgin olive oil) on the soles of the feet at bedtime. Or, add it to a diffuser. When all else fails, this aromatic essence has been proven in scientific studies to induce sleep.

For Women Only

Menstrual Cramps

1. *Try* bromelain, i.e. BromaZyme (uncoated), for halting severe cramps, 2 to 4 tablets every four hours.

2. *Avoid* sugar, as it aggravates the cramps.

3. *Take* edible oil of fennel or rosemary prior to the start of the menses. These herbs greatly relax the pelvic nerves and provide natural, estrogen-like hormones. The hormones in fennel and rosemary are entirely safe, as long as they are used in small amounts like 2 to 10 drops twice daily. High quality, edible fennel and rosemary (wild Mediterranean) are produced by North American Herb & Spice Co.

4. *Realize* that most women with severe menstrual cramps are deficient in several B vitamins. Large doses of all of the B vitamins are indicated.

5. *Add* fish oils if the above isn't effective. Or, regularly consume fatty fish. The oils in these fish help prevent severe menstrual cramping and/or inflammation. Infections within the female organs by yeasts or other organisms may either cause or aggravate menstrual difficulties. Often, cramps will be worse when these infections are active. In such an instance use oil of oregano internally, five drops twice daily. Vaginally, apply oil of myrtle, a few drops twice daily.

Thyroid malfunction is also a common cause of menstrual

problems. Thyroid function may need to be evaluated through blood tests. Nutritional deficiencies may greatly impair the function of this gland, especially iodine deficiency. However, with mild to moderate thyroid dysfunction, routine blood tests for thyroid hormones are seldom abnormal. Another option is to perform self-tests, a subject covered in detail in Dr. Ingram's *Self-Test Nutrition Guide* or via the Web site NutritionTest.com. There are two types of self-tests covered in this book, one written and the other using a thermometer. The combination of these tests is more accurate than blood tests for determining the existence of mild to moderate thyroid disorders.

Nausea (Including Nausea of Pregnancy)

1. *Try* ginger root, whole or ground, or as a tea. Take it several times during the day. Or, use edible Oil of Ginger (in extra virgin olive oil), a few drops in hot water as often as needed. Note: the edible oil of ginger by North American Herb & Spice Co. is entirely safe to use, even by pregnant women.

2. *Avoid* solid foods until nausea clears, eating broths, soups, or juice instead.

3. *Take* HerbSorb, a combination of spices that absorb excess acid and help normalize stomach function.

4. *Eat* brown rice, or, preferably, consume Nutri-Sense as a source of thiamine and other B vitamins.

5. *Avoid* heavy meals, eating 5 to 6 small meals instead.

Vaginal Discharge

1. *Realize* that the most likely cause is yeast infection no matter the previous diagnosis. The second most likely cause is chronic infection from bacteria or parasites such as Trichomonas.

2. *Reduce* or eliminate the intake of sugar and starch.

3. *Rub* the vaginal walls with the lovely, exotic Oil of Myrtle. This is not only soothing, but it is also antiseptic against both bacteria and yeasts. Apply the oil two or three times daily.

4. *Eliminate* all caffeinated beverages.

5. *Increase* your intake of garlic and onions which are especially helpful if they are raw or lightly cooked.

6. *Take* an oregano-garlic supplement. The most effective type for

directly killing yeasts and parasites is one made from uncooked or unprocessed herbs. Oregamax contains wild, unprocessed oregano as well as garlic and onion. Take 2 or more capsules three times daily until the condition clears.

7. *Include* an acidophilus/bifidus supplement, taking a dose every morning and night. Do this regularly for best results.

<u>For Men Only</u>

Prostate Trouble

1. *Take* zinc, 50 to 150 mg per day. Once symptoms are improved, reduce the dosage to 25 to 50 mg daily.

2. *Take* Gene's powerdrops, wild greens formula, about 5 drops twice daily. This is potent, so only small amounts are needed, but it is safe to take more if necessary. These drops provide a wide range of nutrients needed to nourish and revitalize the sex glands. It is aggressive, providing both strength and energy.

3. *Heal* your prostate and urinary tract with chlorophyll. Rich sources of chlorophyll include chlorella, alfalfa, dark green vegetables, and chlorophyll extracts.

4. *Eat* a large handful of pumpkin or squash seeds two or three times daily.

5. *Better yet, add* the tasty and nutritious pumpkinseed oil tonic, Pumpkinol (from the highly nutritious Austrian pumpkin seeds), about one or two tablespoons daily. Or, get the benefits of pumpkinseed oil in a capsule; take ProstaClenz, a special formulation for prostate support, 1 or more capsules daily. ProstaClenz is a special concentrate of pumpkinseed oil which meets the exacting German standards for herbal formulas. It is a 10:1 concentrate and contains herbs which are synergistic in aiding prostate function. Ideally, take both, like a tablespoon of pumpkinseed oil and one or two ProstaClenz caps daily.

Impotence

1. *Eliminate* alcohol, since it causes impotence. The regular consumption of alcohol causes atrophy of the testicles and reduces circulation to the sexual organs.

2. *Increase* your dosage of zinc. You can take between 75 to 100 mg. per day, but, once sexual function returns, reduce the dose, because high amounts of zinc may cause copper deficiency. Ideally, when taking large amounts of zinc, take also copper, 2 to 4 mg daily.

3. *Take* bee pollen, since it contains amino acids and hormones which stimulate sex drive. You need to stay on it for at least 4 months.

4. *Use* the exotic Oil of Myrtle as an aphrodisiac. This is used topically, so rub it all over the body, and it is particularly effective for improving the mood for women.

5. *Add* Royal Kick premium royal jelly, since it stimulates the activity of the sexual glands and boosts the powers of the adrenal glands.

6. *Be* sure to increase your dose of selenium. Take at least 400 mcg. per day.

7. *B vitamins* are important, because they assist all the functions related to the sexual glands. For natural, unprocessed B vitamins, take Nutri-Sense, 3 Tbsp in juice or water daily.

8. *Vitamin E* helps improve circulation to the genitals and increases virility if taken in doses of 800 to 1200 I.U. per day.

9. *Take* Oil of Cilantro/coriander (the edible, natural type), a historically famous aphrodisiac, 20 drops daily.

Receding Hairline

In certain individuals it is possible to stop the hair loss associated with male pattern baldness. In some instances new hair growth can be stimulated. There are innumerable hair treatments, potions, and/or nutritional supplements available for treating this condition, and this can be stultifying. The following protocol will help guide you through this confusion. After several years of trial and error, these are the nutritional agents and lifestyle changes I have found to be the most effective:

1. *Stop* the intake of alcohol if you are a drinker, and if you are a smoker, quit.

2. *Control* your stress, and if you are a worrier, stop worrying. Both cause the muscles in the scalp to tighten, cutting off blood flow to the hair follicles.

3. *Use* a shampoo containing pure herbal extracts. One of the finest is *Shampure*, which is made by the Aveda Corporation. Shampure also contains sources of essential fatty acids such as avocado oil. This oil is valuable for promoting strong healthy hair shafts.

4. *Take* large amounts of essential fatty acids. The more that is consumed, the more aggressive the hair growth will be. It is necessary to take extra doses of B vitamins to help metabolize the fatty acids. You'll need lecithin, primrose oil, cold-pressed vegetable oil, and/or crude Austrian pumpkinseed oil, i.e. Pumpkinol. The best thing to do is make a fatty acid cocktail, and take it morning and night.

5. *Increase* your dosage of zinc to at least 50 mg per day. White spots on the nails indicate a severe zinc deficiency. This may indicate the need to take even higher doses of zinc. Do not exceed 100 mg per day. If taking zinc for prolonged periods, be sure to also take copper, 3 to 5 mg daily.

6. *Try* the highly aromatic, exotic Oil of Bay Berry by North American Herb & Spice Co. This is the newest, most promising breakthrough in hair treatment. Active ingredients include unique herbal oils and fatty acids, which stimulate inactive hair follicles and keep active ones from degenerating. The result is improved sheen, texture, and thickness. For more information contact North American Herb & Spice Co., P.O. Box 4885, Buffalo Grove, IL 60089 (800)243-5242.

7. *Take* Gene's Powerdrops, wild greens formula, a potent source of crude natural vegetable proteins. The nutrients in the powerdrops are severely deficient in people with hair loss.

8. *Increase* your protein intake. Try one of the protein shakes listed in the recipe section. Be sure to take the protein regularly, at least twice per day.

9. *Kill* the fungus that is probably growing on your scalp. Fungal infection is a certainty if you have seborrhea or psoriasis of the scalp. Use Scalp Clenz, an essential oil-based solution, on the scalp at least twice per day. Rub the oil liberally into the scalp at night before bedtime. For additional antifungal power, add a few drops of oil of oregano and massage into the scalp. Take five drops of the oil to kill any fungus growing in the body. This treatment is the most important step. By killing the fungus new hair growth can be stimulated. Also, the oils and vitamins contained within this product nourish the hair follicles. Also, take oil of oregano (edible type) internally, 5 to 10 drops daily.

Maintenance Nutritional Supplement Program

Nutritional supplements are mandatory for anyone who is concerned about his/her health. Ideally, evaluate your own personal needs before beginning supplementation. This can be accomplished by utilizing the written tests in Dr. Cass Ingram's *Self-Test Nutrition Guide*. Through this book you can test yourself to determine specifically what are your deficiencies as well as the degree of the deficiencies. Or, for a more thorough assessment of your specific nutritional status, see the nutritional evaluation system on the World Wide Web, **NutritionTest.com**. This Web site is a convenient means for quickly determining an individual's precise nutritional deficiencies. It is a fee-for-results service, costing between $30.00 to $60.00. However, until this is accomplished the following serves as a basic nutritional program applicable to the majority of individuals:

Nutritional Supplements	**Dosage**
Multiple Vitamin/ Mineral (without iron if you are a non-anemic male or post-menopausal female)	1 to 2 tabs or caps daily
B complex	1-2 tabs or caps daily
Beta Carotene (natural source)	25,000 I.U. daily
Vitamin E (as free tocopherols)	400-800 I.U. daily
Selenium	300-500 micrograms daily, the higher dose being applicable in regions with selenium-deficient soil
Essential Fatty Acids (either as flax seed, borage, or primrose oil)	tablespoon or 6 capsules daily
Cod Liver Oil	teaspoon twice weekly
Fish Oils (EPA/ DHA)	6 capsules daily

Vitamin C

500 to 1000 mg daily. Preferably, use a natural vitamin C flavonoid supplement such as Flavin-C. In this case, small amounts of crude vitamin C are highly protective versus the large amounts needed of synthetic C.

Zinc

30-50 mg daily

Herbal/Food Supplements	**Dosage**
Oregamax wild oregano caps	2 to 4 caps daily
Powerdrops, wild veggie formula	5 to 10 drops daily
Powerdrops, wild berry formula	5 to 10 drops daily
Royal Kick premium royal jelly	2 to 4 caps every morning
Nutri-Sense	3 tablespoons every morning in juice, milk, or water (or on cereal)

This program offers significant protection against the ravages of modern living—pollution, radiation, toxic wastes, ozone, and heavy metals. It is also highly protective against stress. You may have deficiencies of other nutrients than those mentioned. If you can find a nutritionally-oriented health practitioner, he/she might be able to discover these deficiencies. Or, take the nutritional deficiency tests on **NutritionTest.com**. However, the aforementioned regimen offers a baseline, and this will suffice as protective for the majority of individuals.

Individuals who are exposed to even greater amounts of radiation or toxic chemicals need to double or even triple the dose of certain nutrients particularly garlic, beta carotene, chlorella, vitamin E, selenium, and vitamin C. Add edible oil of rosemary and oil of wild sage for additional protection. A partial list of susceptible individuals includes:

artists

auto mechanics

x-ray technicians

radiologists

scientists

painters

printing press operators

workers in chemical plants

airline pilots

flight attendants

frequent flyers

computer operators

machinists

Airline pilots, flight attendants, and frequent flyers should never forgo their daily dose of beta carotene. For this group it is advisable to take at least 50,000 I.U. of natural-source beta carotene daily. Radiologists and x-ray techs should take extra vitamin E and selenium. Cancer is far more prevalent in practitioners of these speciality fields. Why take chances? It would be better to practice overkill; that is, to take antioxidants to an excess rather than skimping on the only substances known to prevent cancer. It is far more dangerous to take too little than to take too much. Natural source beta carotene from algae or other natural sources is the supplement of choice.

Gene's powerdrops™, an extract of fresh raw wild greens and/or berries, is the superior source of antioxidants. This is especially true for those who wish to consume only crude or natural sources of antioxidants, vitamins, minerals, and beta carotene. The powerdrops are crude, unprocessed extracts, so they contain a wide range of flavonoids, carotenes, and antioxidants. They are potent; only a small amount, like 10 drops daily, is necessary.

There are four types of powerdrops: wild greens, wild red, wild purple, and wild berry. All contain a wide range of natural flavonoids, carotenes, and organic acids; all of these substances are potent antioxidants. For optimal results use the wild greens for vitamins, minerals, and beta carotene and the wild berry for crude flavonoids and pigments. Use the wild red as an unprocessed source of the highly potent antioxidant ellagic acid. This oxygen-rich flavonoid is one of the most powerful anti-cancer chemicals known. The wild purple type is ideal for providing the flavonoids needed for optimal vision, but it is also excellent for kidney and heart strength. Wild purple is also an excellent diabetes tonic. The powerdrops are completely natural; there is no concern for interactions with medications, except that the regular intake may decrease the need for drugs. That is a positive side effect.

Powerdrops are easy to take. They come in a tasty liquid form, so no pills are necessary. Simply take a few drops under the tongue as needed. They may be taken at separate times or all at once. They are wild and rare. What's more, they are extracted by a completely natural process. Absolutely no synthetic chemicals are used. Since they are made from wild herbs, vegetation, and berries, only a limited supply is available. The powerdrops may be ordered from the Wild Club by calling 1-800-243-5242. Sign up so you can receive a guaranteed supply.

PART III

For Doctors Only

PART III

For Doctors Only

I. Nutritional Protocols for Selected Diseases

This section lists many of the major diseases seen in North America today along with the nutrients that may be valuable in their treatment. Certainly, there are many other important nutrients, herbs, and remedies beside those mentioned, however, the effort herein is to describe those substances I have found most useful in the reversal of disease.

Note that the remedies for each condition have been divided into 1st and 2nd Priority and that a third category, *Foods and Herbs,* has also been listed. Those found in 1st Priority are the nutrients which have been firmly established by scientific and clinical studies to have a powerful curative effect. Those nutrients listed as 2nd Priority may be useful in improving the disease process and in preventing its progression although they may or may not have been proven through scientific studies. The beneficial effect of some of the substances listed under the category Foods and Herbs has been determined through scientific research, while others are listed as a result of clinical experience. I am a big fan of herbs and medicinal foods and, while vitamin and mineral therapy is crucial, it is the herbs and foods which possess the most magnificent healing properties. I have indicated my favorite remedies with an asterisk after items in this category.

Note that under the herb category essential oils are mentioned frequently. For internal consumption do not use commercial essential oils. Edible plant oils are produced by North American Herb & Spice Co. Items with an asterisk are listed in Appendix B.

Acne

1st Priority

vitamin A

vitamin B$_6$ (especially in
    adolescent acne)

riboflavin

acidophilus

zinc

essential fatty acids

2nd Priority

thiamine

biotin

beta carotene

fiber

Foods and Herbs

wild oregano (as Oregamax caps)*

oil of oregano (topical/internal—use only the edible type)*

oil of myrtle (topical)*

Pumpkinol™ (for essential fatty acids: top tonic for the skin)*

Note: Food allergies should be ruled out and all sources of caffeine
must be eliminated.

Alcohol Addiction

1st Priority

niacin

vitamin C

thiamine

vitamin B$_5$

folic acid

vitamin B$_{12}$

magnesium

zinc

essential fatty acids

glutamine (an amino acid)

2nd Priority

selenium

vitamin A

vitamin E

tyrosine

pantothenic acid

calcium

manganese

silicon

crude chromium (from red grape)

Foods and Herbs

rice bran (as Nutri-Sense™)*   ground flax seed (as Nutri-Sense™)
watermelon   fermented milk products
oil of rosemary   oil of cumin*
Royal Kick™ (for adrenal support)* Resvitanol™ (red sour grape)

Note: Alcoholics are commonly allergic to sugar and/or grains. They may also be allergic to yeasts. If you are an alcoholic aspiring towards abstinence, have your doctor perform the Food Intolerance Test to determine precisely what are your food allergies.

Arthritis

1st Priority	2nd Priority
vitamin C	folic acid
vitamin A	vitamin B_{12}
vitamin E	copper
niacin	manganese
vitamin B_6	PABA
essential fatty acids	thiamine
fish oils	riboflavin
vitamin D	
bioflavonoids	
magnesium	
calcium	
zinc	
selenium	
potassium	
pantothenic acid	

Foods and Herbs

wild oregano (oil/herb)*   garlic
onion   whole goat's milk
alfalfa   kelp(ThyroKelp)*
coriander leaf   raw honey
Gene's Powerdrops™, wild berry   Royal Kick™ premium royal jelly*

Candida Albicans Infection

1st Priority

essential fatty acids
selenium
zinc
vitamin A
magnesium
vitamin B_5
thiamine
biotin
folic acid
riboflavin

2nd Priority

vitamin B_{12}
calcium
vitamin E
beta carotene
bioflavonoids
digestive enzymes

Foods and Herbs

Fung-E-Clenz™
garlic
oil of oregano*

oil of myrtle (esp. yeast vaginitis)*
onion
Oregamax caps*

Cigarette Addiction

1st Priority

tyrosine
calcium
vitamin C
vitamin E
beta carotene
folic acid
vitamin B_{12}
thiamine
niacin

2nd Priority

magnesium
riboflavin
pantothenic acid

Foods and Herbs

Royal Kick premium royal jelly (for the nervous agitation and adrenal support)*
High protein diet (low in sugar)

Note: Few smokers quit with just nutrition alone. There must first be a desire to quit. If you smoke, the programs outlined in this book will not work for you until you quit.

Diabetes

1st Priority	2nd Priority
chromium	selenium
niacin	vitamin E
thiamine	vitamin A
biotin	carnitine
vitamin C	vitamin C
essential fatty acids	vitamin B_{12}
zinc	bioflavonoids
magnesium	fish oils
vitamin B_5	coenzyme Q-10
manganese	potassium

Foods and Herbs

rice bran as Nutri-Sense (rich in chromium and B vitamins)*

extra virgin olive oil (helps prevent circulatory damage)

cucumber

Diabagon™ (edible essential oil complex; proven by Georgetown University)*

Jerusalem or regular artichoke

garlic (helps reduce blood fats)

onion (helps reduce blood fats)

cumin and oil of cumin (potent blood sugar lowering herb)*

Herb-Sorb (a special encapsulated formula with fenugreek, coriander, cumin, and cardamom)*

Glaucoma

1st Priority	2nd Priority
vitamin C (preferably as fresh fruit, vegetables, or a natural	selenium
	zinc

extract— see Appendix B)   choline
bioflavonoids
vitamin B_6
folic acid
chromium
vitamin A
pantothenic acid

Foods and Herbs

Royal Kick premium royal jelly*
oil of sage (only the edible is by North American Herb & Spice)*
parsley
Gene's Wild Berry Powerdrops*

Heart Disease

1st Priority	2nd Priority
niacin	copper
chromium	zinc
vitamin E	vitamin A
fish oils	vitamin B_6
selenium	folic acid
carnitine	essential fatty acids
magnesium	potassium
taurine	
calcium	
manganese	
thiamine	
coenzyme Q-10	

Foods and Herbs

garlic and onions   extra virgin olive oil
Cardio Clenz (edible essential oil complex)*

kelp (as chemical-free
   ThyroKelp)*
Nutri-Sense (for its natural
   B-vitamin content)*

crude Austrian pumpkinseed oil
(alpine source, nutrient-dense)*
rosemary and oil of rosemary*
avocado

High Blood Pressure

1st Priority
potassium
magnesium
calcium
essential fatty acids
niacin
vitamin E

2nd Priority
selenium
vitamin B$_6$
lecithin
vitamin C
bioflavonoids

Foods and Herbs

fermented milk products (the calcium is easier to absorb due to the
   fermentation process)
fish oils and/or fatty fish
turnip, collard, or mustard greens
Essence of Rose Petals (drink an ounce in hot water twice daily as tea)*
oil of rosemary (edible type in olive oil)*
Hercules Strength (wild rosemary/sage/oregano herbal capsules)*
Resvitanol (unprocessed whole grape skin, seed, vine capsule)*

Hypoglycemia

1st Priority
chromium
niacin
thiamine
manganese
vitamin B$_6$
pantothenic acid
lipoic acid

2nd Priority
digestive enzymes
vitamin C
vitamin A
tyrosine
fiber

Foods and Herbs

dessicated liver tablets with or between meals
chlorella tablets taken between meals (for amino acids)
salty, healthy snacks (salted roasted nuts, olives, etc)
stabilized fresh royal jelly (Royal Oil)*
rice bran as Nutri-Sense (rich in B vitamins and chromium)*
Herb-Sorb (spices for blood sugar control)*
Diaba-Gon*

Hypothyroidism

1st Priority

thiamine
riboflavin
niacin
vitamin B_6
zinc
copper
potassium
iodine
tyrosine
essential fatty acids
vitamin A

2nd Priority

selenium
vitamin E
vitamin C
magnesium
calcium

Foods and Herbs

kelp and other iodine-rich sea vegetation (ThyroKelp)*
rice bran as Nutri-Sense (due to its rich thiamine and niacin content)*
fatty fish
seafood, particularly shrimp

Infertility

1st Priority

folic acid
vitamin B_{12}
vitamin A
vitamin E
vitamin C
selenium

2nd Priority

vitamin B_6
niacin
bioflavonoids
amino acids
iodine

zinc
essential fatty acids

Foods and Herbs

royal jelly (Royal Kick)*   bee pollen
oil of oregano (anti-infective)*   kelp (ThyroKelp)*
oil of fennel (edible type in olive oil)*

Osteoporosis

1st Priority	2nd Priority
calcium	copper
magnesium	boron
zinc	vitamin B_{12}
manganese	folic acid
silicon	riboflavin
vitamin A	vitamin K
vitamin D	
vitamin C	
essential fatty acids	
amino acids	

Foods and Herbs

Oregamax (natural source of bone-nourishing trace minerals)*
kelp (natural source of trace minerals)

Parkinson's Disease

1st Priority	2nd Priority
vitamin E	beta carotene
vitamin C	calcium
vitamin B_6	magnesium
selenium	folic acid
thiamine	vitamin B_{12}
tyrosine	lecithin

Foods and Herbs

oil of rosemary*

Hercules Strength (rosemary/sage herbal caps)*

oil of cumin*

Essence of Orange Blossoms (activates neuronal function; relaxes
nerves); add a tablespoon to hot water and drink as a tea twice
daily*

crude fresh/stabilized royal jelly (Royal Oil), as a source of unprocessed
pantothenic acid, biotin, amino acids, and other brain-nourishing
substances*

Stomach or Duodenal Ulcer

1st Priority	2nd Priority
fiber	selenium
vitamin C	vitamin B_1
bioflavonoids	
vitamin A	
zinc	
essential fatty acids	
vitamin U	
folic acid	
vitamin E	

Foods and Herbs

fresh-squeezed cabbage or potato/turnip juice

crude Austrian pumpkinseed oil plus essential oils (Pumpkinol)*

oil of oregano (anti-Helicobacter)*

Oregamax caps*

Herb-Sorb (digestive tonic)

Intesti Clenz (edible essential oil complex)*

II. Interpretation Guide for Routine Blood Chemistry

This section is a guide for both doctors and patients. In particular, the information will help doctors interpret routine blood chemistry in a nutritional manner. The lab figures are given either as milligrams per deciliter or units per liter.

Glucose. . . if high (above 105), this indicates a tendency towards the development of diabetes. If the fasting blood sugar consistently runs high, it is likely that a chromium deficiency exists. Adding chromium to the diet in the form of Brewer's yeast, chromium picolinate, or glucose tolerance factor should help lower the blood sugar. Even more powerful is to take blood sugar lowering herbs such as cumin, fenugreek, and fennel—all of these are found in the anti-diabetic formula, Diabagon. High sugar readings are also seen when the adrenal glands fail to work properly (known as adrenal insufficiency, subclinical Addison's disease, chronic adrenal failure, etc.).

Biotin, as well as thiamine, deficiency is likely. Niacin and pyridoxine help stabilize blood sugar levels. Magnesium helps drive glucose into the cells and this may also be deficient. Fiber intake should be increased. Use Nutri-Sense as a top source of naturally occurring thiamine, niacin, biotin, and magnesium. Increase red meat consumption and eat more avocados to get more natural pyridoxine. Use Royal Kick royal jelly to strengthen the adrenal glands, two capsules twice daily.

Glucose. . . . if low (below 70), hypoglycemic tendencies exist. Again, supplemental chromium and thiamine are indicated. A diet high in protein and low in sweets is suggested. Niacin and pyridoxine will help stabilize blood sugar levels.

If you have low blood sugar, it indicates that the adrenal glands are malfunctioning and are unable to prevent blood sugar levels from dropping. Levels may dip as low as 40 on occasion. Such drops explain mood swings, agitation, depression, fatigue, crying spells, as well as panic attacks, dizziness, and fainting. To regenerate the adrenal glands take Royal Kick, 4 to 6 capsules every morning.

If the above symptoms exist, a glucose tolerance test may be indicated. Also, magnesium levels should be checked in red cells. Magnesium is needed to drive glucose into the cells. Many hypoglycemics are deficient in magnesium as well as zinc. If white spots on the fingernails exist, be sure to give zinc, 50 to 75 mgs. daily.

It is crucial that hypoglycemic patients eat 2 to 3 between meal snacks to help stabilize blood sugar levels. This is in addition to eating three regular meals. Emphasize high protein breakfasts, although fresh fruit, especially the low sugar varieties, is often well tolerated. Snacks must be free of refined sugars, malt, corn syrup, etc.

Creatinine . . . . if high (above 1.2), think of chronic renal insufficiency. Levels over 1.4 usually indicate chronic renal failure. The kidneys can regenerate and, thus, mild elevations in creatinine levels are not always a cause for alarm. However, steadily increasing creatinine levels should be regarded seriously. In males consider stasis of urine due to a swollen, inflamed prostate. In females particularly, consider chronic infection (chronic pyelonephritis), especially if there is a history of bladder and/or kidney infections. The kidneys can be a reservoir for a variety of microbes ranging from E. coli to yeasts and tuberculosis. These germs often cause chronic infections which cannot be diagnosed by routine urine cultures. This is because the microbes are hidden deep within the recesses of the kidney tubules.

In cases involving swollen prostate glands zinc plus essential fatty acids are often curative. The kidneys begin to degenerate in essential fatty acid and/or vitamin A deficiency and, as a result, infection readily becomes established. Take two tablespoons of Austrian pumpkinseed oil, one tablespoon of cod liver oil along with 400 to 800 I.U. of vitamin E daily. Foods rich in potassium should be eaten regularly.

If chronic infection is suspected, do not give antibiotics alone. If the causative organism can be cultured, give antibiotics to which the organism is sensitive along with nutritional agents. In either case use the following nutritional program:

1. Red Sour Grape—6 to 8 capsules daily (for organic acid content)

2. Oregamax (wild oregano) capsules—2 or 3 caps three times daily

3. potassium and magnesium citrate—6 to 12 capsules daily (warning: diarrhea may occur at this dosage)

4. cod liver oil—1 teaspoon twice daily. Take this dosage for the duration of treatment only.

5. Lactobacillus acidophilus/bifidus culture—teaspoon three times daily.

6. essential fatty acids (flax seed oil or cold-pressed sunflower, safflower, soy, or walnut oil)—3 to 4 tablespoons daily.

7. watermelon—eat large quantities or squeeze it into juice. If using juice, drink 10 ounces three times daily. It acts as a mild natural diuretic.

8. fluids—drink a minimum of eight 10 oz. glasses of either water or juice, but avoid orange and grapefruit juices, as they may irritate the kidney/bladder.

9. honey—consume at least 10 ounces of pure raw honey. Honey helps by regulating fluid balance. The sugars within honey, once absorbed, increase the water content of blood by a powerful osmotic effect. This results in an increased rate of urine flow through the kidneys. To get this benefit it is necessary to consume large quantities of it. Ideally, use a honey with antiseptic powers such as wild oregano honey from the Mediterranean such as wild Thistle Honey or Wild Oregano Honey (see Appendix B). Do not be concerned about the sugar content of the honey. Unless the patient has a severe yeast infection, is allergic to sugars, has diabetes, or is severely hypoglycemic, honey is harmless.

10. juices—of special value are the ones rich in potassium which include apricot, tangerine, pomegranate, papaya, beet, and parsley. In addition, most of these juices are rich in vitamin A (beta carotene).

Creatinine....if low (below .7), think of protein deficiency or impaired protein digestion. Lowered levels are often seen in vegetarians. Reduced amounts of hydrochloric acid or impaired secretion of pancreatic enzymes must be considered. Thiamine and niacinamide both increase the secretion of hydrochloric acid and other digestive juices. Digestive enzymes, 2 to 3 tablets with meals, may improve protein assimilation. In addition pyridoxine and zinc are required for adequate protein digestion to proceed. The synthesis of digestive enzymes within the pancreas is dependent upon adequate tissue levels of both of these nutrients. Tissue pyridoxine levels can be assessed with the erythrocyte glutamate pyruvate transaminase test, which is performed at specialty labs only.

Sodium....if high (above 144), think first of dehydration. Kidney disease is possible especially if potassium levels are also elevated. Water softeners or tap water contaminated with sodium can be responsible. If the adrenal glands are producing excess amounts of cortical hormones, blood sodium levels can be elevated. Softened water, which is high in sodium, should be avoided and salt consumption in foods reduced. High doses of vitamin C, pantothenic acid, thiamine, niacin, and vitamin A will relax the adrenal glands and help stop sodium retention.

Sodium....if low (below 139), think first of adrenal cortical insufficiency. The adrenal glands secrete aldosterone—a hormone which conserves sodium. When this hormone is lacking sodium is easily lost through the kidneys. Other causes include acute or chronic diarrhea and kidney disorders. A low sodium level in an individual who is not acutely ill usually means chronic adrenal failure. Symptoms, such as fatigue headaches, indigestion, cold extremities, and constipation, may also be elicited. The adrenal glands secrete over 50 hormones. Thus, the presentation of a person with adrenal insufficiency may be varied and complex. Their symptoms are often vague. Yet, they do fit a pattern, that is if the sodium level remains persistently low. Look for other evidence of adrenal failure such as pigmentation changes, vitiligo, eczema, thin hair, hair loss on the outer third of the legs, and crowding of the lower incisors. Other findings on routine blood chemistry include mild eosinophilia (above 1.5), lymphocytosis, an excessively low cholesterol, and an elevated serum potassium. If you suspect adrenal insufficiency, a 24 hr. urinary ketosteroid and hydroxycorticosteroid determination are indicated.

Potassium....if high (above 5.0), be sure to rule out the more serious causes such as diabetes metabolic acidosis kidney disease or lung disease. As mentioned hypoadrenalism is associated with a high serum potassium. In most cases this potassium elevation is not due to diet or supplements but is caused by a leakage of potassium from the cells into the bloodstream.

Potassium....if low (below 3.7), think first of severe cellular potassium deficiency, since this can lead to fatal cardiac arrhythmia (especially if levels fall below 3.5). If the patient has diarrhea or is vomiting this is the likely cause, since much potassium can be lost through the digestive juices. Use raw honey, 1/3 cup three to four times daily. Many honeys, especially dark ones, are rich in potassium. Honey stops diarrhea by holding water and digestive juices within the gut by helping the immune system eradicate the infection or eliminate the toxin. Imported honeys produced by bees which visit medicinal plants are the ideal type to use. Two examples are Wild Oregano Honey and Wild Thistle Honey. For information on raw honeys and/or mineral-rich dark honeys derived from wild plants see Appendix B.

Be sure to evaluate the patient's diet. Diets high in refined foods eventually induce a potassium deficiency. By the time blood levels become lowered the cells have become extremely deficient. Ask about drug usage. Diuretic use is one of the most common causes of low potassium.

Treatment should consist of potassium supplements as either citrate, acetate, aspartate, or similar amino acid chelates. Avoid potassium chloride tablets (Slow-K, etc.) since their use is associated with a high incidence of gastric and/or intestinal ulcerations. Foods rich in potassium should be added liberally to the diet. These include:

almonds
apricots dried
bananas especially plantain
basil
Brazil nuts
cabbage
cantaloupe
cashews
chestnuts
dates
dill weed
hazelnuts
honey (darker varieties)
honeydew melon
mango
molasses (blackstrap)

papaya
paprika
parsley
parsnips
peaches, dried
peanuts
pecans
pomegranate
prunes
raisins
red pepper
soybean flour
squash (the winter variety is
    particularly high)
tomatoes (especially tomato juice)
turmeric
watermelon

Uric Acid....if high (above 7.5), think of impaired protein synthesis or utilization. Uric acid is a waste product of nucleic acid metabolism. Nucleic acids are the nuclear materials (i.e. RNA and DNA) used by the body to initiate the synthesis of proteins. A high uric acid level may indicate that proteins are being broken down too rapidly. Sugar increases uric acid levels, probably by causing tissue destruction or by increasing the rate at which proteins are broken down. High uric acid may also indicate the need for supplemental folic acid, since this vitamin is involved in the metabolism of nucleic acids. A recent study showed that supplementation with folic acid decreased elevated levels.

Medical conditions associated with elevated uric acid levels include gout, kidney disease, diuretic overuse, diabetes, asthma, rheumatoid arthritis, hyperparathyroidism, and liver disease.

Treatment should include removal of all sources of refined sugar. Foods rich in potassium, magnesium, and folates should be prescribed. Vitamins C, E, A, and other antioxidants should be added. It is interesting to note that uric acid itself has antioxidant-like functions. A large glass of freshly squeezed vitamin A rich vegetable juice, such as carrot-parsley juice, can also be taken daily.

Uric Acid....if low (below 4.0), think first of folic acid deficiency. A lack of uric acid means that not enough nuclear material is being synthesized.

Folic acid, and, to a lesser degree, B_{12} are the key nutrients in this sequence. Adding 5 and up to 20 mgs. of folic acid daily often brings the uric acid to normal. If you see levels as low as 2.5, severe folic acid deficiency is likely. Foods rich in RNA/DNA should be included in the diet, for example:

sardines	other cold water fish
chicken	turkey
liver	wheat or rice germ

Many of the above foods are also rich in antioxidants. Beta carotene, selenium, and vitamin E protect RNA and DNA from damage by radiation and toxic compounds. So do herbal antioxidants such as rosemary, oregano, and sage. The intake of these substances should be increased if uric acid levels are abnormal.

Bilirubin (Total or Direct)....if either of these are elevated, this is evidence of severe liver disease. Viral hepatitis is the first concern, although cancer and other obstructive liver diseases are possible.

Treatment is difficult in the case of obstructive diseases. If the diagnosis of viral hepatitis is confirmed, various foods and herbs which purge bile from the liver may be utilized. Perhaps the most valuable of these is the juice of beets. An 8 oz. glass of beet juice combined with a quarter cup of olive oil and the juice of one whole lemon or lime (that is, if the patient is not citrus intolerant) could help lower bilirubin levels by increasing fecal bile content. As described in Chapter 6 herbal antioxidants, particularly the edible oils of rosemary, cumin, and oregano, halt liver cell damage and prevent further damage from occurring. Large doses of these herbal antioxidants, which are safe for human consumption, stimulates the immune system, helping the body control the growth of the virus as well as assisting the immune system in destroying it. These antioxidants also act to prevent the breakdown of red cell membranes, which will further aggravate the bilirubin levels. In particular, cumin is invaluable, because, in addition to being a potent liver antioxidant, it also dramatically increases bile flow. This is of obvious importance in the event of high bilirubin or biliary stasis.

Bilirubin (Total or Direct)....if decreased (below .2), think first of anemia due to iron deficiency. Less bilirubin is being made because fewer red cells are available for turnover. Barbituates and aspirin derivatives may lower bilirubin measurements.

Bilirubin (Indirect)....if high (above .9), it is likely that more bilirubin is being formed than the body eliminate. Several types of anemia, including hereditary types, like sickle cell and thalassemia, increase indirect bilirubin. In these conditions red blood cells are being rapidly destroyed due to their abnormal shape and function. Inflammatory conditions throughout the body, as well as hepatic inflammation, may also be responsible. If the indirect bilirubin is the only form elevated, it is likely that the patient has a malfunctioning inflamed liver. Treatment is the same as with elevated total bilirubin, with the addition of oil of edible ginger, turmeric, fish oils, and other anti-inflammatory nutrients.

Recent research indicates that certain spice extracts are exceptionally valuable for lowering elevated bilirubin levels. Oils of edible cumin, coriander, rosemary, and oregano have all been shown to improve liver function and increase bile flow. An increase in bile flow is crucial for the reversal of this condition. Liva Clenz is a special formula containing the edible essential oils known to normalize bile synthesis and assist liver function. As a hepatic tonic take 5 or more drops twice daily. Also, take edible oil of ginger, 5 or more drops twice daily.

Triglycerides....if the fasting level is high (above 150), think first of carbohydrate excess and/or alcoholism. I often recommend both fasting and post-prandial (after eating) triglyceride measurements. It is a good idea to see how the body reacts to the norms of life. Levels above 250 after eating indicate severe carbohydrate intolerance. Deficiencies of chromium, niacin, biotin, thiamine, inositol, and magnesium are likely. Essential fatty acid deficiency is another important factor. Hypothyroidism must always be ruled out, since this leads to a defect in how rapidly sugars and starches are metabolized.

Reduce all dietary sources of carbohydrates and watch the triglycerides drop. Carnitine and niacin are most helpful in increasing the rate of fat clearance from the blood stream. They also stimulate its combustion into fuel by the cells. Add to the diet foods rich in carnitine, including avocado, lamb, beef, and chicken. Rice bran or Nutri-Sense is helpful, since it is high in fiber and rich in thiamine and chromium. Chromium, if well absorbed, can cause a dramatic reduction in triglyceride levels.

In stubborn cases check for food intolerance. Allergies to sugar, molasses, malt, etc. can cause elevated triglyceride levels.

Triglycerides....if low (below 50), think of liver malfunction. It is normal to have a certain amount of fat in the blood. Fats are required as a source of fuel for organs such as the heart and kidneys. The liver makes proteins for carrying triglycerides to these organs. Abnormally low triglyceride levels often indicate poor protein synthesis in the liver or impaired hepatic synthesis of fatty acids. Such patients need high doses of essential fatty acids. They also desperately need the B vitamins used in protein and fatty acid synthesis. These include choline, inositol, biotin, niacin, and pantothenic acid, all of which are found in a natural form in Nutri-Sense.

A triglyceride level below 40 is a strong indication of essential fatty acid deficiency. Zinc is needed before essential fatty acids can be properly utilized. Up to 100 mg daily may be helpful. A word of caution—large doses of zinc should not be administered without monitoring the red blood count. In susceptible individuals too much zinc can cause a copper deficiency anemia. This occurs because excess zinc blocks the absorption of copper from the gut. On the other hand, some liver diseases (e.g. Wilson's disease) are associated with extremely high blood and liver levels of copper. In this instance high doses of zinc would be of exceptional value.

Resvitanol, a sour grape extract, is an exceptionally rich source of naturally occurring chromium. Chromium is a powerful substance for lowering triglyceride levels. Plus, Resvitanol is a natural source of the cardiovascular aid, *resveratrol.* Take 3 capsules twice daily.

Cholesterol....if high (above 205), first check for excess dietary carbohydrate. If this is not the case, consider that there exists an increased need for antioxidant protection. Cholesterol is one of the most important antioxidants made by the body. It protects cell membranes from all sorts of noxious insults. An elevated cholesterol level despite a low carbohydrate diet indicates the existence of oxidative damage to cell membranes. As a rule the higher the cholesterol is the greater the free radical activity. When an extremely high cholesterol develops in an individual, I am more concerned about the oxidative damage that is occurring than an imminent heart attack. Try to determine what is causing the elevated free radical activity. Increase dosages of all antioxidants, particularly vitamin E, beta carotene, and selenium. Take herbal antioxidants, such as rosemary, cumin, fenugreek, red sour grape extract, and wild oregano capsules, and watch the cholesterol drop.

Cholesterol is a critical component of cell membranes. It is required for membrane synthesis and repair. Any process which damages cell membranes may cause a secondary rise in cholesterol levels. In other words, the body mobilizes the cholesterol so it can use it in tissue repair.

Nutrients which help reduce cholesterol levels via a sort of fat burning mechanism include niacin, carnitine, vitamin C, taurine, lecithin, and fiber. Garlic, onion, and shiitake mushroom extract all contain substances which help normalize cholesterol synthesis in the liver. Large doses of fish oils (greater than 3.0 grams daily) can be helpful. However, similar results can be achieved by increasing the consumption of fatty fish such as albacore tuna, salmon, sardines, herring, and halibut. The regular consumption of extra virgin olive oil lowers cholesterol levels better than polyunsaturates. However, the most important element is to change the diet and eliminate all sources of refined sugar and starch, including alcohol.

Cholesterol....if decreased (below 160), this may be a sign of immune decline. Think also of adrenal insufficiency. Levels below 130 are highly correlated with cancer. Normalizing low cholesterol levels is often difficult. Squalene is a precursor to cholesterol synthesis. It is found in high amounts in the livers of sharks. Sharks almost never get cancer. Pure extra virgin olive oil also contains squalene. Lowered cholesterol may be an indication of severe manganese deficiency. This could be revealed by a hair analysis or a whole blood manganese level. As of yet there is no first-class test available for assessing manganese nutrition. Regardless, foods rich in manganese should be added to the diet. These include:

almonds	avocados
beets	beet tops
blackberries	blueberries
boysenberries	Brazil nuts
chard, Swiss	chestnuts (fresh)
coconut	figs (dried)
ginger	green beans
lettuce	lima beans
liver	loganberries
navy beans	parsley
peaches, dried	peanuts
pears, dried	persimmons
pineapple	potatoes
raisins	raspberries
rice bran and polishings	soybeans
spices	spinach
strawberries	sunflower seeds
turnip greens	walnuts
wheat germ	whole grain flours

Absorption of manganese from wheat, rye, and oats and other grains may be compromised due to the existence of phytates, which bind minerals so tightly that they cannot be easily absorbed. A similar problem may exist with nuts, which are the richest food source of manganese. Therefore, fruits, vegetables, and meats constitute the best sources, since the manganese they contain is more readily digested and assimilated than the type found in nuts and grains.

Other nutrients important for the metabolism of cholesterol include thiamine, vitamin C, lipoic acid, and essential fatty acids. One of the early signs of essential fatty acid deficiency is an increased cholesterol level. Later, however, the cholesterol often falls well below the normal range. If cholesterol levels are persistently low, check for other signs of essential fatty acid deficiency such as dry skin, constipation, eczema, dry or oily hair, etc.

A significant ill-effect of lowered cholesterol is reduced adrenal hormone synthesis. Without cholesterol, the hormones of the adrenal cortex cannot be produced. The consequences are usually disastrous. Without adequate adrenal cortical hormones a wide range of diseases develops, including arthritis, fungal infections, skin diseases (especially psoriasis and eczema), colitis, chronic pain, hypoglycemia, and even fatal cardiac arrhythmia. There is another serious side effect—immune decay. A complex interaction exists between adrenal hormones and immune function. It is well known that patients with Addison's disease, the extreme type of adrenal failure, are vulnerable to a wide range of infections, particularly fungal infections. If left untreated, such patients can die from infections by opportunistic microorganisms.

A very low cholesterol must not be taken lightly, and in some ways is more ominous than high levels. Anyone with a cholesterol level below 150 to 160 should eat foods rich in cholesterol, including liver, sweetbreads, eggs, beef, lamb, butter, whole milk, and cheese. What's more, sea salt should be regularly consumed, since it helps boost adrenal function by stimulating steroid synthesis. The adrenal gland is the primary organ for conserving salt, and, when it is weakened the body wastes salt. Perhaps the most useful cholesterol-lowering agent is the extract of red sour grape. Known as Resvitanol, this crude grape concentrate contains all of the flavonoids, minerals, and vitamins naturally found in wilderness grapes, because it is made with all components: the skin, seed, vine, and leaf. Plus, it is unique, because it is made from wilderness/mountain-grown grapes, not the genetically modified types as found in commercial grapes. Note: this is not the same as Pycnogenol or grape seed extract, which is chemically treated. Resvitanol is a crude grape supplement, completely unprocessed and free of all chemical residues.

Calcium...if high (above 10.2), think first of the mobilization of excess amounts of calcium from bone (secondary hyperparathyroidism). This can be caused by aluminum toxicity, lithium carbonate therapy, and vitamin D deficiency or even calcium deficiency itself. Often a dose of 1500 to 2000 mg of absorbable calcium with vitamin D (the best source of vitamin D is cod liver oil) will bring the calcium to normal. Other trace minerals, such as magnesium, zinc, copper, and manganese, are needed to maintain bone density, as is vitamin A.

Refined sugar causes the mobilization of calcium and magnesium from bone. This can result in either high or low serum calcium values. Although much ado has been made concerning the possible connection of high protein diets with osteoporosis, refined sugar is the primary culprit. The consumption of refined sugar dramatically increases the mobilization of trace minerals from bone. Do not concentrate on reducing protein intake. Instead, first reduce carbohydrate consumption (especially the refined sugar). A recent study found that adding a protein supplement to the diet, in this case powdered milk, increased bone density. This only makes sense; bone consists primarily of protein bound to minerals.

Calcium....if decreased (below 9.0), a calcium deficiency exists. However this can be caused by a variety of factors, including:

1. low stomach acid output *(hypochlorhydria)*
2. vitamin D deficiency
3. dietary calcium deficiency
4. kidney disease
5. pregnancy (all the calcium is being used up)
6. hypoparathyroidism
7. maldigestion of protein
8. liver dysfunction
9. alcoholic gastritis

The liver makes proteins (e.g. albumin) which act to bind and carry calcium. If the patient does not respond to supplementation with calcium (1500 to 2000 mgs. per day) and vitamin D (two tablespoons of cod liver oil daily), the liver is probably defective in protein synthesis. This would be confirmed by borderline low levels of serum albumin and/or globulin. The answer to this dilemma is to boost albumin and globulin production in the liver. Researchers have determined that herbal antioxidants dramatically enhance the health of the liver cells, improving their capacity to act as synthetic factories. To synthesize a greater amount of albumin/globulin, take the edible oils of rosemary, cumin, and oregano, five drops of each twice daily in juice or water.

The most ideal means to take calcium may not be via megadose pills. Instead, take calcium in the form of calcium-rich wild herbs. As an ideal natural "homeopathic" calcium supplement, take Oregamax, 4 or more capsules twice daily.

Phosphorus....if high (above 4.2), think of dietary excess (soft drinks are high in phosphates, as is red meat). Soft drinks may be the major cause in adolescents, since recent surveys show that teenagers and young adults drink up to twice the volume of soft drinks as water. Persistent elevations may indicate kidney dysfunction, and chronic infection in the kidneys is possible. In addition, both the parathyroid glands and liver manage phosphorus nutrition. Hypofunction of the parathyroids is possible.

Phosphorus....if decreased (below 2.5), think of vitamin D deficiency. Reduced secretion of gastric juices, especially hydrochloric acid, is possible. Low phosphorus is also seen in diabetes and liver disease. Be sure the diet is rich in high phosphorus foods, which include fish, red meat, poultry, eggs, cheese, nuts, seeds, rice bran, soybeans, and peanut butter. In addition, supplement the diet with two tablespoons of cod liver oil daily for at least one month. Increased exposure to sunlight, especially for the elderly, may be necessary.

Alkaline Phosphatase....if elevated (above 110), think first of liver disease. A large concentration of this enzyme is found in the liver, although it is also prevalent in bone and intestinal mucosa. Disease or destruction of any of these tissues leads to elevated levels. In the event of significant elevation the first thought should be either obstructive liver disease or bone disease. Cancer metastases to the bone should be ruled out. However, a wide range of conditions can lead to elevated alkaline phosphatase levels. Be sure also to check the patient's medication list, since drug-induced liver toxicity is a likely cause. The level in children is normally elevated due to bone growth.

Alkaline Phosphatase....if low (below 45), think of zinc deficiency. Zinc is a cofactor for this enzyme, and enzyme synthesis is dependent upon adequate tissue levels of it. Folic acid deficiency may also lead to reduced levels. It is likely that protein digestion in general is impaired. Give 50 to 100 mgs. of zinc and 5 or more mgs. of folic acid daily.

Liver Enzymes (SGOT, SGPT)....if high (above 40), think of inflammation of the liver, i.e. hepatitis. This condition is usually caused by an infection, although toxic chemicals can cause a form of hepatitis. Remember that one of the primary functions of the liver is to detoxify various chemicals and poisons. Whenever there is an exposure to noxious chemicals, they are concentrated specifically in the liver.

    In either case large doses of antioxidants are needed. Beet juice or powder may help heal the liver and decrease enzyme levels. There are many natural substances which have been discovered to heal liver damage and lower elevated enzyme levels. A few of them are mentioned below:

- raw or crude liver extract
- garlic extract

- lipoic acid
- thiamine (as Allithiamine)
- lecithin
- choline
- methionine

- cumin and oil of cumin
- biotin
- oil of rosemary
- cysteine
- selenium

Other herbs which have a protective effect upon liver cells include silymarin, turmeric, licorice root, and ginger. Elevations of SGOT have been associated with selenium deficiency, and increasing tissue stores of this mineral offers significant protection. It is likely that this effect is due to increased synthesis of glutathione peroxidase by hepatocytes.

It is important to note that a significant percentage of the weight of the liver consists of *Kupffer* cells. These are phagocytic cells which clear debris, toxins, and microorganisms before they can do damage. When these cells begin to malfunction, they can become easily overwhelmed, and all sorts of health problems can result. Their proper function is dependent upon an adequate supply of a variety of nutrients. Vitamins A, C, E, B vitamins, selenium, zinc, and essential fatty acids are especially important. If liver enzymes are elevated, Kupffer cells are being overloaded, and viral, bacterial, fungal, and even parasitic infection can run rampant throughout the body and/or within the liver itself. In addition, carbohydrate intolerance may lead to elevated liver enzymes. This damage is a result of the liver being infiltrated by fat. This fatty infiltration results when excess dietary carbohydrates are synthesized into triglycerides and other storage forms of fat. Do not take mild elevations of liver enzymes lightly. At a minimum improve the diet, eliminate the refined carbohydrates, and curtail the booze.

Globulin....if high (above 3.3), think first of hypertrophy of the lymphoid tissue within the bone marrow or lymphatic system. On a more serious scale this could represent the existence of lymphoid tumors, especially if the levels are above 3.5. The liver is also involved in globulin synthesis. Therefore, inflammatory diseases of the liver, especially mononucleosis and hepatitis, should be ruled out. Persistent elevations of globulin levels leads to the suspicion of viral replication within B-lymphocytes, which causes dysfunctional antibody synthesis. Infections by parasites or bacteria are also possible. Large doses of nutrients which nourish the immune system and liver may be needed. Vitamin A (2 to 3 tablespoons of cod liver oil daily) could help squelch the B-lymphocyte proliferation. Selenium, zinc, calcium, magnesium, and manganese are also important, as are the B vitamins, especially B_5, and folic acid.

For greater power in halting the globulin proliferation rely upon the antiseptic herbs. The lymphoctes are likely proliferating due to a stimulus, and the most likely one is infection. To bombard the infection use Oreganol oil of oregano, 5 to 10 drops three times daily in juice or water. Also, take 2 or three drops under the tongue three times daily.

Globulin....if low (below 2.3), think of impaired globulin synthesis by the liver and B-lymphocytes. Most people with low globulin levels are deficient in manganese, zinc, selenium, and other trace minerals needed for protein synthesis. These minerals cannot be properly absorbed or transported in the blood without globulin proteins. This is a monumental problem, because these minerals are required for globulin synthesis. What's more, it is likely that the immune system is under pressure and a chronic viral or yeast infection is almost assured. When globulin levels drop below 2.0, the body becomes vulnerable to invasion by opportunistic microorganisms. This includes colonization of the mucous membranes by Candida albicans or various parasites such as Giardia or amoebas. The liver also becomes much more susceptible to becoming infected, particularly by parasites.

Raising the globulin level often poses a challenge. Liberating the immune system from chronic infections is the prime objective. This can be most readily achieved by consuming the antiseptic herbs, notably oregano, cumin, thyme, garlic, and onion. Attempting to do so with commercial sources of these spices is insufficient. To accelerate the process take oil of oregano and oil of cumin, 5 drops of each three times daily.

Low globulin may indicate dysfunction of the thyroid and adrenal glands. It may also be a sign of systemic vitamin A deficiency. Regarding the latter, look for other signs such as dry or scaly skin, follicular hyperkeratosis (skin that looks like "gooseflesh"), vision disturbances, night blindness, brittle hair, pitted or decayed teeth, chronic diarrhea, etc. Give cod liver oil, 1 tablespoon twice daily, reducing this dosage to a tablespoon weekly once the deficiency is corrected. Be sure to add vitamin E to the cod liver oil after opening to prevent rancidity. In addition, studies have shown that high doses of folic acid and vitamin B_5 (pantothenic acid) raise globulin levels. The likely mechanism is increased globulin synthesis by B-lymphocytes. In this respect it would be wise to add vitamin B_{12}, since it is also required for normal globulin synthesis to proceed.

If a cardiac patient has a low globulin level, beware—his/her ability to transport minerals may be impaired. In such a patient the dose of heart healing minerals, such as calcium, magnesium, copper, zinc, and manganese, must be doubled. These minerals are far more valuable in maintaining the health of the heart than any drug or surgical procedure.

HDL Cholesterol....if low (below 40), think first of liver dysfunction. The liver synthesizes most of the HDL fraction found in the body. Improved liver function will automatically result in an increase in the liver's ability to synthesize proteins such as HDL. In addition, the following is a list of nutrients proven to increase HDL levels:

- chromium
- garlic extract
- red grape extract
- niacin
- vitamin C

- carnitine
- fish oils
- lecithin
- olive oil
- vitamin E

WBC (White blood count)....if high (above 8.9), think of significant infections within the tissues or organs, primarily bacterial and viral infections. Counts above 10.0 usually warn of severe bacterial infection, which may be life-threatening. Extreme—perhaps life threatening—fungal infections may also cause white counts above 10.0.

Often, such massive infections occur, and, yet, it is difficult to determine the site. The foci of infection may be difficult to determine, but likely sites include the teeth, appendix, sinuses, liver, spleen, bloodstream, kidneys, bladder, and pelvic organs. Or, it could be an abscess in such organs which develops after a surgical procedure.

Treatment must be aggressive and may include the need for antibiotics. Natural antiseptics may also be used, particularly oil of oregano (North American Herb & Spice, blue label). Take at least 10 drops three times daily in juice or water. Make a broth of garlic and yellow onions and drink several cups daily. Have your doctor check your white count regularly until it normalizes.

WBC (White blood count)....if low (below 6.0), think of immune suppression as well as malnutrition. The immune suppression is likely caused by chronic infection, notably by viruses and fungi. It is ironic that while bacterial infections raise the white count, yeast and viral infections usually depress it. For viruses the reason is obvious: they thrive by attacking cells, including white blood cells, parasitizing them. To boost the white count the first thing to do is kill the offending organism(s). Take oil of oregano, 5 to 10 drops three times daily in juice or water along with 2 drops under the tongue twice daily. Take Oregamax, 2 or 3 capsules twice daily. For more stubborn infestations double or triple this amount.

White counts below 5.0 indicate severe malnutrition as well as infection. To help nourish and rebuild the white cells take the following nutrients/supplements:

- Nutri-Sense: three heaping tablespoons daily in whole milk or juice
- folic acid: 5 to 10 mg daily
- dessicated liver (fresh organic liver is superior): 8 tabs daily
- Gene's wild greens powerdrops, 10 drops once or twice daily
- fresh meat, especially beef, turkey, and lamb: two large servings daily

RBC (Red blood count)....if high (above 5.9), this is a warning of polycythemia. In this condition excessive amounts of red blood cells clog the blood vessels, leading to impaired circulation. Ultimately, the individual may develop heart and/or lung damage as a result of poor circulation and/or sludging of the blood. To help normalize the blood count the giving of blood may be necessary.

A high count could also result from changing altitude, in other words, individuals who move to areas of high altitude may develop this over a period of years. Eventually, in the majority of individuals the count will stabilize and no harm is done. However, certain individuals may develop a type of chronic mountain sickness, and the primary symptoms are mental confusion, exhaustion, headache, and a ruddy color, some individuals may even develop cyanosis (blueness of the skin) upon exertion. Other causes of high red count include cigarette smoking, prescription steroids (i.e. cortisone/Prednisone), and, more rarely, tumors.

RBC (Red Blood count)....if low (below 4.85), this is an obvious sign of malnourishment. Causes include severe protein deficiency, malabsorption, celiac disease, B vitamin deficiency, hypothyroidism, and iron deficiency. Tapeworm infestation can lead to a low red count; the worms actually eat red blood cells as food. Toxicity can cause low red cell counts, and, if the count is below 4.0, lead poisoning or radiation exposure must be ruled out. Vitamin B_{12} deficiency is the most common nutritional cause of a reduction of red cells. Genetic deficiencies, such as sickle cell anemia and thalassemia, may also be indicated. However, drug toxicity is even a more common cause. Arthritis medications, such as aspirin, Motrin, Naprosyn, and Indocin, are major causes of red blood cell destruction.

To build up the blood eat organic calve's and/or lamb's liver as well as red meat. The best blood building vegetables are avocados, arugula, spinach, beets, and watercress. Certain wild spices build blood, notably cumin, oregano, and mountain sumac (Rhus coriaria). Red Sour Grape, made from the dessicated pure entire grape, including he skin and vine, is the ideal blood builder. Consume 6 or more capsules daily. Take also Oregamax, 6 to 8 capsules daily. Wild oregano is one of the top food sources of natural iron. The iron in oregano is helpful to the body, in other words, it is non-toxic.

Hemoglobin....if high (above 17.0), this may indicate excessive iron in the tissues. It also warns of too many red blood cells (polycythemia). The result of the excess red blood cells is impaired circulation due to sludging of the blood. Vitamin E and fish oils help liquify the blood. However, blood letting may be required.

Hemoglobin....if low (below 14.0), think of massive malnutrition, especially if the levels are below 13.0. The causes include B vitamin deficiency, mineral deficiency, protein deficiency, alcoholism, lead poisoning, arsenic poisoning, and parasite infestation. Hypothyroidism may also cause reduced hemoglobin, especially in women of child bearing age. To build up the blood eat organic calve's or lamb's liver and/or red meat. Consume large amounts of spinach. Excellent blood building supplements are Oregamax, 6 to 8 capsules daily and Resvitanol, 6 to 9 capsules daily. For more information on building the blood see the anemia section in *Supermarket Remedies* (Dr. Cass Ingram, Knowledge House Publishers).

Appendix A

Nutritional Content of Selected Foods

When reviewing these charts, keep in mind one important fact — there is no way to standardize the nutritional content of any given food. The nutritional value of food varies with growing conditions, soil nutrient content, and freshness. The most critical factor is the nutrient content of the soil in which the food is grown. These charts are approximations to the best of human ability. For example, a carrot grown in California will have a selenium or vitamin A content different from one grown in Wisconsin, illustrating that there is no "standardized carrot."

Chart #1

The nutritional benefits of bran has been a hot topic over the past several years. New theories are continuously developing about which bran is the panacea. However, it is the nutritional content that is the true marker for which bran is King. The following chart illustrates the nutritional value of the most popular sources of bran. In this chart wheat germ is listed instead of wheat bran, since its nutritional value is considerably greater. Bran also contains considerable amounts of trace minerals, particularly magnesium, selenium, silicon, chromium, and manganese. However, levels of some of these minerals have yet to be accurately determined.

% of U.S. RDA per equivalent weight	Rice Bran	Wheat Germ	Oat Bran
Thiamine	60	20	20
Riboflavin	6	8	6
Niacin	50	6	1
Vitamin B_6	8	10	Not detectable
Vitamin E	15	8	Not detectable
Iron	15	10	10
Phosphorus	45	25	20
Magnesium	60	15	15
Zinc	10	20	8

This chart illustrates the superiority of rice bran as a source of important nutrients. In addition, rice bran contains a special oil which helps lower cholesterol levels. Both rice and oat bran are rich sources of fiber and can be used as fiber supplements. Get your rice bran plus the germ and polish by consuming Nutri-Sense. To boost the body's levels of natural magnesium and B vitamins, take at least three heaping tablespoons daily.

Chart #2
Foods High in Magnesium

Food sources of magnesium are listed, because the majority of the population is deficient in it. As many as 70% of Americans lack this critical mineral. Symptoms of magnesium deficiency include muscle spasms or twitches, rapid heartbeat, arrhythmia, poor appetite, nausea, back pain, depression, night sweats, excessive body odor, chronic knee/hip pain, kidney stones, muscular exhaustion, and confusion.

Magnesium is found in a vast number of foods, but only the super-rich sources are listed. The following chart lists magnesium in foods as milligrams per equivalent weight.

Rice bran	.785
Coriander leaf, dried	.694
Dillweed, dried	.451
Celery seed	440
Sage	.428
Mustard, dried	.422
Basil	.422
Cocoa powder	.420
Fennel seed	.385
Wheat germ, toasted	.364
Tarragon	.347
Brazil nuts	.318
Soybean flour, defatted	.318
Almonds	.293
Molasses, blackstrap	.258
Spinach, frozen	.104
Chickpeas, dry or canned	.54
Apricots dried	.50

Other excellent sources include black-eyed peas, cashews, pecans, bananas, beet greens, avocados, filberts, tofu, oatmeal, and buckwheat. Foods which are organically grown contain up to 10 times more magnesium than foods that are grown commercially. Using lots of hot, tangy spices is one of the easiest ways to get extra magnesium. A good rule is the hotter the spice is the more magnesium it contains.

Chart #3
Selenium Content of Foods

The selenium content of food varies greatly depending upon where it is grown. This variation is entirely dependent upon the amount of selenium within the soil. The following chart illustrates how incredibly wide of a variation this can be. The figures marked with an @ are foods which were grown in Maryland, a region with relatively low amounts of selenium. Those marked with an * describe foods grown in South Dakota, a high-selenium area. Figures marked with a + describe foods from Venezuela, another region with selenium-rich soils. All foods were analyzed for selenium content by the U.S. Department of Agriculture. You will note that the variation is massive, indicating the danger of relying upon commercial food alone as a source of nutrients.

Selenium Ranges

Food	Amount	(in Micrograms)
Carrots, raw	1	1.8@ to 105 *
Cabbage, shredded	1/2 cup	1.8@ to 316 *
Onion, raw	1/2 cup	1.3@ to 1513 *
Potatoes, raw	1 large	1.0@ to 235 *
Tomatoes, raw	1	0.7@ to 165 *
Cheese	1.5 oz	3.8@ to 18 +
Egg	1 large	5.0@ to 87 +
Chicken breast	4 oz	13.0@ to 79 +

While a head of cabbage from South Dakota and Maryland look alike, their nutrient content is vastly different. If you have lived on the East or Northwestern coast of the United States or in the Great Lakes region for much of your life, you have been getting only a minute amount of selenium from food grown there, *barely enough to keep you alive.* Such individuals should make it a point to include selenium-rich foods in the diet on a daily basis. A selection of selenium rich food includes garlic, organ meats, butter, fish, lobster, crab, clams, lamb, nuts, wheat germ, fresh whole wheat flour, cider vinegar, mushrooms, Swiss chard, radishes, turnips, and mushrooms. However, the mentioned vegetables/fruit are only a viable selenium source if they are grown on selenium-rich soil. Meat can only be a rich source if the animals graze on selenium-rich grass, grain, or fodder.

Chart #4
Highest Food Sources of Vitamin E

Only a few foods contain appreciable amounts of vitamin E. Vitamin E is found in the highest concentration within foods which are naturally rich in oils. In addition, certain vegetables, particularly spinach, tomatoes, and sweet potatoes, contain valuable amounts.

Food	Portion	Vitamin E (I.U.)
Wheat germ oil	1 Tbsp	37.2
Sunflower seeds	1/4 cup	26.8
Wheat germ, raw	1/2 cup	12.8
Sunflower seed oil	1 Tbsp	12.7
Almonds	1/4 cup	12.7
Pecans	1/4 cup	12.7
Hazelnuts	1/4 cup	12.7
Safflower oil	1 Tbsp	12.5
Peanuts	1/4 cup	7.9
Sweet potato	1 small	4.9
Spinach, cooked	1 cup	4.8
Lobster	3 oz	4.5
Salmon steak	3 oz	2.3

The above chart illustrates the difficulty of trying to get adequate amounts of vitamin E through the diet alone. Unless you consume two or more tablespoons of wheat germ oil daily or are eating sunflower seeds by the handful, you need supplemental vitamin E. The minimum recommended dose for most people is 400 I.U. daily.

Chart #5
Food Sources of Biotin

Rich Sources	Good Sources	Fair Sources
• kidney	• cauliflower	• chicken
• liver	• cocoa bean	• carrots
• soybean flour	• eggs	• spinach
	• mushrooms	• most fruits
	• peanuts	• collards
	• peanut butter	• kale

Food Sources of Biotin, continued

Good Sources	Fair Sources
• almonds	• spinach
• beef	• Swiss chard
• veal	• watercress
• halibut	• kiwi fruit
• mackerel	
• sardines	
• lobster	

Chart #6
Food Sources of Folic Acid

Rich Sources	Good Sources	Fair Sources
• liver and other organs	• sunflower seeds	• sweet red peppers
• rice bran and germ	• oranges	• whole wheat flour
• wheat bran	• cantaloupe	• avocados
• spinach	• strawberries	• broccoli
	• salmon	• chicken
	• blue cheese	
	• eggs	
	• wild rice	
	• brown rice	
	• buckwheat flour	
	• lobster	

The folic acid found in eggs and meat is absorbed better than that found in grains, vegetables, and nuts. This should be kept in mind when making food choices based on this chart. Folic acid is easily destroyed by cooking, particularly by boiling. Between 40 to 95% of the original folic acid found in fruits and/or vegetables is lost during canning and cooking primarily because much of the water is discarded, and folic acid is water soluble. However, if the cooking water is retained, as in soup or sauces, or is drunk, much of the folic acid will be recovered.

Chart #7
Food Sources of Pyridoxine (Vitamin B$_6$)

Rich Sources	Good Sources	Fair Sources
• rice bran	• avocados	• eggs
• wheat bran	• bananas	• milk
• sunflower seeds	• corn	• mangos
	• fish	• cantaloupe
	• kidney	• pineapple
	• liver	• figs, dried
	• lean meat	
	• nuts	
	• wild rice	
	• brown rice	
	• soy beans	
	• whole grain flour	

Chart #8
Food Sources of Vitamin B$_{12}$

Vitamin B$_{12}$ is the largest and most complex of all known vitamins. There are few dietary sources of this important vitamin even though little if any is made within the body. Meats and dairy products constitute the majority of dietary intake. This is because vitamin B$_{12}$ originates from bacteria which live in the intestines of animals. These bacteria are found in large amounts primarily in the first stomach (the lumen) of herbivorous animals such as cows, goats, and sheep. Bacteria synthesize this structurally complex vitamin within the lumen from which it is absorbed into the bloodstream to be transported to various organs and tissues. This is why organ meats, muscle meats, eggs, and milk products constitute significant dietary sources. Fish and seafood consume B$_{12}$ through a secondary source—dark green algae, such as chlorella, the richest known plant source of B$_{12}$.

Richest Natural Sources	Excellent Sources	Good Sources
• lamb liver	• roe (fish eggs) from	• catfish
• beef liver	cod, haddock, or herring	• tuna
• lamb kidney	• mackerel	• halibut
• beef kidney	• cod	• lamb
• turkey liver	• crab	• beef
	• eggs	• cheese

Food Sources of vitamin B₁₂, continued

Excellent Sources	Good Sources
• sardines	• veal
• mozzarella cheese	• lobster
• herring	• scallops
• salmon	• oysters
• chlorella	

Chart #9
Food Sources of Vitamin C

Richest Natural Sources	Excellent Sources	Good Sources
• acerola cherry	• guavas	• broccoli
• rose hips	• strawberries	• limes
• wild strawberry leaves	• oranges	• black currants
• crude, unsweetened black currant juice (Currant-C)	• grapefruit	• green peppers
• Gene's Powerdrops™	• lemons	• red peppers
	• red sweet peppers	• parsley
	• kiwi fruit	• turnip greens
		• mustard greens
		• avocados
		• melons
		• papaya
		• Brussels sprouts
		• red cabbage
		• cauliflower
		• collards
		• kale
		• spinach
		• Swiss chard
		• watercress
		• limes
		• basil

Chart #10
Sugar Content of Fruits

Fruit contains the natural sugars fructose and glucose with fructose usually being found in the highest concentration. These sugars are bound to cellulose and other fibers within the whole fruit. This allows the sugars to be released gradually into the bloodstream from which they are delivered to the cells to be used as a source of fuel. The following chart lists the percentages of natural sugar found in fruits:

5-7% Natural Sugar
- cantaloupe
- honeydew
- papaya
- strawberries
- watermelon
- cranberries

8-9% Natural Sugar
- grapefruit
- lemon
- lime

10-12% Natural Sugar
- apricots
- blackberries
- currants
- oranges
- peaches
- tangerines

15-16% Natural Sugar
- apples
- blueberries
- cherries
- grapes
- raspberries
- kumquats
- loganberries
- pineapple
- pears

20% or More Natural Sugar
- apple juice
- bananas
- dates
- figs
- raisins
- grape juice
- orange juice
- prunes and prune juice
- dried cherries

Appendix B
Nutritional Foods and Supplements

Nutritional Products

Useful Facts

Hercules Strength
A special formula of wild herbs famous in ancient Greece–oregano, sage, and rosemary. A synergistic blend for strength and energy.

- For strengthening the body, immune system, and brain
- For improving memory

Oregamax capsules
100% wild, high-mountain oregano, plus Rhus coriaria, a mountain berry, garlic and onion. This blend has been relied upon by humanity for over a thousand years.

- Tremendous formula for supporting immunity, digestion, and elimination
- Has been used successfully for combating allergies
- Bone supplement
- Pain killer

Oreganol gelcaps
Get the same power of the oil of oregano but no taste or heat. Oreganol sealed gelcaps give you seven drops of the oil in a convenient and easy to take form.

- Great for those who need to take large amounts in frequent doses
- Gets into the gut faster with a greater concentration needed for fungus and parasite infestation

---

Oil of Oregano, regular strength
The most powerful herb substance ever. North American Herb & Spice provides guaranteed wild Mediterranean source oregano, the type rigorously researched at Georgetown University. It is also a special species which is hand picked. Strict environmental controls are enacted to protect the source.

- Great for strengthening immunity
- Boost the body's anti-allergy and anti-germ powers with wild oil of oregano
- Not all oregano oils are the same; the research is done on the high-mountain, wild Mediterranean type. Inferior types are Mexican sage, Moroccan, and Spanish, but only the wild oregano of Mediterranean origin is the

Oil of Oregano, regular strength, continued

subject of research at Georgetown University
- Research proves incredibly powerful germ-killing actions, especially against fungi and bacteria

Oreganol Oil of Oregano, SuperStrength
The strongest variety and concentration of Mediterranean wild oregano. Comes from mountains as high as 8,000 feet above sea level. This is the pure wild oregano emulsified in extra virgin olive oil, which makes it edible. Take it internally and apply it topically.

- Research proves anti-viral and anti-parasitic actions
- Use the SuperStrength for the most difficult conditions
- Safe and effective
- Stops pain of burns and sunburn.
- Helps stop bleeding of wounds and pain, and helps heal faster

HerbSorb
(herbs for digestive protection)
When the digestive system needs support and when nothing else works, reach for HerbSorb. This eastern herbal/spice formula contains herbs which fortify the digestive tract and support the absorption of nutrients.

- For the stomach and digestion, this is a reliable herbal formula
- Travel with it; it's preventive
- Use for diarrhea parasites and food poisoning episodes
- Aroma and taste are delightful-open capsule and add to recipes

Royal Kick premium royal jelly
This is a special type of high quality royal jelly, containing a greater amount of active ingredients than any other. Rely upon premium grade royal jelly for a tremendous increase in strength and energy.

- Use it to gain the control and power you need
- Fortified with pantothenic acid
- Royal jelly helps balance the hormone system
- Useful for hot flashes/menstrual complaints
- Reduces fatigue

Royal Oil
(stabilized fresh royal jelly)
This is the only fresh royal jelly available in a stabilized form. Since royal jelly is highly vulnerable to spoilage and degradation, stabilized fresh royal

- Gives the hormone system the youth and vigor everyone needs
- Balance your hormones quickly and easily with this tasty and powerful formula
- Gain energy quickly
- Feel calmer fast; safe and effective for kids, too

jelly provides the immense benefits of royal jelly fresh everyday, without the need for refrigeration.

- Use as often as needed Especially helpful during high stress episodes

Flavin-C
Get your vitamin C from completely natural sources, not even a milligram of synthetic or genetically engineered vitamin C is added. Crude, natural Vitamin C is easier on the body than the synthetic type.

- Natural vitamin C is the safest type to consume. Plus, the natural bioflavonoids are needed to make the vitamin C work better. It is utilized better and stays in the body longer
- Six caps provide over 100% of the RDI

BromaZyme
proteolytic plant enzymes
BromaZyme is a combination of the highest quality bromelain and papain, guaranteed to be the most powerful strength available.

- Plant enzymes have been proven in modern research to fight inflammation, pain, and swelling
- Digest protein and clear out toxins and poisons with the powers of highest potency plant enzymes

Pure kelp (ThyroKelp™)
This is a kelp supplement for supporting the function of the thyroid gland. ThyroKelp is harvested from wild kelp beds in the far Northern Pacific in deep cold waters. This area is rich in nutrients and the cleanest source of kelp.

- Virtually all commercially available kelp is contaminated with heavy metals
- Tests show ThyroKelp is free of heavy metals
- This kelp is a top source of naturally occurring iodine and trace minerals

Wild Power Tea
A special tea and cleansing tonic made from wild herbs and flowers. Contains wild borage flowers, wild hibiscus petals, and wild strawberry leaves.

- Wild flowers and petals make the most powerful and useful herbal tea ever
- Use this tea to release the body of poisons and excess fluid
- Strengthen the kidneys and heart immediately with this lovely and nutritious herbal tonic
- Great natural diuretic

Oil of Myrtle
Myrtle is a Mediterranean plant with respected medical properties.

- Doctors are impressed with myrtle because of its anti-diabetic and anti-fungal

It is a sweet smelling oil and is gentle on the skin; in fact, it helps nourish and sooth skin, plus it exhibits anti-aging properties.

properties
- It's a love potion too. Rub it anywhere on the body for an exotic effect
- As a tonic for supporting the immune system and pancreas take 5 drops twice daily

Oil of Cumin
Historically cumin extract was used to block diabetes, stimulate liver function, and eradicate parasites. Note: stools may naturally darken to a rich brown color after taking this oil.

- This pungent spice is one of the most ancient of all known herbal medicines
- A few drops twice daily offer tremendous liver and pancreatic support
- Increase production of protective glutathione enzyme

Oil of Sage
Edible oil of sage provides power for adrenal function, plus it helps reverse nervous stress. Use only edible oil of sage, not the aromatherapy type, which has not been screened for edibility. North American Herb and Spice has the edible oils.

- Support your adrenal and nervous system with the powers of wild sage
- The ancients used sage for physical strength as well as for calming the nerves
- A super-strong antioxidant for preserving the skin and other tissues

Oil of Rosemary
This is the supreme of all antioxidants, protecting the body from toxic damage and aging. Take a few drops daily in juice or water to give the body a feeling of balance impossible to achieve with any other substance.

- Rosemary is a lovely addition to facial soaps and body washes
- Rosemary also soothes the nerves and supports brain function by preventing aging, memory loss, etc.
- Also useful for balancing adrenal function
- A far more powerful and useful antioxidant than vitamins C or E

Oil of Bay Berry
Made of the natural extract of wild bay berries plus myrtle and rosemary. This is a face and hair tonic.

- Strengthen the facial skin, enrich it, and thicken/enrich the hair
- Useful for scalp disorders and dry skin. Add to pump or body soaps for an exotic effect

Oil of Cilantro-plus
Made from high mountain

- An easy to use tonic for digestion
- Use the oil of cilantro to balance

Cilantro. Cilantro gently cleanses the liver by increasing the activity of its detoxification enzymes.

- the entire digestive process
- Lovely gentle flavor enhances many recipes

Oil of edible Fennel

Mountain grown fennel is a unique spice/herb with valuable therapeutic powers. Take it to balance the hormones and to combat hot flashes. Settles stomach complaints fast. Use only high mountain fennel from the edible spice. Beware of imitations.

- Researchers have also found that fennel fights fluid retention
- It is perhaps the most powerful of all natural diuretics
- Has been used for centuries as a digestive aid
- As a hormone tonic it is useful for supporting a wide range of female functions

Oil of Ginger

Made from the whole ginger plant. This powerhouse provides all of the immense value of ginger but in a far superior form than the dried capsule or even fresh. This is edible ginger, providing hundreds of uses.

- Ginger fights nausea, upset stomach, and intestinal/colon complaints
- Use it for digestive enhancement like nothing else
- Add it to any food or marinade
- Fill a capsule and take for stomach pain

Oil of Wild Mint

Made from wild mint which grows naturally on mountain soil. Wild mint is more powerful than farm-raised.

- A great flavoring substance.
- German researchers have determined that mint is valuable for reversing spastic bowel and colitis
- Modern research also indicates that it fights diabetes
- Wild mint tones the entire intestinal system
- It is anti-parasitic

Oil of edible Cinnamon

Cinnamon is an antiseptic that tastes great. It has a naturally sweet and spicy taste. North American Herb and Spice uses real cinnamon from the edible portion, which is difficult to find.

- A wonderful flavoring, this is the ideal immune tonic for children
- Add it to any food or beverage, especially cider and oatmeal
- Great on sweet potatoes, pumpkin, and squash
- Add to ice cream for added taste

Oil of Wild Lavender
Completely different than the commercial types, this wild and high-mountain lavender is pungent, aromatic, and, most importantly, edible. Other lavenders are made from hybridized or genetically engineered plants, which are not the true lavenders. North American Herb and Spice provides this rare and safe oil.

- Research proves a valuable role for lavender in reversing skin injury (particularly burns), fighting infections, and for relaxing the nerves
- This exotic oil can be rubbed anywhere on the body, but take it internally as well
- Add it to atomizers or vaporizers
- To sweeten the air in the home add a few drops to a pump spray bottle and spray into the air

Juice of Oregano
Cleanse your intestines of all impurities with with this potent digestive tonic. Completely natural and free of all solvents/chemicals.

- Relished in the Mediterranean as a daily health tonic, the oregano juice is a source of natural oxygen from the high mountain wild oregano plant Helps us stay healthy/live longer

Juice of Rosemary
Rosemary is made from the leaves of mountain-grown, wild rosemary. Excellent for memory.

- Protects and nourishes the brain and nervous system
- Activates the nerves to activate the health of the entire body

Essence of Orange Blossoms
This is the most luscious and nourishing tea and tonic imaginable. Made from the medicinal-like bitter orange blossom. Taste is exotic.

- Known in eastern Europe/Middle East as "White Coffee"
- Gives that natural healthy feeling without the caffeine
- Its the guilt-free and healthy natural high

Essence of Rose Petals
This is the most aromatic drink ever imaginable. Full of the naturally occurring essential oil, this is the true rose petal essence, extracted from mountain-grown damascene rose petals. Made strictly from mountain grown rose petals. Natural antibiotic properties.

- Use as a tonic, beverage, tea, and aromatic boost
- Drink it plain in hot water or with a teaspoon of orange blossom honey
- Great for immune support and to balance hormones and mood
- Calm your nerves immediately with the power of rose petal essence

Resvitanol™ (Red Sour Grape)
What a nourishing type of grape extract this is; the only one with measurable amounts of key nutrients like potassium, vitamin C, and chromium. This is the true grape flavonoid in a capsule. Made from natural grapes, never genetically engineered.

- Offers immense support for heart and artery function
- Strengthen the entire circulatory system with this high mountain grape concentrate
- Resvitanol's chromium is a completely natural type found only in grapes

Nutri-Sense
The key formula for naturally rebuilding the nutritional needs of the body. The natural source of crude, unprocessed B vitamins and trace minerals.

- Boost vitamin/mineral status naturally
- Nutri-Sense is great added to cereal, soup, or in shakes/malts
- A tremendous source of natural niacin, pantothenic acid, magnesium, and thiamine.
- Great for weight loss. Simply add to juice or water and consume as a breakfast; it is more nourishing than any typical breakfast

Pumpkinol™
The most nutrient-dense of all food oils, this is a nutritional treasure chest, filled with a wide range of difficult-to-procure nutrients. Its a super-tonic, containing dozens of nutrients, polyphenols, vitamin E, iron, and essential fatty acids, all in a natural form. It's a liquid; simply consume one or more teaspoons daily.

- Natural polyunsaturate speeds weight loss
- Halts desire for sweet or harmful foods
- Nourishing and supportive for prostate function
- Highly nourishing for children
- Helps nourish and build healthy skin-provides natural E
- Great on salads, cheese, and soups
- Ideal for healthy skin, hair, and nails

ProstaClenz
Clenz yourself from the inside out with this first ever herbal & essential fatty acid tonic. Made from a special type of pumpkinseed oil from pumpkins growing in the hills of south central Austria.

- The active ingredient is concentrated 10:1 for extra value
- Other prostate-cleansing herbs, including rosemary and oregano, are added to potentiate the action

**Flavin-C
(natural crude vitamin C)**
Natural vitamin C is rare, since virtually all supplements use the synthetic. The problem is the synthetic is genetically engineered. Or, it is made synthetically, usually from extracts of corn, which may contain pesticide residues.

- Millions of people are allergic to corn, which is the raw material for synthetic vitamin C
- Natural vitamin C is easier on the body and more readily utilized
- There are no side effects with natural vitamin C

Fung-E-Clenz
A combination of wild/edible essential oils, including oils of oregano, sage, cumin, and bay leaf. Clenz yourself from the inside out with the powers of wild essential oils and essences.

- Formulated as a result of research by fungal disease expert, Marc Bielski, M. D.
- Contains spice and herbal essential oils proven in research to possess anti fungal action.

ViraClenz
Hundreds of different kinds of viruses may attack the body. When viruses attack, the immune system needs major support. Get the immune strength you need with ViraClenz. A combination of various edible essential oils, including oils of cinnamon, oregano and bay leaf.

- Specifically formulated for strengthening the antiviral defenses
- Take a few drops under the tongue as often as possible

LivaClenz
A healthy liver is mandatory for optimal health. This is a special formula of edible essential oils specifically for cleansing the liver. A combination of cumin, coriander, cilantro, and oregano oils.

- Gently aids the body's detoxification processes through completely natural methods
- Add it to olive oil and lemon juice for a liver cleanse

Safer sweeteners and honeys[*]

Pomegranate Sauce
Made from mountain-grown vine ripened pomegranates. It is a concentrate of pomegranate make in a crude fashion. Why labor with the difficult to eat fruit? Simply take a teaspoon of the syrup daily.

- Mentioned in all of the holy books, now researchers know why this tart fruit is so important: it contains natural substances which combat cancer and strengthen immunity
- Use it in cooking, especially in meat or rice dishes
- Make a tasty pomegranate lemonade. Simply add a tablespoon of the syrup to 12 ounces of ice water; stir and drink ice cold. Beware of the froth, because when you stir it, the froth can overflow the glass.

Red Grape Molasses
It is impossible to find a more tasty and nourishing sweetener. Far more digestible than refined or raw sugar, use this wonderful Mediterranean treat raw or in cooking to provide much-needed natural carbohydrates.

- Grape molasses is made from Mediterranean mountainous grapes and is free of pesticides residues and other chemicals.
- A highly digestible and "safe" sweetener for children

Carob Molasses
Made from the wild-growing Carob pods, possibly the manna of the Bible. Not excessively sweet but wonderful in taste. None of the negatives of chocolate but all of the rich taste.

- This is a highly useful and digestible sweetener, especially for children
- Use it as a topping for any rich dessert

Date Molasses
Made from vine-ripened dates. Dates are super-rich in trace minerals, especially potassium.

- Far more digestible and useful than regular sugar
- Use this in cooking and on cereals and for a natural potassium source

[*]Use only after the first 90 days on this diet.

Wild Oregano Honey

You can tell if a honey is crude/raw if it is extremely thick; that is, if it sticks to spoons or utensils aggressively and it sinks to the bottom of a cup of hot tea and stays there. In other words, you have to stir it aggressively to get it to mix in the hot water. The value is high and, thus, it is of the most superior grade and value possible.

- Use this crude, wild honey as a tonic for digestion, immunity, and overall health
- Wild oregano honey is rare, crude, and raw
- The bees are never fed sugar; therefore, it is a medicinal grade of honey

Wild Thistle Honey

You can tell if a honey is crude/raw if it is extremely thick, that is so thick that the following occur: it sticks to spoons or utensils aggressively and it sinks to the bottom of a cup of hot tea and stays there. In other words, you have to stir it aggressively to get it to mix in the hot water. Thistle honey is rare, crude, and raw. The value is high, and thus, it is of the most superior grade possible.

- Use this crude wild honey as a tonic for digestion, immunity, and overall health
- The bees are never fed sugar. Thus, it is a medicinal grade type of honey
- A tremendous digestive tonic
- The most rare honey; limited supply available
- German research indicates that thistle extracts boost liver function

Neroli Orange Blossom Honey

A rare honey, derived from the highly aromatic Mediterranean orange blossom. It is completely different than the commercial type made from hybrid/American orange groves.

- It is easy to digest, not excessively sweet, and wonderful to taste
- Add to hot herbal tea or spread on toast/bagels
- easy to digest, ideal sweetener for children. Add to hot or cold cereals

Other Unique Products

Royal Oil
Royal is the first and only stabilized royal jelly without added honey or sweeteners. Royal jelly is credited with miraculous rejuvenating and regenerating properties. For improving hormone balance, fighting fatigue, stress, nervousness or panic attacks, royal jelly is essential.

- Abundant in vitamins D, E & Bs as well as niacin, riboflavin, biotin and pantothenic acid
- Modern research shows royal jelly has powerful effect upon adrenal function
- For an energy boost take it under the tongue, or add it to smoothies, shakes, juice or warm cereals

Currant—C
(Crude Black Currant Juice)
From the Alpine foothills comes the most lovely currant berries, growing high in the mountainous organic soil. Currants are the best berry source of vitamin C, plus they are super-rich in bioflavonoids. Correct your vitamin C / bio-flavonoid deficiencies naturally with Currant–C.

- Wonderful mixed in ice or seltzer water—for a superb treat mix in cream or whole milk
- Each ounce contains over 50% of the minimum daily requirement

Gene's Powerdrops ™
(wild greens formula)
There is nothing like this in the world—This is the only wild greens juice available, packing the power that only wild greens offer. The wild greens blend consists of a combination of wilderness greens, including wild dandelion greens and nettles.

- Use it as a natural source of riboflavin, folic acid and vitamin C, potassium, calcium, and more
- Gene's Powerdrops are never pasteurized or heated—they're preserved by natural oils. This is why it is super-rich in vitamins and minerals; it is a completely natural, wild food.

Diabagon ™
(crude edible essential oils)
Researched at Georgetown University, Diabagon has been proven (in experimental animals) to naturally lower blood sugar and blood pressure. It is a highly unique formula containing oils of fenugreek, ginger, cumin, and more.

- Great tonic for pancreas/liver support
- Add it to food and beverages
- Great for improving carbohydrate tolerance
- A natural way to support the blood sugar mechanism
- Researched/tested/guaranteed

Appendix C

Books, Cassettes, and Internet

#1 *How to Eat Right and Live Longer*—$21.95 (Completely revised edition of the former *Eat Right to Live Long*)

345 pages   6 x 9 inch softbound

Dr. Ingram's most comprehensive book on diet and nutrition. Describes the treatment of a wide range of illnesses through diet and nutritional supplementation. Emphasis is on the nutritional treatment of heart disease, high cholesterol, high triglycerides, diabetes, obesity, allergies, arthritis, neurological disorders, and alcoholism. Step-by-step nutritional protocols, dietary instruction, personalized nutritional/blood analysis, and 100 recipes included.

#2 *Self-Test Nutrition Guide*—$24.95

330 pages   5 1/2 x 8 1/2 inch hardbound

Test yourself to determine your nutritional deficiencies from *A to zinc*. Other tests show evidence of possible health problems such as adrenal insufficiency, chemical toxicity, thyroid insufficiency, intestinal malabsorption, liver dysfunction, and premature aging. Sugar, caffeine, sulfite, and MSG overload are also evaluated. Each test is followed by specific and thorough nutritional recommendations. Find out what you are lacking.

#3 *Who Needs Headaches?*—$13.95

164 pages   6 x 9 inch softbound

A nutritional approach to solving the migraine dilemma. Emphasizes food allergies, nutritional deficiencies, and hormonal disturbances and how to diagnose them as well as how to reverse them nutritionally. Chapter on structural therapy for tension headaches included.

#4 *Tea Tree Oil: the Natural Antiseptic* (formerly *Killed on Contact: The Tea Tree Oil Story*) $13.95

110 pages   5 1/2 x 8 1/2 inch softbound

Some things need to be killed: bacteria, viruses, fungi, parasites, and parasitic insects. Learn how to battle infectious disease with tea tree oil, one of Nature's most versatile and potent antiseptics. Information particularly valuable for homemakers, travelers, wilderness buffs, fishermen, and athletes.

#5 *How to Survive Disasters with Natural Medicines*—$13.95

137 pages   5 1/2 x 8 1/2 inch softbound

Natural disasters, toxic waste spills, fires, parasite infestations, accidents, radiation leakage, and water contamination all demand immediate action. Learn to deal with both major and minor disasters using only natural remedies which are both safe and effective. Destroy ticks, stop wound infection, end the pain of toothache, neutralize animal/insect bites, abort diarrhea and/or dysentery, treat burns/cuts — all with natural substances.

#6 *Supermarket Remedies for Better Health*—$29.95

340 pages   5 1/2 x 8 1/2 inch softbound

Reverse health problems with foods, herbs, and spices. Learn to shop for your ailments at the supermarket, health store, and farmer's market. A supermarket juice that reverses heart disease, a vegetable that halts depression, a berry which eliminates stomachaches, a fruit which lowers cholesterol, a berry for poor vision, a protein for great energy, a spice which kills germs and much more. Use supermarket remedies for hundreds of ailments.

#7　The Cure is in the Cupboard: How to Use Oregano for Better Health— 19.95
　　170 pages, 51/2 x 81/2 inch softback
Oregano helps you regain your health and then stay healthy. This is what saved Dr. Ingram's life. Learn how to use oregano and its essential oil for fighting infection and eliminating pain. Combat skin disorders, injuries, wounds, and dental problems. Particularly valuable for fungal infections.

#8　Lifesaving Cures—$19.95
　　300 pages　6 x 9 inch softbound
You'll need help to survive in the 21st century and to reverse everyday illnesses. With this book of natural cures you have the answers for stress, viral syndromes, food poisoning, epidemics, water contamination, deadly bacteria parasites, and radiation poisoning.

#9　The Diabetes Cure—price yet to be determined (For info call 1-800-243-5242)
　　200 pages, 5 1/2 x 8 1/2 softback
The most powerful diabetes solutions ever. Special program gives precise guidance for diet plus dozens of recipes. Find out the most powerful home remedies for reversing diabetes-especially the potent spice extract Diabagon. Unique diet included. Gives the latest research on what really works. Special section on reversing hypoglycemia included.

> NOTE: Order any 4 books and receive a free copy of either
> *The Cure is in the Cupboard* or *Lifesaving Cures*, your choice.

Cassette Tapes and Programs

#1　The Survivor's Nutritional Pharmacy—$29.95
Learn exactly how to survive major disasters and everyday injuries that could threaten your health and life. Simple and inexpensive remedies such as honey, garlic, onion, vinegar, and enzymes may save your life. Information different from the book.

#2　How to Use Oregano for Common Illnesses—$9.95
A must addition for oregano lovers. Contains detailed information not found in the book. Specific protocols for dozens of illnesses and diseases plus case histories. Learn hundreds of uses for wild oregano oil and herb—from the Doctor himself.

#3　Selected Interviews and Lectures: The Best of Dr. Cass Ingram—$44.95
　　4 tapes　Total time: 4 hours (approximate)
Hear Dr. Ingram tell it like it is during his information-packed interviews. Over three hours of tapes give information on how to eat right, herbal science, nutritional therapy, and much more. Entertaining and informative. Makes a perfect gift.

#4　Professional/Advanced Series—$89.95*
　　The Warning Signs of Nutritional Deficiency
　　4 tapes Total time: 4 hrs　Manual: 100 pages, with Judy Kay Gray, M. S.
Master Dr. Ingram's knowledge about nutritional deficiency and natural medicine. Find out how to discern your specific deficiencies; become proficient in spotting nutritional deficiencies in others. Includes lifesaving information on the treatment of disease with nutritional medicine. Become an expert.

* Normal price for this program is $129.95. Save $40.00 when you order from this book.

ORDER FORM

Item	Quantity	Amount

BOOKS

#1 *How to Eat Right and Live Longer* _____ _____

#2 *Self-Test Nutrition Guide* _____ _____

#3 *Who Needs Headaches?* _____ _____

#4 *Tea Tree Oil—the Natural Antiseptic* _____ _____

#5 *How to Survive Disasters With Natural Medicines* _____ _____

#6 *Supermarket Remedies* _____ _____

#7 *The Cure Is in the Cupboard* _____ _____

#8 *Lifesaving Cures* _____ _____

#9 *The Diabetes Cure* _____ _____

TAPES

#1 *The Survivor's Nutritional Pharmacy* _____ _____

#2 *How to Use Oregano for Common Illnesses* _____ _____

#3 *Selected Interviews and Lectures:*
The Best of Dr. Cass Ingram _____ _____

#4 *The Warning Signs of Nutritional Deficiency*
Professional/Advanced Series _____ _____

Sub-Total _____

Sales Tax (if any) _____

Shipping* _____

TOTAL _____

*Shipping Charges: $6.00 for single books—add $1.00 for each additional book.
For cassette tapes only, add $4.00 shipping charge.
Payment by check, money order, or credit card.

Make checks payable to: NAHS
P.O. Box 4885
Buffalo Grove, Illinois 60089
Phone: (800) 243-5242 • Fax: 847 473-4780

For Visa/Mastercard orders provide the following information:

Card#_____ Exp. Date_____

Signature_____

Name_____

Address_____

City_____ State_____ Zip_____

Bibliography

1. Aaseth, J., et al. 1980. Decreased levels of selenium in alcoholic cirrhosis. *N.E.J.M.* Oct 16.

2. Abdullah, T.H., Kandil, O., ElKadi, A., et al. 1988. Garlic revisited: therapeutic for the major diseases of our times? *Nat'l Med. Assoc.* 80(4):43945.

3. Ackerman, I.A., Weinstein, I.B., Kaplan, H.S. 1978. Cancer of the esophagus. In: *Cancer in China* (eds. H.S. Kaplan and A. Tsuchitani). New York: A.R. Liss, pp. 111-36.

4. Adetumbi, M.A., Lau, B.H.S. 1983. Allium Sativum (garlic)—a natural antibiotic. *Medical Hypotheses* 12:227-37.

5. Agharanya, J.C., Alonso, R., Wurtman, R.J. 1981. Changes in catecholamine excretion after short-term tyrosine ingestion in normally fed human subjects. *Am. J. Clin. Nutr.* 34:82-87.

6. Agharanya, J.C., Wurtman, R.J. 1982. Effect of acute administration of large neutral amino acids on urinary excretion of catecholamines. *Life Sciences* 30(9):739-46.

7. Airola, P. 1978. *The Miracle of Garlic.* Health Plus Publishers, Phoenix.

8. Alexander, M., et al. 1985. Oral beta carotene can increase the numbers of OKT4+ cells in human blood. *Immunology Letters* 9:221.

9. Ambrosio, G., Weisfeldt, M.L., Jacobus, W.E. 1987. Evidence for a reversible oxygen radical-mediated component of reperfusion injury: reduction by recombinent human superoxide dismutase administered at the time of reflow. *Circulation* 75(1): 282-91.

10. Amella, M., Bonner, C., Briancon, F. et al. 1985. Inhibition of mast cell histamine release by flavonoids and bioflavonoids. *Planta Medica* 51: 16-20.

11. Ames, B. 1983. Dietary carcinogens and anti-carcinogens. *Science* 221:1256-64.

12. Anonymous. 1987. Second opinions reduce by-pass surgery. *Am. Med. News* Oct. 2, p. 72.

13. Augustine, G.J., Jr., Levitan, H. 1980. Neurotransmitter release from a

vertebrate neuromuscular synapse affected by a food dye. *Science* 207: 1489-90.

14. Azuma, J., et al. 1985. Therapeutic effect of taurine in congestive heart failure: a double-blind crossover trail. *Clin. Cardiol.* 8:276:82.

15. Balentine, J.D. 1982. *Pathology of Oxygen Toxicity.* Academic Press, New York.

16. Beck, W.S. 1988. Cobalamin and the nervous system. *N.E.J.M.* 318:1752-54.

17. Becker, C.E., et al. 1976. Diagnosis and treatment of amanital phalloides-type mushroom poisoning: use of thioctic acid. *West. J. Med.* 125:100-09.

18. Beisel, W.R., Edelman, R., Nauss, K., Suskind, R. 1981. Single nutrient effects on immunologic function. *J.A.M.A.* 245:53.

19. Belizan, J.M., et al. 1983. Reduction of blood pressure with calcium supplementation in young adults. *J.A.M.A.* 249:1161-5.

20. Belman, S. 1983. Onion and garlic oil inhibit tumor growth. *Carcinogenesis* 4(8):1063-65.

21. Belsheim, J.A., Gnarpe, G.H. 1981. Antibiotics and granulocytes. Direct and indirect effects on granulocyte chemotaxis. *Acta. Path. Micro. Scand.* 89:217-21.

22. Benda, L., Dittrich, H., Ferenzi, P., et al. 1980. The influence of therapy with silymarin on the survival rate of patients with liver cirrhosis. *Wiener Klinishee Wochenschrift* Oct. 10, p. 678.

23. Berkow, S., Palmer, S. 1986. Nutrition in medical education: current status and future directions. *Amer. Inst. Nutr.* (study completed by the National Research Council for Food and Nutrition—National Academy of Sciences, 2101 Constitution Avenue N.W. Washington. D.C. 20418).

24. Bertram, J., Peng, A., Rundhaug, J. 1988. Carotenoids have intrinsic cancer chemopreventive action in 10TI cells. *F.A.S.E.B.J.* 2:1413

25. Beutler, E., et al. 1985. Plasma glutathione in health and in patients with malignant disease. *J. Lab. Clin. Med.* 105:581-84.

26. Bever, B.O., Zahnd, G.R. 1979. Plants with oral hypoglycemic action. *Quar. J. Crude Drug Res.* 17: 139-96.

27. Bishop, J.E. 1977. Deaths of 2 liquid protein dieters tied to unusual heart rhythm abnormalities. *The Wall Street Journal* Dec. 1, p. 8.

28. Bjarnason, 1., et al. 1987. Blood and protein loss via small intestinal inflammation induced by non-steroidal anti-inflammatory drugs. *Lancet* 2:711.

29. Bjerve, K.S., Thoresen, L., Borsting, S. 1988. Linseed and cod liver oil induce rapid growth in a 7-year old girl with n-3 fatty acid deficiency. *J. Parent. Ent. Nutr.* 12:521-25.

30. Bland, J. 1978. *The Use of the Clinical Laboratory in Preventive Medicine.* Bellevue Redmond Medical Labs Inc., Tacoma, Wash.

31. Bland, J. 1982. *The Accessory Food Factors in Health Promotion.* Vol. 2. Keats Publishing Inc.~ New Canaan, Conn., pp. 1-25.

32. Bland, J. 1985. *Nutraerobics.* Harper & Row, San Francisco.

33. Bland, J. (ed.). 1985. *Yearbook of Nutritional Medicine.* Keats Publishing, Inc., New Canaan, Conn.

34. Blau, L.W. 1950. Cherry diet control for gout and arthritis. *Tex. Rep. Bio. Med.* 8:309-11.

35. Bliznakov, E.G. 1986. *The Miracle Nutrient—Coenzyme Q-10.* Bantam Books.

36. Bloom, W.L., Flinchum, D. 1960. Osteomalacia with pseudofractures caused by the ingestion of aluminum hydroxide. *J.A.M.A.* 174:1327.

37. Blume, E. 1986. Aflatoxin. *Nutrition Action Healthletter.* Vol. 13(8). Center for Science in the Public Interest, Washington, D.C.

38. Bombardelli, E., Cirstoni, A., Carruthers, M. 1982. The effect of acute and chronic (Panax) ginseng saponins treatment on adrenal function; biochemical and pharmacological. *Proceedings of 3rd International Ginseng Symposium* pp. 9-16.

39. Bonjour, J.B. 1977. Biotin in man's nutrition and therapy: a review. *Int. J. Vit. Nutr. Res.* 47: 107- 18.

40. Bordia, A., Bansal, H.C., Arora, S.K., et al. 1975. Effect of the essential oils of garlic and onion on alimentary hyperlipidemia. *Atherosclerosis* 21: 15.

41. Bordia, A. 1981. Effect of garlic on blood lipids in patients with coronary heart disease. *Am. J. Clin. Nutr.* 34:2100.

42. Breneman, J.C. 1978. Basics of Food Allergy. Charles C. Thomas, Springfield, ILL.

43. Brittelli, M., Culik, R., Dashiell, O., et al. 1979. Skin absorption of hexafluoroacetone: teratogenic and lethal effects in the rat fetus. *Tox. Appl. Pharm.* 47:35-39.

44. Brock, K., Berry, G., Mock, P., et al. 1988. Nutrients in diet and plasma and risk of in situ cervical cancer. *J. Nat. Canc. Inst.* 80:580-85.

45. Bruce, W.R., Dion, P.W. 1981. Studies relating to a fecal mutagen. *Am. J. Clin. Nutr.* 35:2511-12.

46. Buist, R.1984. *Food Intolerance: What It is and How to Cope With It.* Harper & Row, Sydney, Australia.

47. Burke, W.B. Jr. 1982. *Inositol: Nature's Anxiety Fighter.* Hawkes Publishing, Inc., Salt Lake City, Utah.

48. Burr, M., et al. 1987. Atrophic gastritis and vitamin C status in two towns with different stomach cancer death rates. *Br. J. Canc.* 56: 163-67.

49. Burto, G.W., Foster, D.O., Perly, B., et al. 1985. Biological antioxidants. *Philos. Trans. R. Soc.* B. London (ed.) 311:565-78.

50. Burton, J. 1989. Dietary fatty acids and inflammatory skin disease. *Lancet* I :27-31.

51. Busse, W.W., Kopp, D.E., Middleton, E. 1984. Flavonoid modulation of human neutrophil function. *J. Allergy Clin. Immunol.* 73:801-9.

52. Calabarese, E.J. 1981. *Nutritional and Environmental Toxicity: the Influence of Nutritional Status on Pollutant Toxicity and Carcinogenicity.* Vol. 1-2. John Wiley & Sons, Chichester.

53. Caporaso, N. , Smith, S. M . , Eng, R. H. K. 1 983 . Anti-fungal activity in human serum after ingestion of garlic allium-sativum. *Antimicrob. Agents Chemother.* 23(5):700-02.

C54. Arrol, J.E. Brooke, M.H., Shumate, J.B. 1981. Carnitine intake and excretion in neuromuscular diseases. *Am. J. Clin. Nutr.* 34:2693-8.

55. Chanarin, 1., Stephenson, E. 1988. Vegetarian diet and cobalamin deficiency: their association with tuberculosis. *J. Clin. Path.* 41 :759-62.

56. Chen, L. 1988. Effects of diuretics on riboflavin status and urinary excretion. *F.A.S.E.B.J.* 2:1573.

57. Cheney, G. 1949. Rapid healing of peptic ulcers in patients receiving fresh cabbage juice. *California Medicine* 70(1): 10-14.

58. Cheney, G. 1950. The nature of the antipeptic-ulcer factor. *Stanford Med. Bull.* 8(3):145-59.

59. Chow, C.K. 1979. Nutritional influence on cellular antioxidant defense systems. *Am. J. Clin. Nutr.* 32:1066-81.

60. Clark, D. 1957. The endocrine approach to the treatment of allergy. *Ann. West. Med. Surg.* 2(9):404-07.

61. Clark, A.J., Mossholder, M.S., Gates, R. 1987. Folacin status in adolescent females. *Am. J. Clin. Nutr.* 46:302-6.

62. Clausen, J. 1988. Chromium induced clinical improvement in symptomatic hypoglycemia. *Bio. Tr. Elem. Res.* 17:229-36.

63. Cleave, T.L., Campbell, G.D. 1969. *Diabetes, Coronary Thrombosis and the Saccharine Disease.* John Wright & Sons Bristol, England.

64. Cloarec, M.J., et al. 1987. Alpha tocopherol: effect on plasma lipoproteins in hypercholesterolemic patients. *Isr. J. Med. Sci.* 23(8):869-72.

65. Cody, V., Middleton, E., Harborne, J.B. (eds.) 1986. *Plant Flavonoids in Biology and Medicine—Biochemical, Pharmacological, and Structure-activity Relationships.* A.R. Liss, New York.

66. Coggeshall, J.C. , Heggers, J. P. , Robson, M.C. , et al. 1 985 . Biotin status and plasma glucose in diabetics. *Annal. N. Y. Acad. Sci.* 447:38992.

67. Collins, E.B., Ardt, P. 1980. Inhibition of C. Albicans by lactobacilli and lactobacillic fermented dairy products. *F.E.M.S.* Micro. Rev. (Sept.), 46:343-56.

68. Cook, J.D., et al. 1974. Serum ferritin as a measure of iron in normal subjects. *Amer. J. Clin. Nutr.* 27:9681-87.

69. Coombs, R.R.A., Oldham, G. 1981. Early rheumatoid-like joint lesions in rabbits drinking cow's milk. *Int. Arch. Allergy Appl. Immunol.* 64:287.

70. Cornell, R., Walker, W.A. Isselbacher, K.J. 1971. Intestinal absorption of horseradish peroxidase. A cytochemical study. *Lab. Invest.* 25:42-8.

71. Cousins, N. 1986. Panic—the ultimate disease. *Holistic Medicine.* March/April.

72. Cox, R.A., Hoppel, C.l. 1973. Biosynthesis of carnitine and 4-N-trimethylaminobutyrate from lysine. *Biochem. J.* 136: 1075-82.

73. Crittenden, P.J. 1948. Studies on the pharmacology of biotin. Arch. *Int. Pharmacodyn. Ther.* 76:263-75.

74. Cruikshank, J. M., Thorp, T.M., Zacharias, J.F. 1987. Benefits and potential harm of lowering high blood pressure. *Lancet* 1:581-83.

75. Curtis, A.C., Baliner, R.S. 1939. The prevention of carotene absorption by liquid petrolatum. *J.A.M.A.*113:1785.

76. Damrau, F. 1961. The value of bentonite for diarrhea. *Medical Annals District Columbia* 30 (6) pp. 326-28.

77. Darsee, J.R., Heymsfield, S.B. 1981. Decreased myocardial taurine levels. *N.E.J.M.* 304:129.

78. Davies, I.J. 1972. *The Clinical Significance of the Essential Biological Metals.* Charles C. Thomas, Publisher.

79. Davies, S., Stewart, A. 1987. *Nutritional Medicine.* Pan Books, London.

80. Dawson-Hughes, B., Seligson, F.H., Hughes, V.A. 1986. Effects of calcium carbonate and hydroxyapatite on zinc and iron retention in postmenopausal women. *Am. J. Clin. Nutr.* 44:83-88.

81. Dean, R., Cheeseman, K. 1987. Vitamin E protects against free radical damage in lipid environments. *Bioc. Biop. R.* 148: 1277-82.

82. Diamond, H. and Diamond, M. 1985. *Fit for Life.* Warner Books, Inc. New York.

83. Dillard, C.J., et al. 1978. Effects of exercise, vitamin E, and ozone on pulmonary function and lipid peroxidation. *J. Appl. Physiol.* 45:927-32.

84. DiLuzio, N.R. 1973. Antioxidants, lipid peroxidation, and chemical-induced liver injury. *Fed. Proc.* 32:1875-81.

85. DiMagno, E.P., et al. 1977. Fate of orally ingested enzymes in pancreatic insufficiency. *N. E.J. M.* 296(23): 1318-22.

86. DiPerna, P. 1984. Leukemia strikes a small town. *New York Times Magazine,* pp. 100-08.

87. Donahue, R.P., et al. 1987. Central obesity and coronary heart disease in men. *Lancet* 1:821.

88. Dormandy, T.L. 1978. Free radical oxidation and antioxidants. Lancet 1:647-50.

89. Drasar, B.S., Hill, M.J. 1972. Intestinal bacteria and cancer. *Amer. J. Clin. Nutr.* 25:1399-1404.

90. Dreizen, S. 1979. Nutrition and the immune response—a review. *Int. J. Vit. Nutr. Res.* 49:220.

91. Droull, J. 1982. *Drinking Water and Health.* Vol. 4. National Academy of Sciences Press, Washington, D.C.

92. Duke, J.A. 1985. *Handbook of Medicinal Herbs.* CRC Press, Boca Raton, FL.

93. Eaton, S.~ Konner, M. 1985. Paleolithic nutrition. *N.E.J.M.* 312(5) Jan. 31.

94. Edington, J., Geekie, M., Charter, R., et al. 1987. Effect of dietary cholesterol on plasma cholesterol concentration in subjects following reduced fat, high fiber diet. *Br. Med. J.* 294:333-36.

95. Elwood, P.C., et al. 1984. Greater contribution to blood lead from water than from air. *Nature* 310:13840.

96. Ensminger, A.H., et al. 1983. *Foods and Nutrition Encyclopedia.* Vol. 1&2. Pergus Press, Clovis, CA.

97. Fannelli, O. 1978. Carnitine and acetyle-carnitine, natural substances endowed with interesting pharmacological properties. *Life Sci* 23:2563-70.

98. Farber, E. 1981. Chemical carcinogenesis. *N.E.J.M.* 305:1379.

99. Fernandes, K.M., Shahani, M.A. 1987. Therapeutic role of dietary lactobacilli and lactobacillic fermented dairy products. *F.E.M.S. Micro. Rev.* (Sept.) 46:343-56.

100. Florence, T.M. 1984. Cancer and aging: the free radical connection. *Int. Clin. Nutr. Rev.* 4 (1) pp 6-19.

101. Foldi, M. 1972. Vitamin P and Lymphatics. *Angiologica* 9(3):375-89.

102. Folkers, K.~ Yamamuran Y. (eds). 1986. *Biomedical and Clinical Applications of Coenzyme* Q-10. Bantam Books.

103. Fox, M. 1984. *Healthy Water for a Longer Life.* Healthy Water Research Institute. Las Vegas, Nevada.

104. Francis, A., Shetty, T., Bhattach, R. 1988. Modifying role of dietary factors on the mutagenicity of aflatoxin Bl: in vitro effects of trace minerals. *Mutat. Res.* 199:85-93.

105. Freeman, B.A., Crapo, J.D. 1982. Biology of disease: free radicals and tissue injury. *Lab. Invest.* 47:412426.

106. Fritz, I.B. 1963. Carnitine and its role in fatty acid metabolism. *Adv. Lipid Res.* 1:285-334.

107. Frost, D.V., Lish, P.M. 1975. Selenium in biology. *Ann. Rev. Pharm.* 75(15): 259-84.

108. Fujita, T., et al. 1987. Effects of increased adrenomedullary activity and taurine in patients with borderline hypertension. *Circulation* 75:525.

109. Fujisawa, K., Suzuki, H., et al. 1984. Therapeutic effects of liver hydrolysate preparation on chronic hepatitis—a double blind, controlled study. *Asian Med. J.* 26:497-526.

110. Fulder, S.J. 1981. Ginseng and the hypothalamic-pituitary control of stress. *Am. J. Chin. Med.* 9:112-8.

111. Gettis, A. 1987. Serendipity and food sensitivity: a case study. *Headache Journal* 27:73-75.

112. Gibson, G.E, et al. 1988. Reduced activities of thiamine-dependent enzymes in the brains and peripheral tissues of patients with Alzheimer's disease. *Archives of Neurology* 45:836-40.

113. Glavind, L., Zeuner, E. 1986. The effectiveness of a rotary electric toothbrush on oral cleanliness in adults. *J. Clin. Periodont.* 13(2):135-38.

114. Goldberg, I.K. 1980. L-tyrosine in depression. *Lancet* 2:364.

115. Goldman, I.S., Kantrowitz, N.E. 1982. Cardiomyopathy associated with selenium deficiency. *N.E.J.M.* 305:701.

116. Goldstein, G.W. 1977. Lead encephalopathy: the significance of lead inhibition of calcium uptake by brain mitochondria. *Brain Res.* (Netherlands) 136(1):185-188.

117. Grant, E.C. 1979. Food allergies and migraine. *Lancet* 5:966.

118. Griffith, R., et al. 1987. Success of L-lysine therapy in frequently recurrent herpes simplex infection. *Dermatolog.* 175:183-90.

119. Grundy, S., Florentin, L., Nix, D., et al. 1988. Comparison of monounsaturated fatty acids and carbohydrates for reducing raised levels of plasma cholesterol in man. *Am. J. Clin. Nutr.* 47:966-69.

120. Gupta, S., Agarwal, L.B., Epstein, G., et al. 1980. Panax: a new mitogen and interferon producer. *Clin. Res.* 28:504A.

121. Gutteridge, J.M., et al. 1982. Superoxide-dependent formation of hydroxyl radicals and lipid peroxidation in the presence of iron salts. *Biochem. J.* 206:605-09.

122. Hackney, J.D., et al. 1975. Experimental studies on human health effects of air pollutants. 11 *Ozone Arch. Envir. Hlth* 30:379-84.

123. Hall, K. 1976. Allergy of the nervous system: a review. *Ann. Allergy* 36:49.

124. Halliwell, B., Gutteridge, J.M.C. 1984. Lipid peroxidation, oxyge radicals, cell damage, and antioxidant therapy. *Lancet* 1396-97.

125. Harris, J.B., et al. 1967. Lipoic acid: essential cofactor for gastric secretion. *Fed. Proc.* 26:273.

126. Havsteen, B. 1983. Flavonoids, a class of natural products of high pharmacological potency. *Biochem. Pharm.* 32:1141-8.

127. Heimburger, D., et al. 1987. Improvement in bronchial squamous

metaplasia in smoker treated with folate and B$_{12}$. *Am. J. Clin. Nutr.* 45:866.

128. Hicks, J.T. 1964. Treatment of fatigue in general practice: a double-blind study. *Clin. Med. J.* pp. 85-90.

129. Hikino, H., Kiso, Y., Wagner, H., et al. 1984. Antihepatotoxic actions of flavonolignans from Silybum marianum fruits. *Planta Medica* 50:248.

130. Hill, M.J., Drasar, B.S., Aries, V., et al. 1971. Bacteria and the etiology of cancer of the large bowel. *Lancet* 1:95-100.

131. Hirayama, S., Kishikawa, H., Kume, T., et al. 1978. Therapeutic effect of liver hydrolysate on experimental liver cirrhosis. *Nisshin Igaku* 45:528-33.

132. Hollander, D., Tarnawski, H. 1985. Aging-associated increase in intestinal absorption of macromolecules. *Gerontology* 31: 133-37.

133. Hollman, J., et al. 1983. Coronary artery spasm at site of previous angioplasty. *J. Amer. Coll. Card.* 2:1039-1045.

134. Horrobin, D.F., Manku, M.S. 1983. Essential fatty acids in clinical medicine. *Nutrition and Health* 2: 127-34.

135. Horwitt, M.K. 1980. Relative biological values of D-alpha-tocopheryl acetate and all-rac-A tocopheryl acetate in man. *Am. J. Clin. Nutr.* 33:1856-1860.

136. Horwitt, M.K. 1980. Therapeutic uses of vitamin E in medicine. *Nutr. Rev.* 38(3).

137. Hoyumpa, A.M. 1983. Alcohol and thiamine metabolism. *Alcoholism: Clinical and Experimental Research* 7(1).

138. Isaacs, J.P., Lamb, B.S. 1974. Trace metals, vitamins, and hormones in ten-year treatment of coronary atherosclerotic heart disease. *Texas Heart Institute Symposium* Feb. 21.

139. Isselbacher, K.J. 1977. Metabolic and hepatic effect of alcohol. *N.E.J.M.* March 17, 296(11).

140. Jamal, G.A. , Carmichael, H. , Weir, A. l. 1 986. Gamma-linoleic acid in diabetic neuropathy. *Lancet* May 10, letter to the editor.

141. Jacques, P., et al. 1987. Vitamin intake and senile cataract. *J. Am. Col. Nutr.* 6:435.

142. Jayaraj, A.P., Tovey, F.I., Clark, C.G. 1980. Possible dietary protective factors in relation to the distribution of duodenal ulcer in India and Bangladesh. *Gut* 21: 1068-76.

143. Jensen, B. 1987. *Chlorella: Gem of the Orient.* Bernard Jensen Publisher, Escondido, CA.

144. Johns, D.R. 1986. Migraine provoked by aspartame. *N.E.I.M.* 315:456.

145. Johnson, F.C.1979. The antioxidant vitamins. *CRC Crit. Rev. Food Sci Nutr.* 11:217-309.

146. Jones, A.V., Shorhouse, M., McLaughlan, P., et. al. 1982. Food intolerance: a major factor in the pathogenesis of irritable bowel syndrome. *Lancet* Nov. 20.

147. Jones, L.A.O., Gould, J.H. 1980. Elemental content of predigested liquid protein products. *Amer. J. Clin. Nutr.* 33:2545.

148. Jones, M.H. 1984. *The Allergy Self-Help Cookbook.* Rodale Press, Inc., Emmanus, Penn.

149. Kabacoff, B.L., et. al. 1963. Absorption of chymotrypsin from the intestinal tract. *Nature* 199:815.

150. Kagawa, K., et. al. 1986. Garlic extract inhibits the enhanced peroxidation and production of lipids in carbon tetrachloride-induced liver injury. *Jap. J. Pharm.* 42:19.

151. Kamm, J.J., Dashman, T., Connely., A., et. al. 1975. Effect of ascorbic acid on amine nitrite toxicity. *Ann. New York Acad. Sci.* 258: 169-74.

152. Kamm, J.J., Dashman, T., Newmark, H., et. al. 1977. Inhibition of amine nit rite hepatotoxicity by alpha-tocop herol. *Toxicol. Appl. Pharm.* 41:575-83.

153. Kandil, O.M., et. al. 1987. Garlic and the immune system in humans: its effect on natural killer cells. *Fed. Proc.* 46:441.

154. Kannel, W.B., Pearson, G., McNamara, M. 1969. Obesity as a force of morbidity and mortality. F.P. Herald (ed). *Adolescent Nutrition and Growth.*

155. Karkkainen, P., et. al. 1986. Alcohol intake correlated with serum trace elements. *Alc. Alcohol* 23:279-82.

156. Kaul, T.N., Middleton, E., Ogra, P.L. 1985. Anti-viral effect of flavonoids on human viruses. *J. Med. Virol.* 15:71-9.

157. Kelsay, J.L., et. al. 1979. Effect of fiber from fruits and vegetables on metabolic responses of human subjects. *Am. J. Clin. Nutr.* 32:1876.

158. Kendler, B. 1987. Garlic and onion: a review of their relationship to cardiovascular disease. *Prev. Med.* 16:670-85.

159. Kennedy, M.J., Volz, P.A. 1985. Ecology of candida albicans gut colonization: inhibition of candida adhesion, colonization, and dissemination from the gastrointestinal tract by bacterial antagonism. *Infection and Immunity* 49(3):654-63.

160. Kikuchi, Y., Koyama, T. 1983. Cholesterol-induced impairment in red cell deformability and its improvement by vitamin E. *Clin. Hemorh.* 3:375.

161. Kiso, Y., Suzuki, Y., Watanabe, N., et. al. 1983. Antihepatotoxic principles of Curcuma longa rhizomes. *Planta Medica* 49: 185-7.

162. Kligman, A., Mills, O., Leyden, J., et. al. 1981. Oral vitamin A in acne vulgaris. *Int. J. Derm.* 20:278-85.

163. Knapp, H.R., Reilly, 1., Alessandrini, P., et. al. 1986. In vivo indexes of platelet and vascular function during fish-oil administration in patients with atherosclerosis. *N.E.J.M.* Apr. 10 p. 93742.

164. Kok, F.J., et. al. 1989. Decreased selenium levels in acute myocardial infarction. *J.A.M.A.* 261(8):1161-64.

165. Kondoh, M., Ohe, M., Akifumi, O., et. al. 1984. Effect of sodium saccharin on rat pancreatic enzyme secretion. *J. Nutr. Sci. Vitaminol.* 30:569-76.

166. Konishi, F., et. al. 1985. Anti-tumor effect induced by a hot water extract of chlorella vulgaris (CE): resistance to meth-A tumor growth mediated by CE-induced polymorphonuclear leukocytes. *Cancer Immunol. Immunother.* 19:73-78.

167. Kopaladze, R.A., Turova, N.F. 1985. Correction of impaired oxygen supply with antioxidants. Izv. *Akad. Gruz. SSR. Ser. Biol.* 11 :324-9.

168. Kornhauser, A., et. al. 1986. Protective effects of beta carotene against psoralen toxicity: relevance to protection against carcinogenesis. *Anti-Mutagenesis and Anticarcinogenesis Mechanisms.* Plenum Press, New York.

169. Korovka, L.S. 1976. Ascorbic acid content in wild growing edible plants of Komi-Permiak National Okrug, USSR. *Vopr. Pitan.* (6):76-77.

170. Korpela, H., Kumpulainen, J.T., Sotaniemi, E.A. 1985. The role of selenium deficiency in the pathogenesis of alcoholic liver disease. *Nutrition Research,* Suppl. I; pp. 424-25. Pergamon Press, LTD.

171. Krause, M.V., Mahan, L.K. 1984. *Food, Nutrition, and Diet Therapy.* W.B. Sanders Co., Philadelphia, Penn.

172. Krinsky, N., et. al. 1982. Interaction of oxygen and oxy-radicals with carotenoids. *J. Can. Res. Clin. Onco.* 69:205.

173. Kromhout, D., Coulander, C. 1982. Dietary fiber and 10 year mortality from coronary heart disease, cancer and all causes. *Lancet* Sept. 4:518.

174. Kuhnau, J., 1976. The flavonoids: a class of semi-essential food components: their role in human nutrition. *Wld Rev. Diet* 24:117-91.

175. Kuller, L. 1969. Sudden death in atherosclerotic heart disease. The case for preventive medicine. *Amer. J. Card.* 24:617.

176. Lahman, S. 1970. Studies on placental transfer: trichloroethylene. *Ind. Med.* 39:46-9.

177. Langer, S.E., Scheer, J.F. 1984. *Solved: The Riddle of Illness.* Keats Publishing, Inc., New Canaan, Conn.

178. Langsjoen, P.H., Vadhanavikit, S., Folkers, K. 1985. Response of patients in classes 111 and IV of cardiomyopathy to therapy in a blind and crossover trial with coenzyme Q-10. *Proc. Natl. Acad. Sci.* 82:4240.

179. Lau, B.H.S., et. al. 1987. Effect of an odor-modified garlic preparation on blood lipids. *Nutr. Res.* 7:139.

180. Lau, B.H.S., et. al. 1983. Allium sativum (garlic) and atherosclerosis: a review. *Nutr. Res.* 3:119.

181. Laurent, J., Rostoker, R., Robeva, C., et. al. 1987. Is adult idiopathic

nephrotic syndrome food allergy? value of oligoantigenicdiets. *Nephron* (Sept.) 47:7-11.

182. Lawson, M., Bunker, V., Clayton, B., et. al. 1987. The effect ofdietary fibre on apparent absorption of zinc, copper, iron and manganese in the elderly. *P. Nutr. Soc.* 46:53A.

183. LeGrady, D., et. al. 1987. Coffee consumption and mortality in the Chicago Western Electric Company. *Am. J. Epidem.* 126:803-812.

184. Lessof, M.H. (ed.) 1983. *Clinical Reactions to Foods.* John Wiley & Sons, Chichester.

185. Levine, S.A., Kidd, P.M. 1987. *Antioxidant Adaptation: Its Role in Free Radical Pathology.* Biocurrents Division, Allergy Res. Group, Publisher.

186. Levine, S.A., Kidd, P.A. 1985. Biochemical pathologies initiated by free radical oxidant compounds in the etiology of food hypersensitivity disease. *Int. Clin. Nutr. Rev.* 5(1):5-23.

187. Lindenbaum, J., Healton, E., Savage, D., et. al. 1988. Neuropsychiatric disorders caused by cobalamin deficiency in the absence of anemia or macrocytosis. *N.E.J.M.* 318: 1720-28.

188. Littarru, G.P., Ho, L., Folkers, K. 1972. Deficiency of coenzyme Q-10 in human heart disease. Part 11. *Internat. J. Vit. Res.* 42:413.

189. Lonsdale, D. 1987. Thiamine and its fat soluble derivatives as therapeutic agents. *Int. Clin. Nutr. Rev.* 7(3): 114-25

190. Maebashi, M. 1978. Lipid-lowering effect of carnitine in patients with type IV hyperlipoproteinaemia. *Lancet* 1:805.

191. Malkinson, F. 1964. Permeability of the stratum corneum. In: W. Montagna, W.E. Lobit, Jr. (eds): *The Epidermis.* Academic Press. New York.

192. Mallos, T. 1979. *The Complete Middle East Cookbook.* McGraw-Hill, New York.

193. Massey, L., et. al. 1988. Acute effects of dietary caffeine and aspirin on urinary mineral excretion in pre- and postmenopausal women. *Nutr. Res.* 845-51.

194. Marshall, A.W., et al. 1982. Treatment of alcohol-related liver disease

with thioctic acid: a six month randomized double-blind trial. *Gut* 23: 1088-93.

195. McClain, C.J., Su, L. 1983. Zinc deficiency in the alcoholic: a review. *Alcoholism: Clinical and Experimental Research* 7(1).

196. McLennan, P., Abeywardena, M., Charnock, J. 1988. Dietary fish oil prevents ventricular fibrillation following coronary artery occlusion and reperfusion. *Am. Heart J.* 116:709-17.

197. Meck, W., Church, R. 1987. Nutrients that modify the speed of internal clock and memory storage processes. *Behav. Neuro.* 101 :465-75.

198. Mengel, C.E. 1968. Rancidity of the red cell. Peroxidation of red cell lipid. *Amer. J. Sci.* June 255:34145.

199. Michaelson, G., Juhlin, L., Vahlquist, A. 1977. Effects of oral zinc and vitamin A in acne. *Arch. Derm.* 113:31-6.

200. Michaelson, G., Vahiquist, A., Juhlin, L. 1977. Serum zinc and retinol binding-protein in acne. *Br. J. Derm.* 96:283-6.

201. Middleton, E. 1984. The flavonoids. trends in pharmaceutical science. *Science* 5:335-8.

202. Miller, D.S., Parsonage, S. 1975. Resistance to slimming: adaptation or illusion? *Lancet* Apr. 5, p. 773.

203. Miller, J.D. 1982. The new pollution: ground water contamination. *Environment* 24:8.

204. Misiewicz, G. 1972. Gastrointestinal manifestations of stress and the psychopathic personality. *Medicine* 3:183-88.

205. Mock, D., Johnson, S., Holman, R. 1988. Effects of biotin deficiency on serum fatty acid composition: evidence for abnormalities in humans. *J. Nutr.* 118:34248.

206. Monro, J., Brostoff, J. 1980. Food allergy in migraine. *Lancet* July 5:1014

207. Morley, J.E. 1982. Food peptides—a new class of hormones? *J.A.M.A.* 17:2379-80.

208. Moses, H.A. 1979. Trace elements: an association with cardiovascular

diseases and hypertension: *J. Nat'l. Med. Assoc.* 71(3):227-28.

209. Mueller, L.J., et. al. 1987. Rotary electric toothbrushing— clinical effects on the presence of gingivitis and supragingival dental plaque. *Dental Hygiene* 61(12):546-50.

210. Mussalo-Rauhamaa, H., et. al. 1987. Decreased serum selenium and magnesium levels in drunkenness arresters. *Drug Al. Dep.* 20:95-103.

211. Nakazono, K. 1985. Active oxygen and factors scavenging it in synovial fluid in rheumatoid arthritis. *Nigata Igakkai Zasshi* 99:489-501.

212. Nely, J. R.~ Morgen, H. E. 1 974. Relationships between carbohydrates and lipid metabolism and the energy balance of the heart muscle. *Ann. Rev. Physical.* 36: 413460.

213. Niki, E., Tsuchiya, J., Yoshikawa, Y., et al. 1986. Oxidation of lipids. XIII. Antioxidant activities of alpha-, beta-, gamma-, and delta-tocopherols. *Bull Chem. Soc. Jpn* 59:497-501.

214. Novi, A.M., Flokke, R. Stukenkemper, M. 1982. Glutathione and aflatoxin Bl-induced liver tumors: requirement for an intact glutathione molecule for regression of malignancy. In R. Baserga (ed). Cell proliferation, Cancer, and Cancer Therapy a conference in honor of Ann Goldfeder. *New York Academy of Sciences Annals* 397:62-71.

215. Oelgetz, A.W., et al. 1935. The treatment of food allergy and indigestion of pancreatic origin with pancreatic enzymes. *Amer. J. Dig. Dis. Nutr.* 2:422-26.

216. Oelgetz, A.W., et al. 1939. Pancreatic enzymes and food allergy. *Med. Rec.* 150:276-79.

217. Offenbacher, E., Stunyer, F. 1980. Beneficial effect of chromium-rich yeast on glucose tolerance and blood lipids in elderly patients. *Diabetes* 29:919-25.

218. 218. Opie, L.H. 1977. Role of carnitine in fatty acid metabolism of normal and ischemic myocardium. *Am. Heart J.* 3:375.

219. Oram J.F., Wenger, J.I., Neely, J.R. 1975. Regulation of long chain fatty acid activation in the heart muscle. *J. Biol. Chem.* 250:73-78.

220. Orengo, I., et al. 1988. The influence of dietary menhaden oil upon photocarcinogenesis. *Clin. Res.* 36:85A.

221. Orengo, I., Black, H., Kettler, A., et al. 1988. Influence of dietary menhaden oil upon carcinogenesis and related responses to UV-radiation. (meeting abstract). *J. Inv. Derm.* 90:594.

222. Pauling, L. 1986. *How to Live Longer and Feel Better.* W.H. Freeman and Co. New York.

223. Pereira, M.A., et al. 1982. Trihalomethanes as inhibitors and promoters of carcinogenesis. *Envir. Hlth Persp.* 46: 151-56.

224. Petersdorf, R. (ed). 1983. *Harrison's Principles of Internal Medicine.* 10th ed. McGraw Hill, New York.

225. Peticone, F., et al. 1988. Protective magnesium treatment in ischemic dilated cardiomyopathy (meeting abstract). *J. Am. Col. Nutr.* 7:403.

226. Pothier, L., et al. 1987. Plasma selenium levels in patients with advanced upper gastrointestinal cancer. *Cancer* 60:2251-2260.

227. Prasad, K.N. 1982. Effects of tocopherol on morhological alterations and growth inhibition in melanoma cells in culture. *Cancer Res.* 42:550.

228. Prasad, K.M.~ Bholaz N.R.1984. *Nutrition and cancer. In Yearbook of Nutritional Medicine,* J. Bland (ed). 1:178-89.

229. Pryor, W.A. fed). 1976. *Free Radicals in Biology.* Vow. 1-3. Academic Press, New York.

230. Puddey, I.B. 1987. Regular alcohol use raises blood pressure in treated hypertensive subjects. *Lancet* 10:647-651.

231. Pye, V.I., Patrick, R. 1983. Ground water contamination in the United States. *Science* 221:713-18.

232. Randi, A., et al. 1987. Orally administered vitamin B_6 prolongs the bleeding time and inhibits platelet aggregation in human volunteers. *Thromb. Haem.* 58:176.

232. Reading, C M., Meillon, R.S. 1988. *The Family Tree Connection.* Keats Publishing, Inc. New Canaan, Conn.

233. Rebouche, C.J., Engel, A.G. 1980. Tissue distribution of carnitine biosynthetic enzymes in man. *Biochem. Biophvs. Acta.* 630:22-29.

234. Reed, L.J. 1953. Metabolic functions of thiamin and lipoic acid. *Physical*

Rev. 33:544-59.

235. Reid, K., et al. 1987. Double-blind study of yohimbine in treatment of psychogenic impotence. *Lancet* 2:241.

236. Reiser, S., et al. 1987. Effect of copper intake on blood cholesterol and its lipoprotein distribution in men. *Nutr. Rep. In.* 36:641-49.

237. Reiter, L., et al. 1987. Vitamin B_{12} and folate intakes and plasma levels of black adolescent females. *J. Am. Diet. Assoc.* 87.

238. Resnik, L. 1987. Interrelation of calcium and magnesium with renin-sodium factors in essential hypertension. *J. Am. Coll. Nutr.* 6:62-63.

239. Riales, R., Albrink, M. 1981. Effects of chromium chloride supplementation on the glucose tolerance and serum lipids, including HDL, in adult men. *Am. J. Clin. Nutr.* 34:2670-8.

240. Rice, S. L. , Eiten Miller, R. R. , Koehler, P.E. 1976. Biologically active amines in food: a review. *J. Milk. Food Technol.* 39(5):353-8.

241. RobsVn, J.R.K., et al. 1977. Metabolic response to food. *Lancet* Dec. 24 & 31, p. 1267.

242. Roe, D.A. 1983. *Drug-Induced Nutritional Defeiences.* A.V.I., Westport, Conn.

243. Rogers, S. 1985. Sugar and health. *Lancet* Feb. 23.

244. Rosenberg, E., Belew, P. 1982. Microbial factors in psoriasis. *Arch. Derm.* 118:1434-44.

245. Rosenberg, L., et al. 1982. Breast cancer and alcoholic beverage consumption. *Lancet* Jan 30:267.

246. Rossi, C.S., Siliprandi, N. 1982. Effect of carnitine on serum HDL cholesterol: report of two cases. *John Hopkins Med. J.* 150:51-54.

247. Rowe, N.A., Gorlin, R.J. 1959. The effect of vitamin A deficiency upon experimental oral carcinogenesis. *J. Dent. Res.* Jan-Feb, pp. 72-83.

248. Ruddel H., et al. 1987. Effect of magnesium supplementation in patients with labile hypertension. *J. Amer. Col. Nutr.* 6:445.

249. Saffiotti, J., Montesano, R., Sellakumar, D.V.M., et al. 1967.

Experimental cancer of the lung. Inhibition by vitamin A of induction of tracheobronchial squamous metaplasia. *Cancer* May, pp. 857-63.

250. Sakula, A., et al. 1980. Vitamin A and cancer. *Lancet* 2:1029.

251. Salonen, J., et al. 1988. Relationship of serum selenium and antioxidants to plasma lipoproteins, platelet aggregability and prevalent ischaemic heart disease in Eastern Finnish men. Atherosclerosis 70:155-60.

252. Salmi, H.A., Sarna, S. 1982. Effect of silymarin on chemical, functional, and morphological alterations of liver. A double-blind controlled study. Scand. *J. Gastroenterol.* 17:517-21.

253. Samuni, A., et al. 1981. Unusual oxygen-induced sensitization of the biological damage due to superoxide radicals. *J. Biol. Chem.* 256:12632.

254. Sandhu, D.K., Warraich, M. K., Singh, S. 1980. Sensitivity of yeasts isolated from cases of vaginitis to aqueous extract of garlic. *Mykosen* 23(12):3169-73.

255. Sandine, W.E. 1979. Roles of lactobacillus in test intestinal tract. *Journal of Food Protection* 42:259-62.

256. Scholar, E., et al. 1988. Effects of diets enriched in cabbage and collards on metastasis of BALB/c mammary carcinoma (meeting abstract). *P. Am. Assoc. Ca.* 29:149.

257. Schrauzer, G.N. 1976. Selenium and cancer: a review. *Bioinorganic Chemistry* 5:275.

258. Schrauzer, G.N. 1977. Cancer mortality correlation studies ILL. Statistical associations with dietary selenium intakes. *Bioinorganic Chemistry* 7:23

259. Schrauzer, G.N., White, D.A. 1978. Selenium in human nutrition: dietary intakes and effects of supplementation. *Bioinorganic Chemistry* 8:303-18.

260. Schroeder, H.A. 1973. *The Trace Elements and Man.* Devin-Adair Co., Old Greenwich, Conn.

261. Schroeder, H.A. 1974. *The Poisons Around Us.* Indiana Univ. Press, London.

262. Schwarz, K.S. 1970. The cellular mechanisms of vitamin E action: direct and indirect effects of alpha-tocopherol on mitochondrial respiration.

Ann. N. Y. Acad. Sci.

263. Scragg, R., et al. 1982. Birth defects in household water supply. Epidemiological studies in the mount Gambier region of South Australia. *Med. J. Austr.* 2:577-79.

264. Scriver, C.R., Rosenberg, L.E. 1973. Amino acid metabolism and its disorders. Alex Schaffer (ed). *Major Problems in Clinical Pediatrics.* W.B. Saunders Co., Philadelphia.

265. Seelig, M. S. , Heggtveit, H .A. 1 974. Magnesium interrelationships in ischemic heart disease: a review. *Am. J. Clin. Nutr.* 27:59.

266. Seiss, W., Roth, P.P., Scherer, B.C., et al. 1980. Platelet membrane fatty acids, platelet aggregation and thromboxane formation during mackerel diet. *Lancet* March pp.441-44.

267. Shamberger, R.J. 1976. Selenium in health and disease. *Proc. Symp. Selen. Tell Envir.* Industrial Health Foundation, Inc. Pittsburgh, Penn.

268. Shariff, R., et al. 1988. Vitamin E supplementation in smokers. *Clin. Res.* 36:A770.

269. Shaw, D.M., et al. 1984. Senile dementia and nutrition. (Letter to the editor). *Brit. Med. J.* 288:792-93.

270. Shaw, J.H. 1987. Causes and control of dental caries. *N.E.J.M.* 317:996.

271. Shaw, S., Lieber, C.S. 1983. Plasma amino acids in the alcoholic: nutritional aspects. *Alcoholism: Clinical and Experimental Research* 7(1).

272. Siccardi, A., Fortunato, A., Marconi, M., et al. 1981. Defective bactericidal reaction by the alternative pathway of complement in atopic patients. *Infect. Immun.* 33:701-3.

273. Snook, J.T., Palmquist, D.L., et al. 1983. Selenium status of a rural (predominately Amish) community living in a low-selenium area. *Am. J. Clin. Nutr.* 38:620.

274. Sohler, A., Kruesi, M., Pfeiffer, C.C. 1977. Blood lead levels in psychiatric outpatients reduced by zinc and vitamin C. *J. Orthomol. Psy.* 6(3):272-276.

275. Solinan, M.A., Fahmy, S.A., et al. 1970. Liver cell regeneration in prophylaxis and treatment of carbon tetrachloride hepatotoxicity. *J.*

Egypt. Med. Assoc. 53(3):214-22.

276. Spallholz, J.E. 1981. Anti-inflammatory, immunological, and carcinostatic attributes of selenium in experimental animals. *Adv. Exp. Med. Biol.* 135:43-61.

277. Stampfer, M.J., Hennekens, C.H. 1982. Carotene, carrots, and white blood cells. *Lancet* Sept. 11:615.

278. Steenblock, D. 1987. *Chlorella: Natural Medicinal Algae.* Aging Research Institute, El Toro, Calif.

279. Stevens, R., et al. 1988. Body iron stores and the risk of cancer. *Am. J. Clin. Nutr.* 319:1047-52.

280. Stevenson, D. 1979. Food allergies and migraine. *Lancet* July 14:103.

281. Stewart, R., Dodd, H. 1964. Absorption of carbon tetrachloride, trichloroethylene, tetrachloroethylene, methylene chloride, and 1, 1, I-trichloroethane through human skin. *Ind. Hyg. J.* Sept. - Oct. pp. 439-46.

282. Suda, D., et al. 1986. Inhibition of experimental oral carcinogenesis by topical beta carotene. *Carcinogenesis* 7:711

283. Suekawa, M., Ishige, A., Yuasa, K., et al. 1984. Pharmacological studies on ginger. I. Pharmacological actions of pungent constituents, (6)-gingerol and (6)-shogaol. *J. Pharm. Dyn.* 7:836-48.

284. Sugino, K., Kiyohiko, D., Yamoda, K., et al. 1987. The role of lipid peroxidation in endotoxin-induced hepatic damage and the protective effect of antioxidants. *Surgery* June l; Vol. 6.

285. Sugiyama, S., Kitazawa, M., Ozawa, K., et al. 1980. Antioxidative effect of coenzyme Q- 10. *Experiontia* 36: 1002.

286. Sullivan, J.L. 1981. Iron and the sex difference in heart disease risk. *Lancet* June 13, p. 1239.

287. Sullivan, J.L. 1983. Vegetarianism, ischemic heart disease, and iron. (letter to the editor). *Am. J. Clin. Nutr.* 37:882-86.

288. Suzuki, Y., Kamikawa, T., Yamazaki, N. 1980. Protective effects of I-carnitine on ischemic heart. *Carnitine Biosynthesis, Metabolism, and Functions.* Academic Press, pp. 341-52.

289. Swain, A., Truswell, A.S., Loblay, R.H. 1984. Adverse reactions to food. *Food Technology in Australia.* 36(10): 467-71.

290. Swain, A., Dutton, S.P., Truswell, A.S. 1985. Salicylates in foods. *J. Amer. Diet. Assoc.* 85(8):950-60.

291. Szejnwald-Brown, H., Bishop, D.R., Rowan, C.A. 1984. The role of skin absorption as a route of exposure for volatile organic compounds (VOCs) in drinking water. *Amer. J. Pub. Hlth* 74(S):479-83.

292. Tanaka, K. 1981. New light on biotin deficiency. *N.E.J.M.* 304:839-40.

293. Tappel, A.L. 1973. Lipid peroxidation damage to cell components. *Fed. Proc.* 32:1870-74.

294. Tappel, A.L. 1980. On antioxidant nutrients: how they may protect you from smog and other environmental pollutants and some aging reactions. *Executive Health Magazine.*

295. Tappel, A.L. 1980. Measurement of and protection from in vivo lipid peroxidation. W.W. Pryor (ed). *Free Radicals in Biology* 4:2-47.

296. Tarayre, J.P., Lauressergies, H., et al. 1977. Advantages of a combination of proteolytic enzymes, flavonoids, and ascorbic acid in comparison with non-steroidal anti-inflammatory agents. *Arznein-Forsch. Drug Res.* 27(1): 1144.

297. Tengroth, B.* Ammitzboll, T. 1984. Changes in the content and composition of collagen in the glaucomatous eye—basis for a new hypothesis for the genesis of chronic open angle glaucoma. *Acta Opthamol* 62:999-1008.

298. Thomsen, M., et al. 1978. Improved pacing tolerance of the ischemic human myocardium after administration of carnitine. *Am. J. Cardiol.* 43:304.

299. Towns, S.J., Mellis, C.M. 1984. Role of acetyl salicylic acid and sodium metabisulphite in chronic childhood asthma. *Pediatrics* 73(5):631 -7.

300. Trivellato, M., et al. 1984. Carnitine deficiency as the possible etiology of idiopathic mitral valve prolapse: case study with speculative annotation. *Texas Heart Institute Journal* 11(4):370

301. Tuchweber, B., Trost, W., Salas, M., et al. 1976. Prevention of praseodymium-induced hepatotoxicity by silybin. *Toxicol. Appl. Pharmacol.* 38:559-70.

302. Ulrey, D.E. 1976. Selenium in animal nutrition: health implication. *Proc. Symp. Selen. Tell. Envr.* Industrial Health Foundation Inc., Pittsburgh, Penn.

303. Upadhyay, M.P., Manadhar, K.L., Shrestha, R.B. 1980. Anti-fungal activity of garlic against fungi isolated from human eyes. *J. Gen. Appl. Microbiol* 26(6):421-24.

304. Vahouny, G., Kritchevsky, D. 1982. *Dietary Fiber in Health and Disease.* Plenem Press, New York.

305. Vander, A.J. 1981. *Nutrition, Stress and Toxic Chemicals.* University of Michigan Press, Ann Arbor, Mich.

306. Vanderhoek, J.Y., Makheja, A. H., Bailey, J.M. 1980. Inhibition of fatty-acid oxygenases by onion and garlic oils evidence for the mechanism by which these oils inhibit platelet aggregation. *Biochem. Pharmacol.* 29(23):3169-73.

307. Wald, N., et al. 1988. Serum beta-carotene and subsequent risk of cancer: results from the BUPA study. *Br. J. Canc.* 57:428-33.

308. Waldbott, G.L. 1978. *Health Effects of Environmental Pollutants.* 2nd ed. C.V.Mosby Co., St. Louis.

309. Wald, N., et al. 1987. Serum vitamin E and subsequent risk of cancer. *Br. J. Canc.* 56:69-72.

310. Walker, W.A. 1981. *Intestinal Transport of Macromolecules. Physiology of the Gastrointestinal Tract.* L.R. Johnson (ed). Raven Press, New York.

311. Walker, W.A. 1982. Mechanisms of antigen handling by the gut. *Clinics in Immunology and Allergy* 2(1): 15-35.

312. Wang, L.F., Lin, J.K., Tung, Y.C. 1979. Protective effect of chlorella on hepatic damage induced by ethionine in rats. *J. Formosan Med. Assoc.* 78:1010-19.

313. Ward, R., Peters, D.P. 1987. Nutritional and vitamin E status of alcohol abusers with and without chronic skeletal muscle myopathy. *Alc. Alcohol* 22:A6.

314. Watson, R., Leonard, T. 1986. Selenium and vitamins A, E, and C: nutrients with cancer prevention properties. *J. Am. Diet. Assoc.* 86:505-10.

315. Webster, P., Dyckner, T. 1987. Magnesium and hypertension. *J. Am. Coll. Nutr.* 6:321-8.

316. Webster, R., Maibach, H. 1977. Percutaneous absorption in man and animal: A perspective. In: U. Drill and P. Lazar (eds) *Cutaneous Toxicity.* Academic Press, New York.

317. Weisberger, A.S. 1958. Tumor inhibition by a sulfhydryl blocking agent related to an active principle of garlic. *Cancer Research* Dec. 18:1301-8.

318. Weiss, S.J., Lampert, M.B., Test, S.T. 1983. Long-lived oxidants generated by human neutrophils. *Science* 222:626.

319. Werbach, M.R. 1987. *Nutritional Influences on Illness.* Third Line Press Inc., Tarzana, CA.

320. Westrick, E. Shapiro, A., et al. 1988. Dietary tryptophan reverses alcohol-induced impairment of facial recognition but not verbal recall. *Alc. Clin. Exp.* 12:531 -33.

321. Whitacre, M.E., Combs, G.F. 1983. Selenium and mitochondrial integrity in the pancreas of the chick. *J. Nutr.* 113:1972.

322. White, J.W., Jr. 1976. Relative significance of dietary source of nitrate and nitrite. J. Agri. Food. Chem. 23:886-891.

323. White, J.W., Jr. 1976. Correlation relative significance of dietary source of nitrate and nitrite. *J. Agri. Food. Chem.* 24:202.

324. Wilkins, J.R.ILL, Reiches, N.A., Kruse, C.W. 1979. Organic chemical contaminants in drinking water and cancer. *Am. J. Epidemiol.* 110:420-448.

325. Willett, W., et al. 1976. Selenium and human health. *Nutr. Rev.* 34(11):347.

326. Williams, S.R. 1973. *Review of Nutrition and Diet Therapy.* C.V. Mosby Co., St. Louis.

327. Williams, R.J. 1971. *Nutrition Against Disease.* Pitman, New York.

328. Williams, R.J. 1980. *Alcoholism—The Nutritional Approach.* Univ. Texas Press, Austin.

329. Wimhurst, J.M., Manchester, K.L. 1972. Comparison of abilityof Mg and Mn to activate the key enzymes of glycolysis. *F.E.R.S. Letters* 27:321-6.

330. Winitz, M., et al. 1964. Effect of dietary carbohydrate on serum

cholesterol levels. *Archives of Biochemistry and Biophysics* 108:576-79.

331. Wissler, R.W.1976. Current status of regression studies. *Athero. Rev.* 3:213.

332. Wissler, R.W. 1979. Evidence for regression of advanced atherosclerotic plaques. *Arteriosclerosis* 5:398.

333. Wolf, G. 1982. Is dietary carotene an anti-cancer agent? *Nutr. Rev.* 40:257.

334. Wright, A., et al. 1986. Food allergy or intolerance in severe recurrent aphthous ulceration of the mouth. *Br. Med. J.* 292(6530): 1237-8.

335. Wurtman, J.J., Zeisel, S.H. 1982. Carbohydrate craving in obese people. *Inter. J. Eat. Dis.* 1:4.

336. Wurtman, R.J., Wurtman, J.J. 1983. Physiological and Behavioral Effects of Food Constituents. *Nutrition and the Brain.* Vol. 6. Raven Press, N.Y.

337. Wynder, E. 1987. Amount and type of fat/fiber in nutritional carcinogenesis. *Prev. Med.* 16:451459.

338. Yanick, P., Jaffe, R. 1988. *Clinical Chemistry and Nutrition Guidebook: a Physician's Desk Reference.* Vol. I T&H Publishing.

339. Yudkin, J., Edelman, 1., Hough, L. (eds.) 1971. *Sugar: Chemical, Biological, and Nutritional Aspects of Sucrose.* Daniel Davey, Hartford, Conn.

340. Yudkin, J. 1957. Diet and coronary thrombosis. Hypothesis and fact. *Lancet* 11:155-62.

341. Yudkin, J., et al. 1986. Dietary sucrose affects plasma HDL cholesterol concentrations in young men. *Ann. Nutr. Metab.* 30(4):261-66.

342. Ziegler, R., et al. 1984. Dietary carotene, vitamin A and risk of lung cancer among white men in New Jersey. *J. Nat.'l. Can. Inst.* 73:1429.

343. Zimmerman, B. 1979. Do onions and garlic prevent thrombi? *Mod. Med.* 23.

344. Zioudrou, C., Klee, W.A. 1979. Possible roles of peptides derived from food proteins in brain function. *Nutrition in the Brain* 4: 125-52.

Index

363

D

W—Z

ORDER FORM

Item	Quantity	Amount

BOOKS

#1	*How to Eat Right and Live Longer*	_____	_____
#2	*Self-Test Nutrition Guide*	_____	_____
#3	*Who Needs Headaches?*	_____	_____
#4	*Tea Tree Oil—the Natural Antiseptic*	_____	_____
#5	*How to Survive Disasters With Natural Medicines*	_____	_____
#6	*Supermarket Remedies*	_____	_____
#7	*The Cure Is in the Cupboard*	_____	_____
#8	*Lifesaving Cures*	_____	_____
#9	*The Diabetes Cure*	_____	_____

TAPES

#1	*The Survivor's Nutritional Pharmacy*	_____	_____
#2	*How to Use Oregano for Common Illnesses*	_____	_____
#3	*Selected Interviews and Lectures: The Best of Dr. Cass Ingram*	_____	_____
#4	*The Warning Signs of Nutritional Deficiency Professional/Advanced Series*	_____	_____

	Amount
Sub-Total	_____
Sales Tax (if any)	_____
Shipping*	_____
TOTAL	_____

*Shipping Charges: $5.00 for single books—add $1.00 for each additional book.
For cassette tapes only, add $4.00 shipping charge.
Payment by check, money order, or credit card.

Make checks payable to: NAHS
P.O. Box 4885
Buffalo Grove, Illinois 60089
Phone: (800) 243-5242 • Fax: 847 473-4780

For Visa/Mastercard orders provide the following information:

Card#_____ Exp. Date_____

Signature_____

Name_____

Address_____

City_____ State_____ Zip_____

For more information see pages 333-334.

ORDER FORM

Item	Quantity	Amount
BOOKS		
#1 *How to Eat Right and Live Longer*		
#2 *Self-Test Nutrition Guide*		
#3 *Who Needs Headaches?*		
#4 *Tea Tree Oil—the Natural Antiseptic*		
#5 *How to Survive Disasters With Natural Medicines*		
#6 *Supermarket Remedies*		
#7 *The Cure Is in the Cupboard*		
#8 *Lifesaving Cures*		
#9 *The Diabetes Cure*		
TAPES		
#1 *The Survivor's Nutritional Pharmacy*		
#2 *How to Use Oregano for Common Illnesses*		
#3 *Selected Interviews and Lectures: The Best of Dr. Cass Ingram*		
#4 *The Warning Signs of Nutritional Deficiency Professional/Advanced Series*		

	Amount
Sub-Total	
Sales Tax (if any)	
Shipping*	
TOTAL	

*Shipping Charges: $5.00 for single books—add $1.00 for each additional book.
For cassette tapes only, add $4.00 shipping charge.
Payment by check, money order, or credit card.

Make checks payable to: NAHS
P.O. Box 4885
Buffalo Grove, Illinois 60089
Phone: (800) 243-5242 • Fax: 847 473-4780

For Visa/Mastercard orders provide the following information:

Card#_____ Exp. Date_____

Signature_____

Name_____

Address_____

City_____ State_____ Zip_____

For more information see pages 333-334.

ORDER FORM

Item	Quantity	Amount

BOOKS

#1 *How to Eat Right and Live Longer*	_____	_____
#2 *Self-Test Nutrition Guide*	_____	_____
#3 *Who Needs Headaches?*	_____	_____
#4 *Tea Tree Oil—the Natural Antiseptic*	_____	_____
#5 *How to Survive Disasters With Natural Medicines*	_____	_____
#6 *Supermarket Remedies*	_____	_____
#7 *The Cure Is in the Cupboard*	_____	_____
#8 *Lifesaving Cures*	_____	_____
#9 *The Diabetes Cure*	_____	_____

TAPES

#1 *The Survivor's Nutritional Pharmacy*	_____	_____
#2 *How to Use Oregano for Common Illnesses*	_____	_____
#3 *Selected Interviews and Lectures: The Best of Dr. Cass Ingram*	_____	_____
#4 *The Warning Signs of Nutritional Deficiency Professional/Advanced Series*	_____	_____

Sub-Total	_____
Sales Tax (if any)	_____
Shipping*	_____
TOTAL	_____

*Shipping Charges: $5.00 for single books—add $1.00 for each additional book.
For cassette tapes only, add $4.00 shipping charge.
Payment by check, money order, or credit card.

Make checks payable to: NAHS
P.O. Box 4885
Buffalo Grove, Illinois 60089
Phone: (800) 243-5242 • Fax: 847 473-4780

For Visa/Mastercard orders provide the following information:

Card#_____ Exp. Date_____

Signature_____

Name_____

Address_____

City_____ State_____ Zip_____

For more information see pages 333-334.

ORDER FORM

Item	Quantity	Amount

BOOKS

#1 *How to Eat Right and Live Longer* _____ _____

#2 *Self-Test Nutrition Guide* _____ _____

#3 *Who Needs Headaches?* _____ _____

#4 *Tea Tree Oil—the Natural Antiseptic* _____ _____

#5 *How to Survive Disasters With Natural Medicines* _____ _____

#6 *Supermarket Remedies* _____ _____

#7 *The Cure Is in the Cupboard* _____ _____

#8 *Lifesaving Cures* _____ _____

#9 *The Diabetes Cure* _____ _____

TAPES

#1 *The Survivor's Nutritional Pharmacy* _____ _____

#2 *How to Use Oregano for Common Illnesses* _____ _____

#3 *Selected Interviews and Lectures:*
The Best of Dr. Cass Ingram _____ _____

#4 *The Warning Signs of Nutritional Deficiency*
Professional/Advanced Series _____ _____

Sub-Total _____

Sales Tax (if any) _____

Shipping* _____

TOTAL _____

*Shipping Charges: $5.00 for single books—add $1.00 for each additional book.
For cassette tapes only, add $4.00 shipping charge.
Payment by check, money order, or credit card.

Make checks payable to: NAHS
P.O. Box 4885
Buffalo Grove, Illinois 60089
Phone: (800) 243-5242 • Fax: 847 473-4780

For Visa/Mastercard orders provide the following information:

Card#_____ Exp. Date_____

Signature_____

Name_____

Address_____

City_____ State_____ Zip_____

For more information see pages 333-334.

ORDER FORM

Item	Quantity	Amount

BOOKS

#1 *How to Eat Right and Live Longer* _____ _____

#2 *Self-Test Nutrition Guide* _____ _____

#3 *Who Needs Headaches?* _____ _____

#4 *Tea Tree Oil—the Natural Antiseptic* _____ _____

#5 *How to Survive Disasters With Natural Medicines* _____ _____

#6 *Supermarket Remedies* _____ _____

#7 *The Cure Is in the Cupboard* _____ _____

#8 *Lifesaving Cures* _____ _____

#9 *The Diabetes Cure* _____ _____

TAPES

#1 *The Survivor's Nutritional Pharmacy* _____ _____

#2 *How to Use Oregano for Common Illnesses* _____ _____

#3 *Selected Interviews and Lectures:*
The Best of Dr. Cass Ingram _____ _____

#4 *The Warning Signs of Nutritional Deficiency*
Professional/Advanced Series _____ _____

Sub-Total _____

Sales Tax (if any) _____

Shipping* _____

TOTAL _____

*Shipping Charges: $5.00 for single books—add $1.00 for each additional book.
For cassette tapes only, add $4.00 shipping charge.
Payment by check, money order, or credit card.

Make checks payable to: NAHS
P.O. Box 4885
Buffalo Grove, Illinois 60089
Phone: (800) 243-5242 • Fax: 847 473-4780

For Visa/Mastercard orders provide the following information:

Card#_____ Exp. Date_____

Signature_____

Name_____

Address_____

City_____ State_____ Zip_____

For more information see pages 333-334.

ORDER FORM

Item	Quantity	Amount

BOOKS

#1 *How to Eat Right and Live Longer* _____ _____

#2 *Self-Test Nutrition Guide* _____ _____

#3 *Who Needs Headaches?* _____ _____

#4 *Tea Tree Oil—the Natural Antiseptic* _____ _____

#5 *How to Survive Disasters With Natural Medicines* _____ _____

#6 *Supermarket Remedies* _____ _____

#7 *The Cure Is in the Cupboard* _____ _____

#8 *Lifesaving Cures* _____ _____

#9 *The Diabetes Cure* _____ _____

TAPES

#1 *The Survivor's Nutritional Pharmacy* _____ _____

#2 *How to Use Oregano for Common Illnesses* _____ _____

#3 *Selected Interviews and Lectures:*
The Best of Dr. Cass Ingram _____ _____

#4 *The Warning Signs of Nutritional Deficiency*
Professional/Advanced Series _____ _____

Sub-Total _____

Sales Tax (if any) _____

Shipping* _____

TOTAL _____

*Shipping Charges: $5.00 for single books—add $1.00 for each additional book.
For cassette tapes only, add $4.00 shipping charge.
Payment by check, money order, or credit card.

Make checks payable to: NAHS
P.O. Box 4885
Buffalo Grove, Illinois 60089
Phone: (800) 243-5242 • Fax: 847 473-4780

For Visa/Mastercard orders provide the following information:

Card#_____ Exp. Date_____

Signature_____

Name_____

Address_____

City_____ State_____ Zip_____

For more information see pages 333-334.

ORDER FORM

Item	Quantity	Amount
BOOKS		
#1 *How to Eat Right and Live Longer*	_____	_____
#2 *Self-Test Nutrition Guide*	_____	_____
#3 *Who Needs Headaches?*	_____	_____
#4 *Tea Tree Oil—the Natural Antiseptic*	_____	_____
#5 *How to Survive Disasters With Natural Medicines*	_____	_____
#6 *Supermarket Remedies*	_____	_____
#7 *The Cure Is in the Cupboard*	_____	_____
#8 *Lifesaving Cures*	_____	_____
#9 *The Diabetes Cure*	_____	_____
TAPES		
#1 *The Survivor's Nutritional Pharmacy*	_____	_____
#2 *How to Use Oregano for Common Illnesses*	_____	_____
#3 *Selected Interviews and Lectures: The Best of Dr. Cass Ingram*	_____	_____
#4 *The Warning Signs of Nutritional Deficiency Professional/Advanced Series*	_____	_____

Sub-Total	_____
Sales Tax (if any)	_____
Shipping*	_____
TOTAL	_____

*Shipping Charges: $5.00 for single books—add $1.00 for each additional book.
For cassette tapes only, add $4.00 shipping charge.
Payment by check, money order, or credit card.

Make checks payable to: NAHS
P.O. Box 4885
Buffalo Grove, Illinois 60089
Phone: (800) 243-5242 • Fax: 847 473-4780

For Visa/Mastercard orders provide the following information:

Card#_____ Exp. Date_____

Signature_____

Name_____

Address_____

City_____ State_____ Zip_____

For more information see pages 333-334.